Cardiology

Ragavendra R. Baliga, MD, MBA, FRCP, FACC
Clinical Professor
Director of Cardiology, Ohio State University Hospital East
Ohio State University
Columbus, Ohio

Student authors

Daniel Becker
University of Michigan School of Medicine
Ann Arbor, Michigan

David Corteville
University of Michigan School of Medicine
Ann Arbor, Michigan

Michael D. Nauss
University of Michigan School of Medicine
Ann Arbor, Michigan

UK edition authors **Anjana Siva and Mark Noble**

UK series editor Wilf Yeo

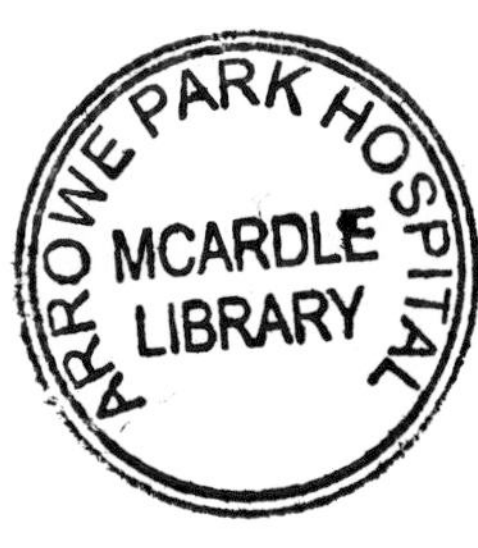

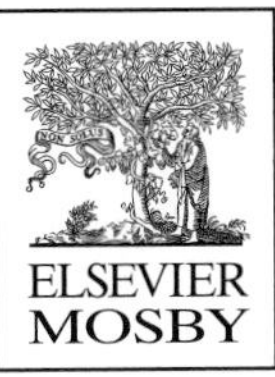
ELSEVIER
MOSBY

ELSEVIER
MOSBY

1600 John F. Kennedy Blvd.
Ste 1800
Philadelphia, PA 19103-2899

CRASH COURSE: CARDIOLOGY ISBN 0-323-03564-7

First Edition 1999.

Notice

Knowledge and best practice in this field are constantly changing. As new research and experience broaden our knowledge, changes in practice, treatment and drug therapy may become necessary or appropriate. Readers are advised to check the most current information provided (i) on procedures featured or (ii) by the manufacturer of each product to be administered, to verify the recommended dose or formula, the method and duration of administration, and contraindications. It is the responsibility of the practitioner, relying on their own experience and knowledge of the patient, to make diagnoses, to determine dosages and the best treatment for each individual patient, and to take all appropriate safety precautions. To the fullest extent of the law, neither the Publisher nor the Authors assume any liability for any injury and/or damage to persons or property arising out or related to any use of the material contained in this book.

The Publisher

Library of Congress Cataloging-in-Publication Data

Baliga, R. R.
Cardiology/Ragavendra Baliga; student authors, David Corteville, Daniel Becker, Michael D. Nauss.–1st ed.
p. ; cm.–(Crash course)
ISBN 0-323-03564-7
1. Heart–Diseases–Diagnosis. I. Title. II. Series.
[DNLM: 1. Heart Diseases. 2. Physical Examination. WG 201 B186c 2005]
RC683.B325 2005
616.1'2075–dc22 2004063173

Acquisitions Editor: Alex Stibbe
Project Development Manager: Stan Ward
Publishing Services Manager: David Saltzberg
Design: Andy Chapman
Cover Design: Richard Tibbets
Illustration Manager: Mick Ruddy

Printed in China

Last digit is the print number: 9 8 7 6 5 4 3 2 1

Dedicated to
Jayashree, Anoop, and Neena

Preface

Crash Course Cardiology is designed to help medical students in their internal medicine and clinical clerkship. In addition, it will help students preparing for the USMLE Steps 2 and 3.

Part I is focused on the approach to the patient, depending on symptoms. Part II includes history, clinical examination, and common investigations in patients with cardiovascular disease, and Part III discusses specific diseases, including diagnosis and treatment. The strengths of this text include the liberal use of diagrams and "hints" to highlight essential information that is expected from every medical student.

The book is best used soon after examining a patient with cardiovascular disease. This approach allows students to go back to the patient to compare their clinical findings with the text. In my experience, clinical medicine is best learned by using the 4-step Baliga **ERRD** technique: **e**licit, **r**ead, **r**eview, and **d**iscuss. To elaborate:

1. **E**licit the history, clinical features, and relevant investigations.
2. **R**ead relevant medical literature immediately.
3. Then go back to the patient to **r**eview history, clinical features, and diagnostic tests.
4. Finally, **d**iscuss with peers, seniors, or the attending physician.

Therefore, I encourage students to take this book to the hospital during their internal medicine or cardiology clinical clerkship so that it is readily available for use soon after they have examined a cardiovascular patient.

Finally, this book is a primer, and follow-up texts for further reading include the third edition of *250 Cases in Clinical Medicine* by R. R. Baliga (W.B Saunders) and *Practical Cardiology* by Eagle and Baliga (2003).

Ragavendra R. Baliga, MD, MBA, FRCP (Edin), FACC

Acknowledgments

I thank Anjana Siva and Mark Noble for allowing me to adapt their British book for U.S. medical students.

I thank Daniel Becker, David Corteville, and Michael Nauss for critically reviewing this book and giving me three separate perspectives from the view of a medical student. They were third- and fourth-year medical students at University of Michigan Medical School when they worked on this project. Dan is now a resident at Brigham & Women's Hospital and Harvard Medical School, Dave is a resident at University of California, San Francisco (UCSF), and Mike is a resident at University of Cincinnati. I have no doubt that they all will continue to excel in their field of endeavor. It was a pleasure to work with them.

Finally, I thank my wife Jay for doing my share of the domestic chores and my children Anoop and Neena for their patience while I worked on this book.

Contents

THE PATIENT PRESENTS WITH

1. Chest Pain

Differential diagnosis of chest pain

Chest pain is one of the most common presenting complaints seen any physician, including cardiologists to emergency medicine physicians, and family practitioners. It is important to remember that:

- There are many causes of chest pain.
- Some are life-threatening and require prompt diagnosis and treatment, whereas others are more benign.
- In order to be diagnosed with a MI a patient must have two of the following three: chest pain, EKG changes suggestive of ischemia or infarction, or elevation of cardiac enzymes.

The first differentiation to be made is between cardiac and noncardiac chest pain (Fig. 1.1)

History to focus on differential diagnosis of chest pain

Because the differential diagnosis is so diverse a thorough history is very important.

Presenting complaint

Differentiation depends upon a detailed history of the pain with particular emphasis on the following characteristics of the pain (Fig. 1.2):

- Continuous or intermittent.
- Duration (if the patient can tell you the when the pain started down to the exact minute, think dissection).
- Frequency.
- Whether the patient has had this chest pain before.
- Position of the pain—central or lateral/posterior.
- Exacerbating factors—exertion, emotion, food, posture, movement, breathing.
- Radiation of the pain—to neck, arms, head.
- Quality of pain—crushing, burning, stabbing.
- If the patient has had an episode of chest pain previously, how is this episode alike and different from the typical episode of chest pain?

Past medical history

This may provide important clues:

- History of coronary artery disease.
- History of peptic ulcer disease or of frequent ingestion of nonsteroidal anti-inflammatory drugs/steroids.
- History of gastroesopheagal reflux disease (GERD).
- Recent operations—cardiothoracic surgery may be complicated by Dressler's syndrome, mediastinitis, coronary artery disease, or pulmonary embolus (PE).
- History of immunosuppression: consider herpes zoster for chest pain.
- Pericarditis may be preceded by a prodromal viral illness.
- Pulmonary embolus may be preceded by a period of inactivity (e.g., recent operation, illness, or long journey).
- Hypertension is a risk factor for both coronary artery disease and dissection of the thoracic aorta.

Remember that pneumonia can present with chest pain. The elderly can present without a fever or bad cough despite a lung infection. Always look at the chest X-ray. The white blood cell (WBC) count is not that helpful because it can be raised secondary to an infection or heart attack.

Drug history, family history, and social history

Other risk factors for coronary artery disease such as a positive family history and smoking should be excluded.

A history of heavy alcohol intake is a risk factor for gastritis, peptic ulcer disease, and pacreatitis.

When a patient presents as a hospital emergency with cardiac chest pain, contact the cardiac catheterization laboratory immediately. If cardiac cardiac catheterization is not available, try to differentiate diagnoses for which thrombolysis is contraindicated from those for which it is indicated. Thrombolysis is contraindicated in pericarditis and dissection of the thoracic aorta. If pulmonary embolism (PE) is suspected, request spiral CT of chest using PE protocol.

Differential diagnosis of chest pain	
System involved	**Pathology**
Cardiac	Myocardial infarction Angina pectoris Pericarditis Prolapse of the mitral valve Tampanode
Vascular	Aortic dissection
Respiratory (all tend to give rise to pleuritic pain)	Pulmonary embolus Pneumonia Pneumothorax Pulmonary neoplasm
Gastrointestinal	Esophagitis due to gastric reflux Esophageal tear Peptic ulcer Biliary disease Pancreatitis
Musculoskeletal	Cervical nerve root compression by cervical disc Costochondritis Fractured rib
Neurological	Herpes zoster
Psychogenic	Anxiety Panic disorder Conversion disorder Malingering

Fig. 1.1 Differential diagnosis of chest pain.

Examination of patients who have chest pain

Points to note on examination of the patient who has chest pain are shown in Fig. 1.3.

Inspection

On inspection, look for:

- Signs of shock (e.g., pallor, sweating)—may indicate myocardial infarction (MI), dissecting aorta, PE.
- Labored breathing—may indicate MI leading to congestive ventricular failure (CHF) or a pulmonary cause.
- Signs of vomiting—suggests MI or an esophageal cause.
- Coughing—suggests LVF, pneumonia; ask the patient about color of sputum and hemoptysis.

Cardiovascular system

Note the following:

- Pulse and blood pressure—any abnormal rhythm, tachycardia, bradycardia, hypotension, hypertension. Inequalities in the pulses or blood pressure between different extremities are seen in aortic dissection.
- Mucus membranes—pallor could suggest angina due to anemia; cyanosis suggests hypoxia.
- Any increase in jugular venous pressure—a sign of right ventricular infarction or pulmonary embolus.
- Carotid pulse waveform—a collapsing pulse is seen with aortic regurgitation, which can complicate aortic dissection. It is slow rising if angina is due to aortic stenosis.
- Displaced PMI (point of maximal impulse), abnormal cardiac impulses (e.g., paradoxical movement in anterior myocardial infarction).
- On auscultation—listen for a pericardial rub, third heart sound (a feature of CHF), mitral or aortic regurgitation (features of myocardial infarction or dissection respectively), aortic stenosis (causes angina).

Respiratory system

Note the following signs:

- Breathlessness or cyanosis.
- Unequal hemithorax expansion—a sign of pneumonia and pneumothorax.
- Abnormal dullness over lung fields—a sign of pneumonia.
- Any bronchial breathing or pleural rub—signs of pneumonia and pleurisy.

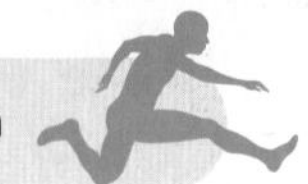

Characteristic	Myocardial ischemia	Pericarditis	Pleuritic pain	Gastrointestinal disease	Musculoskeletal	Aortic dissection
Quality of pain	Crushing, tight, or bandlike	Sharp (may be crushing)	Sharp	Burning	Usually sharp but may be dull ache	Sharp, stabbing, tearing
Site of pain	Central anterior chest	Central anterior	Anywhere (usually very localized pain)	Central	May be anywhere	Retrosternal. Interscapular
Radiation	To throat, jaw, arms, or neck	Usually no radiation	Usually no radiation	To throat	To arms or around chest to back	Usually no radiation
Exacerbating and relieving factors	Exacerbated by exertion, anxiety, cold; relieved by rest and sublingual NTG	Exacerbated when lying back; relieved by sitting forward	Exacerbated by breathing, coughing, or moving; relieved when breathing stops	Peptic ulcer pain often relieved by food and antacids (cholecystitis and esophageal pain are exacerbated by food)	May be exacerbated by pressing on chest wall or moving neck	Constant with no exacerbating or relieving factors
Associated features	Patient often sweaty, breathless, and shocked; may feel nauseated	Fever, recent viral illness (e.g., rash, arthralgia)	Cough, hemoptysis, breathlessness; shock with pulmonary embolus	Flatulence, burping	Other affected joints; patient otherwise looks very well	Unequal radial and femoral pulse and blood pressure; aortic regurgitant mumur may be heard on auscultation

Fig. 1.2 Characteristics of different types of chest pain. (NTG, nitroglycerin.)

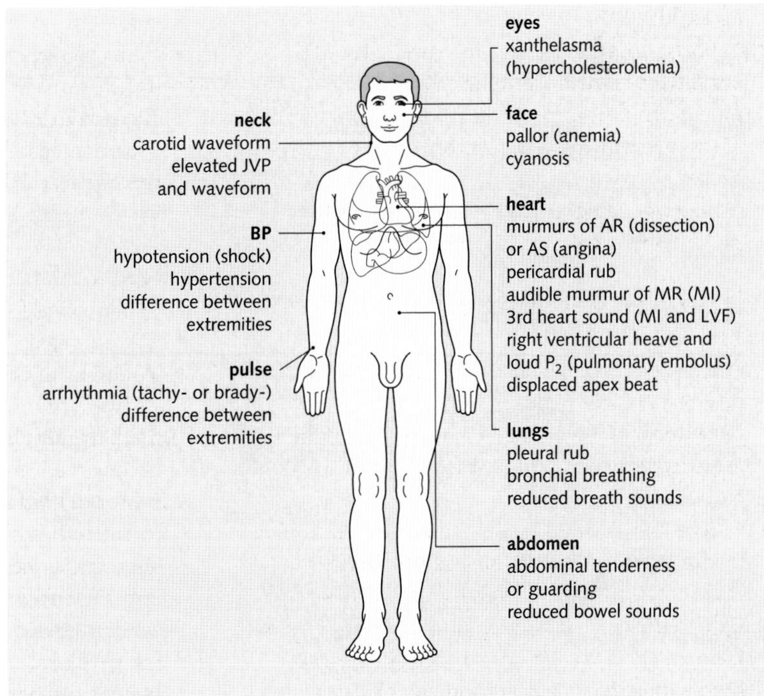

Fig. 1.3 Points to note when examining a patient who has chest pain. (AR, aortic regurgitation; AS, aortic stenosis; BP, blood pressure; JVP, jugular venous pressure; LVF, left ventricular failure; MI, myocardial infarction; MR, mitral regurgitation; P_2, pulmonary component of the second heart sound.)

Gastrointestinal system

Specifically look for:

- Abdominal tenderness or guarding.
- Scanty or absent bowel sounds—suggests an ileus (e.g., due to perforated peptic ulcer and peritonitis).

Investigation of patients who have chest pain

A summary of tests used to investigate chest pain is shown in Fig. 1.4, and an algorithm is shown in Fig. 1.5.

Blood tests

These include:

- Myoglobin, which rises within an hour (faster than CK-MB) following cardiac injury.
- Serum troponins, and CK-MB—may be elevated in MI from 4 hours after the onset of infarction.
- Complete blood count (CBC)—anemia may exacerbate angina. WBC count may rise after MI.
- Renal function and electrolytes—may be abnormal if the patient has been vomiting, leading to dehydration and hypokalemia, or due to diuretic therapy.
- Arterial blood gases—hypoxia is a sign of PE and CHF; hypocapnea is seen with hyperventilation.
- Liver function tests, serum amylase and serum lipase—deranged in cholecystitis and peptic ulcer disease.

Electrocardiography

Findings may include:

- Bundle-branch block (BBB)—if new, this may be due to MI; if it is old, MI cannot be diagnosed from the ECG.
- ST elevation in absence of BBB indicates acute MI (rarely it is due to Prinzmetal's angina).
- Diffuse ST elevation in chest and limb leads: acute pericarditis.
- Fully developed Q waves—indicate old MI (i.e., over 24 hours old); Q waves indicate dead myocardium.
- Atrial fibrillation secondary to coronary artery disease or any pulmonary disease.
- ST depression in absence of BBB—indicates myocardial ischemia. At rest this equates with unstable angina or non-Q wave infarction; on exertion this equates with effort-induced angina pectoris or tachyarrhythmias.

In the event of a large PE the classic changes to be seen are:

- Sinus tachycardia (or atrial fibrillation).
- Tall P waves in lead II (right atrial dilatation).
- Right axis deviation and right bundle-branch block.
- S wave in lead I, Q wave in lead III, and inverted T wave in lead III (S1Q3T3 pattern); seen only with very large PE.

Chest radiograph

The following signs may be seen:

- Cardiomegaly.
- Widening of the mediastinum in aortic dissection. Of note, trauma films often make the mediastinum look falsely wide. This happens because they are taken as an AP film (anterior to posterior) rather than the PA view normally taken by the radiology department. In an AP film the heart and great vessels are farther away from the film and therefore look slightly wider. If you are concerned about dissection, get a CT.
- Lung lesions.
- Pleural and pericardial effusions.

First-line tests to exclude a chest pain emergency

Text	Diagnosis
Arterial blood gases	In dyspneic patients severe hypoxemia suggests pulmonary embolus, CHF, or pneumonia
Cardiac enzymes	May be normal in first 4 hours after MI, but CK-MB will then increase
D-dimer	In suspected PE
ECG	Normal EKG does not exclude non-ST elevation MI (NSTEMI)
CXR	Widened mediastinum suggests aortic dissection; may show pleural effusion or pulmonary consolidation
CT scan	Carry out urgently for suspected aortic dissection; PE protocol

Fig. 1.4 First-line tests to exclude a chest pain emergency. CK-MB, creatine kinase composed of M (muscle) and B (brain) subunits, which is found primarily in cardiac muscle; D-dimer in suspected PE. CT, computed tomography; CXR, chest radiography; EKG, electrocardiography; CHF, congestive heart failure; MI, myocardial infarction.)

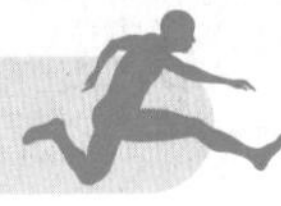

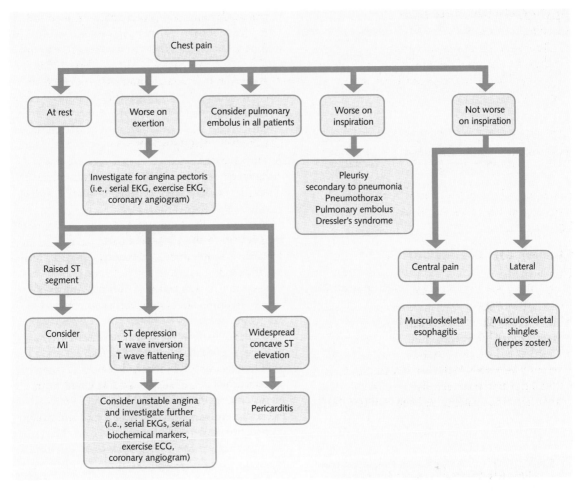

Chest pain

At rest

Worse on exertion

Consider pulmonary embolus in all patients

Worse on inspiration

Not worse on inspiration

Investigate for angina pectoris (i.e., serial EKG, exercise EKG, coronary angiogram)

Pleurisy secondary to pneumonia
Pneumothorax
Pulmonary embolus
Dressler's syndrome

Raised ST segment

Central pain

Lateral

Consider MI

ST depression
T wave inversion
T wave flattening

Widespread concave ST elevation

Musculoskeletal esophagitis

Musculoskeletal shingles (herpes zoster)

Consider unstable angina and investigate further (i.e., serial EKGs, serial biochemical markers, exercise ECG, coronary angiogram)

Pericarditis

Fig. 1.5 Algorithm for investigation of chest pain. (MI, myocardial infarction; UA, unstable angina.)

- Decreased vascular markings in PE.
- Pulmonary edema.

Echocardiography

This may reveal:

- Pericardial effusion—suggests pericarditis or dissection.
- Regional myocardial dysfunction (e.g., hypokinesis—a poorly contracting heart)—a feature of myocardial infarction or ischemia.
- Aortic dissection with false lumen.
- Aortic or mitral valve abnormalities.

Computed tomography (CT) and magnetic resonance imaging (MRI)

These are the most sensitive methods for excluding aortic dissection and should be performed urgently if this diagnosis is suspected. Often spiral CT for pulmonary embolism is useful when V/Q scan is not helpful or there is underlying structural lung disease.

Ventilation/perfusion (V/Q) scan

This excludes PE in most cases if performed promptly. If the scan is negative and PE is strongly suspected, a more sensitive test is a pulmonary angiogram. The landmark study PIOPED (Prospective Investigation of Pulmonary Embolism Diagnosis) showed that using clinical judgement along with V/Q scans could result in better diagnosis of PE. V/Q scans are not useful in patients with underlying structural lung damage such as COPD, interstitial lung disease.

Exercise tolerance test or myocardial perfusion scan

This may be performed if angina is suspected.

Acute substernal chest pain at rest

This situation represents a medical emergency requiring rapid diagnosis and treatment. It is necessary in this situation to distinguish among:

- MI (see Chapter 14).
- Unstable angina.
- Pericarditis.
- Dissection of thoracic aorta.
- PE.
- Mediastinitis secondary to esophageal tear (Boerhaave's syndrome).
- Noncardiac chest pain.

Cardiac catheterization

Urgent cardiac catheterization is the treatment for MI with an onset less than 24 hours previously. The pain of MI is characteristically a tight, crushing band-like pain that may radiate to the jaws or arms. At hospitals without facilities for percutaneous coronary angioplasty (PTCA) and stenting of the coronary artery, thrombolysis should be considered. PTCA/stent should be considered for those who have two out of the following three findings:

- New EKG changes such as new LBBB or ST elevations. Non-ST elevation MI (NSTEMI) is also an acute indication.
- Clinical picture consistent with classic angina—especially in those who have known CAD or appropriate risk factors such as advanced age, male sex, smoking, diabetes mellitus, hyperlipidemia, hypertension.
- Positive cardiac markers: CK, CK-MB, troponin.

Conditions for which thrombolysis is contraindicated

Thrombolysis can be lethal in:

- NSTEMI—thrombolysis can cause harm in such patients.
- Pericarditis.
- Dissection of thoracic aorta.

Pericarditis

- The patient may have a prodromal viral illness.
- Pain may be exacerbated by breathing movements.
- There may be concomitant indications of infection.

Examination may reveal a pericardial rub—an added sound (or sounds) in the cardiac area on auscultation, which has a scratchy quality and seems close to the ears.

If complicated by pericardial effusion, there may be:

- An impalpable cardiac impulse.
- An increased cardiothoracic ratio on the chest radiograph, with a globular-shaped heart shadow.
- The ECG shows characteristic concave-upward, raised ST segments in all leads except limb lead AVR. Thrombolysis is contraindicated because it causes hemopericardium.

Dissection of the thoracic aorta

The pain is acute, sharp, and tearing. There is often radiation of the pain to the back (as with the pain of pancreatitis). There may be a previous history of or current hypertension. Patients often can recall the exact moment the pain started.

On examination, the patient may be in shock, and there may be delays between the major pulses (e.g., right brachial vs. left brachial, brachial vs. femoral).

Chest radiography may show a widened mediastinum. The ECG will not show ST elevation unless the coronary ostia are dissected. Confirmation may require high-resolution spiral CT scanning, transesophageal echocardiography, or MRI (which is the best investigation when available; Fig. 1.6).

Thrombolysis is contraindicated because it causes massive bleeding from the aorta.

Mediastinitis

This is unusual and need not usually be considered unless there is a possibility of an esophageal leak (e.g., after endoscopy or esophageal surgery). Rarely can esophageal rupture come from trauma (Boerhaave's syndrome).

Pulmonary embolus

Pulmonary emboli may present as acute chest pain in an ill patient or as intermittent chest pain in a relatively well patient. For this reason it is crucial to suspect PE in all patients who have chest pain that is not typically anginal. When your attending asks for a differential diagnosis for anyone having any sort of chest pain or shortness of breath, PE should always be on your list.

The pain of a PE may be pleuritic or tight in nature and may be located anywhere in the chest. It may be accompanied by the following symptoms and signs:

Overview of dissection of the thoracic aorta	
Predisposing factors	Hypertension Bicuspid aortic valve Pregnancy Marfan, Turner's, Noonan's syndrome Connective tissue diseases—SLE, Ehlers-Danlos syndrome Men > women Middle age
Pathophysiology	Damage to the media and high intraluminal pressure causing an intimal tear Blood enters and dissects the luminal plane of the media, creating a false lumen
Classification	Stanford classification: type A, all dissections involving the ascending aorta; type B, all dissections not involving the ascending aorta
Symptoms	Central tearing chest pain radiating to the back Further complications as the dissection involves branches of the aorta: coronary ostia—myocardial infarction; carotid or spinal arteries—hemiplegia, dysphasia, or paraplegia; mesenteric arteries—abdominal pain
Signs	Shocked, cyanosed, sweating Blood pressure and pulses differ between extremities Aortic regurgitation Cardiac tamponade Cardiac failure
Investigation	CXR—widened mediastinum with or without fluid in costophrenic angle EKG—may be ST elevation CT/MRI—best investigations, show aortic false lumen Transesophageal echo if available also very sensitive Echocardiography—may show pericardial effusion if dissection extends proximally; tamponade may occur
Management	Pain relief—morphine Intravenous access—central and arterial line Fluid replacement—initially colloid, then blood when available—crossmatch at least 10 units Blood pressure control—intravenous labetalol, or an esmolol, diltiazem, or nitroglycerin drip—keep blood pressure at 120/80 mmHg Surgery for all type A dissections Medical management and possibly surgery for type B

Fig. 1.6 Overview of dissection of the thoracic aorta. (CT, computed tomography; CXR, chest radiography; EKG, electrocardiography; MRI, magnetic resonance imaging.)

Conditions predisposing to deep venous thrombosis	
Condition	**Examples**
Smoking	
Immobility	Prolonged bed rest for any reason, long air journeys
Postoperative status	Abdominal and pelvic surgery, leg and hip surgery
Hemoconcentration	Diuretic therapy, polycythemia
Hypercoagulable states	Malignancy, oral contraceptive pill, protein C/protein S deficiency, factor V Leiden, etc.
Venous stasis (poor flow of venous blood)	Congestive heart failure, atrial fibrillation (formation of thrombus in the right ventricle may result in PE)

Fig. 1.7 Conditions predisposing to deep venous thrombosis. Keep in mind Virchow's triad (immobility, hypercoagulable, vascular injury).

- Dyspnea.
- Dry cough or hemoptysis.
- Tachycardia.
- Hypotension and sweating.
- Sudden collapse with syncope.

Massive PE will cause collapse with cardiac arrest. The EKG may show ventricular tachyarrhythmias or sinus rhythm with pulseless electrical activity (PEA).

Patients will often experience a sense of "impending doom" or profound anxiety.

Conditions predisposing to clot formation in the deep veins of the leg are associated with a high incidence of PE (Fig. 1.7).

The mortality rate resulting from PE is approximately 10%. Appropriate investigations to exclude PE should be carried out promptly, and anticoagulation should be initiated with either intravenous heparin as an infusion or an appropriate low-molecular-weight heparin preparation subcutaneously. If PE is confirmed, warfarin therapy should be commenced.

2. Dyspnea

Dyspnea is an uncomfortable awareness of one's own breathing. It is considered abnormal only when it occurs at a level of physical activity not normally expected to cause any problem.

Differential diagnosis of dyspnea

Dyspnea is the main symptom of many cardiac and pulmonary diseases. A working knowledge of the differential diagnosis is required to be able to differentiate acute life-threatening conditions from those that do not require immediate treatment (Fig 2.1).

Any diagnosis of dyspnea should focus on anything that interrupts the process of breathing between the brain and the lungs or the ability to carry and distribute oxygen. For example:

- Brain.
- Peripheral nerves.
- Respiratory muscles/chest wall.
- Lungs/bronchioles/alveoli.
- Heart.
- Blood/amount of hemoglobin.

History to focus on the differential diagnosis of dyspnea

Differentiation depends upon a detailed history of the dyspnea (Fig. 2.2) with particular emphasis on the following details:

- Acute or chronic.
- Continuous or intermittent.
- Exacerbating and relieving factors—such as exertion, lying flat (suggests orthopnea in pulmonary edema), sleep (suggests paroxysmal nocturnal dyspnea, PND, which is waking from sleep gasping for breath in left ventricular failure (LVF)). Shortness of breath associated with lack of sleep suggests sleep apnea.
- If bronchodilators relieve symptoms, the patient may have reactive airways disease.
- Associated features such as cough—ask for details of sputum production. Determine how much sputum is produced in a day. Ask about the color: yellow–green sputum suggests pneumonia or exacerbation of chronic obstructive pulmonary disease (COPD); pink frothy sputum suggests LVF; hemoptysis can be a feature of pneumonia, pulmonary embolus (PE), and carcinoma of the lung.
- Chest pain—ask for details of location, nature of pain, radiation, etc. (see Chapter 1).
- Palpitations/lightheadedness—ask about rate and rhythm.
- Ankle edema—suggestive of congestive heart failure; swelling usually worse at the end of the day and best first thing in the morning.
- Wheeze—suggestive of airways obstruction (i.e., asthma, COPD, or neoplasm of the lung causing airway obstruction). Wheeze can also occur during left ventricular failure.

Examination of dyspneic patients

As usual, a thorough examination is needed because the differential diagnosis is potentially wide (Fig. 2.3).

Inspection

Note the following:

- Fever—suggests infection (PE or myocardial infarction may be associated with a low-grade fever).
- Signs of shock—pallor, sweating; suggests acute LVF, pneumonia, PE.
- Inspect for labored or obstructed breathing (any intercostal retractions?), tachypnea, or cyanosis. One or more usually present with resting dyspnea.
- Cough—suggests acute LVF, pneumonia; note the appearance of the sputum (always ask to look in the sputum cup if it is present).
- Appearance of hands and fingers—such as clubbing, asterixis (sign of carbon dioxide retention).

Differential diagnosis of dyspnea	
System involved	**Pathology**
Cardiac	Cardiac failure Coronary artery disease Valvular heart disease—aortic stenosis, aortic regurgitation, mitral stenosis/regurgitation, pulmonary stenosis Cardiac arrhythmias
Respiratory	Pulmonary embolus Airway obstruction—COPD, asthma Pneumothorax Pulmonary parenchymal disease (e.g., pneumonia, interstitial lung disease, lung neoplasm) Pleural effusion Chest wall limitation—myopathy, neuropathy (e.g., Guillain–Barré disease), rib fracture, kyphoscoliosis
Other	Obesity (limiting chest wall movement or sleep apnea) Anemia Psychogenic hyperventilation, panic attack, anxiety Acidosis (e.g., aspirin overdose, diabetic ketoacidosis)

Fig. 2.1 Differential diagnosis of dyspnea. (COPD, chronic obstructive airways disease.)

- Appearance of chest—a barrel-shaped chest is a feature of emphysema; kyphoscoliosis causes distortion.

Cardiovascular system

Check the following:

- Pulse and blood pressure—any abnormal rhythm, tachycardia, bradycardia, hypotension, hypertension?
- Mucus membranes—pallor suggests dyspnea in anemia; cyanosis suggests hypoxia in heart failure, COPD, PE, pneumonia, and lung collapse.
- Carotid pulse waveform and jugular venous pressure (JVP)—JVP is elevated in cardiac failure and conditions causing pulmonary hypertension (e.g. PE, COPD). Pay attention to the lung exam when JVP is noted. PE, pneumothorax, and cardiac tamponade can present with clear lungs and JVP. JVP stemming from LVF will cause pulmonary edema before causing JVP resulting in crackles on physical examination.
- Point of maximal impulse (PMI)—displacement suggests cardiac enlargement, and a right ventricular heave suggests pulmonary hypertension.
- Heart sounds—note any audible murmurs or added heart sound. Third heart sound in heart failure; mitral regurgitation or aortic valve lesions may cause LVF.
- Peripheral edema.

Respiratory system

Check the following:

- Expansion—unequal thorax expansion is a sign of pneumonia or pneumothorax.
- Vocal fremitus—enhanced vocal fremitus is a sign of consolidation; reduced vocal fremitus is a sign of effusion and pneumothorax.
- Abnormal dullness over hemithorax with reduced expansion—suggests pneumonia.
- Stony dullness at one or both lung bases—suggests pleural effusion.
- Hyperresonance over hemithorax with less expansion— suggests pneumothorax. (Remember, if the patient has a tension pneumothorax do *not* get a CXR. Treat first by placing an angiocatheter in the second intercostals space, then get a CXR).
- Bilateral hyperresonance with loss of cardiac dullness—suggests emphysema.
- Bronchial breathing—suggests pneumonia.
- Crackles—suggests pneumonia, pulmonary edema, pulmonary fibrosis.
- Wheeze—asthma, COPD, cardiac asthma in LVF.
- Peak flow test—this is part of every examination of the respiratory system. You should always ask to do this, particularly in an outpatient clinic. Explain the technique to the patient clearly and then perform three attempts and take the best out of three. Peak flow will be reduced in active asthma and COPD. This test is useful in monitoring response to therapy.

Gastrointestinal system

Examine for hepatomegaly and ascites—seen in congestive heart failure or isolated right-sided failure.

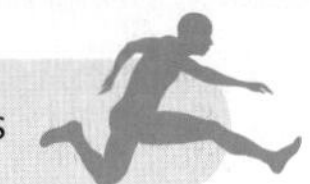

Presenting history for different diseases causing dyspnea					
	Cardiac failure	**Coronary artery disease**	**Pulmonary embolus**	**Pneumothorax**	**COPD and asthma**
Acute or chronic	May be acute or chronic	Acute	Acute (less commonly, recurrent small PEs may present as chronic dyspnea)	Acute	Acute or chronic
Continuous or intermittent	May be continuous or intermittent	Usually intermittent, but an acute MI may lead to continuous and severe LVF	Continuous	Continuous	Continuous or intermittent; these disorders range from the acute, life-threatening exacerbations to chronic, relatively mild episodes
Exacerbating and relieving factors	Exacerbated by exertion and lying flat (orthopnea and PND may occur) and occasionally by food; relieved by rest, sitting up, oxygen, and NTG	Exacerbated by exertion, cold; may be relieved by oxygen			Exacerbated by exertion, pulmonary infections, allergens (e.g., pollen, animal danders); relieved by bronchodilator inhalers
Associated features	May be chest pain (ischemia may cause LVF); palpitations—arrhythmias may precipitate LVF; cough with pink, frothy sputum	Chest pain (central crushing pain radiating to left arm or throat) and sweating; occasionally palpitations—atrial fibrillation may be precipitated by ischemia	Pleuritic chest pain (sharp, localized pain worse on breathing and coughing) and bright red hemoptysis; atrial fibrillation may occur	Pleuritic chest pain; there may be a history of chest trauma	Cough with sputum; pleuritic chest pain if associated infection; wheeze

Fig. 2.2 Presenting history for different diseases causing dyspnea. (COPD, chronic obstructive airways disease; NTG, nitroglycerine; LVF, left ventricular failure; CHF, congestive heart failure; MI, myocardial infarction; PE, pulmonary embolus; PND, paroxysmal nocturnal dyspnea.)

Investigation of dyspneic patients

A summary of first-line tests to exclude emergencies is shown in Fig. 2.4.

Blood tests

These include:

- Complete blood count—may reveal anemia or leukocytosis (in pneumonia).
- Basic metabolic panel—deranged due to diuretic treatment of cardiac failure, possible syndrome of inappropriate antidiuretic hormone secretion in pneumonia.
- D-dimer—when PE is suspected.
- Cardiac enzymes (troponin, CK, CK-MB)—elevated if dyspnea secondary to myocardial infarction.
- Liver function tests—deranged in hepatic congestion secondary to congestive cardiac failure.
- Arterial blood gases (Fig. 2.5).

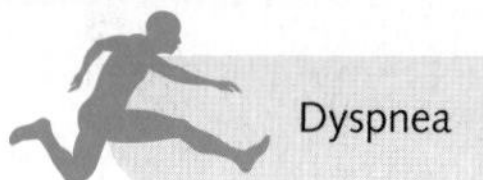

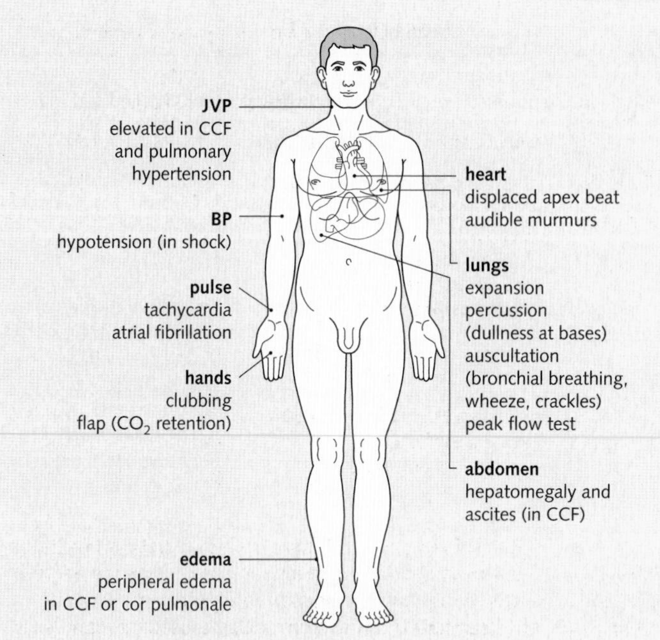

Fig. 2.3 Points to note when examining a dyspneic patient. (BP, blood pressure; CHF, congestive heart failure; JVP, jugular venous pressure.)

Notes on blood gases:

- Hypoxia and hypocapnea are seen in LVF and pulmonary embolus (this shows a drop in pCO_2 due to hyperventilation as a response to hypoxia).
- Hypoxia and hypercapnea may occur in COPD and severe asthma. In the former condition, this is because the respiratory center has readjusted to he chronic hypoxia and oxygen therapy causes the blood pO_2 to rise and the respiratory drive to fall, so ventilation is reduced and the blood pCO_2 rises. In asthma, exhaustion causes the ventilatory drive to fall off and the pCO_2 to rise, this precedes respiratory arrest and is an indication for mechanical ventilation of the patient).
- Arterial pH—in acute conditions such as acute LVF, pulmonary embolus, pneumothorax, and early asthma a respiratory alkalosis occurs (i.e., a low pCO_2 and a high pH of 7.4). The kidneys have not yet compensated by excreting bicarbonate.
- In COPD with chronic CO_2 retention the pH is normal as metabolic compensation has occurred and bicarbonate levels rise due to renal retention of bicarbonate (this takes a few days to occur).
- In severe asthma with acute CO_2 retention the pH falls as the pCO_2 rises as there has been insufficient time for metabolic compensation to occur.

Electrocardiography

This may show:

- Ischemic changes may be seen in patients with coronary artery disease.
- Sinus tachycardia with S1, Q3, T3 in patients who have had a large PE.
- Atrial fibrillation—may be seen secondary to any lung pathology or ischemia.

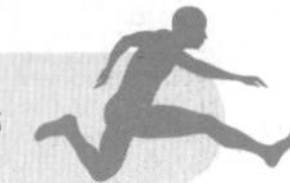

First-line tests to exclude a dyspneic emergency

Test	Diagnosis
CXR	Acute LVF—pulmonary edema with or without large heart shadow Acute asthma—clear overexpanded lungs Pneumothorax—absence of lung markings between lung edge and chest wall Pneumonia—consolidation
EKG	Look for evidence of MI, ischemia, pulmonary embolus
Arterial blood gases	Normal pH excludes uncompensated acute hyperventilation or respiratory failure; hypoxia suggests LVF or significant lung disease (use the level of hypoxia and pCO_2 to guide the need for oxygen therapy or mechanical ventilation)
Peak flow	Reduced in airway obstruction (asthma, COPD), but may also be reduced in sick patients because of weakness (it is an effort-dependent test)

Fig. 2.4 First-line tests to exclude a dyspneic emergency. (COPD, chronic obstructive airways disease; CXR, chest radiography; EKG, electrocardiography; LVF, left ventricular failure; MI, myocardial infarction.)

Arterial blood gas results in dyspneic patients

	pO_2 (mmHg)	pCO_2 (mmHg)	pH
Normal range	80–100	35–45	7.36–7.44
Ventilatory failure (e.g., chronic obstructive airways disease, severe asthma with exhaustion)	<60	>60	7.30
Acute hyperventilation	>100	<30	7.48
Hypoxia (e.g., left ventricular failure, pulmonary embolus)	<60	30	7.41

Fig. 2.5 Examples of arterial blood gas results in dyspneic patients. The low pH in ventilatory failure is secondary to an acute retention of carbon dioxide. The high pH in acute hyperventilation results from an acute loss of carbon dioxide (respiratory alkalosis). The case of hypoxia shown here has led to hyperventilation and a fall of carbon dioxide and must have been present for some time because the pH is compensated to normal by renal excretion of bicarbonate.

Chest radiography

Note the following:

- Cardiomegaly in cardiac failure. Pulmonary edema may also be seen.
- Focal lung consolidation in pneumonia (shadowing of a lung segment with an air bronchogram).
- Pleural effusion—suggests PE, infection, or cardiac failure.
- Hyperexpanded lung fields in emphysema (ability to count more than six rib spaces over the lung fields); bullae may be seen in emphysema.
- Presence of a pneumothorax—ask for a film in full expiration if this is suspected.
- Oligemic lung fields in PE.

Echocardiography

This may reveal:

- Left ventricular failure.
- Valve lesions.
- Left atrial myxoma.
- Right ventricular hypertrophy and pulmonary hypertension.

Ventilation/perfusion scan

This may be used to exclude PE—a mismatched defect with good ventilation and no perfusion is diagnostic of a PE; matched defects are due to pneumonia or COPD or pulmonary scar tissue.

If the V/Q scan is negative or equivocal in a high-risk patient, it is reasonable to proceed to pulmonary angiography. This is the most sensitive test for a PE.

Computed tomography (CT)

CT is used to obtain detailed visualization of pulmonary fibrosis, parenchymal disease, pleural effusion, or small peripheral tumors that cannot be reached with a bronchoscope. CT angiography may be used to evaluate for PE. A high-resolution CT scan gives good definition of lung parenchyma and may prevent the need for a biopsy in some diseases.

Pulmonary function tests

These tests are used to investigate:

- Lung volumes—increased in COPD, reduced in restrictive lung disease.
- Flow volume loop—scalloped in COPD.
- Carbon monoxide transfer (DLCO)—reduced in the presence of normal airway function in restrictive lung diseases and pulmonary edema.

Notes on dyspnea and arterial blood gases:

- Life-threatening cardiopulmonary conditions, respiratory failure, and carbon monoxide poisoning may not cause prominent dyspnea but may present as coma or semi-coma or obtundation.
- Severe hypoxia or tissue underperfusion causes metabolic acidosis (low pH with normal or low pCO_2).
- Most importantly—arterial blood gases must be performed for all dyspneic patients at presentation.

Dyspnea at rest of recent onset

This situation represents a cardiopulmonary emergency requiring rapid diagnosis and treatment. It is necessary in this situation to distinguish between the life-threatening causes:

- Tension pneumothorax.
- Life-threatening asthma.
- Acute LVF.
- PE.
- Fulminant pneumonia.

Pneumothorax

Pneumothorax (or air in the pleural space) may cause acute or chronic dyspnea. There are a number of possible causes, all creating a connection between the pleural space and the atmosphere (either via the chest wall or the airways). These include:

- Trauma (e.g., a blow to the chest resulting in fracture of the ribs or insertion of a central venous cannula).
- Rupture of bullae on the surface of the lung—this occurs in some otherwise healthy young patients (more commonly in men than in women) or in patients who have emphysema. The typical patient who has a spontaneous pneumothorax is a tall, thin male smoker. Patients usually present with acute chest pain. Of note, this can also happen in marijuana smokers when they perform the Valsalva maneuver and hold their breath (increasing the intrathoracic pressure). If a patient with spontaneous pneumothorax complains more about being hungry than about chest pain, ask about drug use.

Tension pneumothorax can occur if the air continues to accumulate in the pleural cavity, resulting in a progressive increase in pressure and displacement of the mediastinum away from the side of the lesion. This is characterized by the following clinical signs:

- Severe and worsening dyspnea.
- Displaced trachea and PMI.
- Hyperresonance on the affected side with reduced breath sounds and vocal fremitus.
- Progressive hypotension due to reduced venous return and therefore reduced filling of the right ventricle.
- Eventually collapse and cardiac arrest and possibly electromechanical dissociation.

Treatment should be immediate. Insertion of a needle into the pleural space (usually second intercostals) results in gas spontaneously escaping from the pleural cavity. A chest tube should then be inserted and connected to a low-intensity suction device.

Acute asthma

This is another medical emergency requiring prompt diagnosis and treatment. Signs suggestive of a severe asthma attack include:

- Inability of the patient to talk in full sentences due to dyspnea.
- Patient sitting forward and using accessory muscles of respiration—prominent diaphragmatic movements and pursing of the lips on expiration.
- Tachycardia.
- Peak flow 30% of normal or less (not usually used for diagnosis of acute asthma).
- Pulsus paradoxus—a drop in systolic blood pressure of more than 10mmHg on inspiration.
- Silent chest due to severe airflow limitation. If the patient suddenly stops wheezing, you should do one of two things. Either congratulate yourself for a successful treatment or get ready your laryngoscope to intubate the patient. The disappearance of wheezing in asthmatic patients may signal that they can no longer move enough for the flow to create a wheezing noise.

Hypercapnea on blood gas analysis (or "normalization" of pCO_2 from a low baseline) suggests that the patient is becoming exhausted and respiratory arrest may be imminent. This may occur before there is severe hypoxia. The patient should be considered for intubation and mechanical ventilation.

Appropriate treatment with intravenous hydrocortisone, oxygen therapy, nebulized bronchodilators, and intravenous fluids should be commenced immediately.

Acute left ventricular failure

The detailed management of acute left ventricular failure is discussed in more detail in Chapter 19. The patient needs urgent treatment or will die from asphyxiation. Classic signs of left ventricular failure include:

- Severe dyspnea.
- Central cyanosis.
- Patient sits upright.
- Bilateral basal fine end-respiratory crackles (in severe LVF the crackles extend upward to fill both lung fields).
- Hypotension secondary to poor left ventricular output (common).

Blood gases show hypoxia and often hypocapnea due to hyperventilation. There is usually a metabolic acidosis as a result of poor tissue perfusion.

Treatment includes sitting the patient up, 100% inhaled oxygen via a mask, and intravenous furosemide, morphine, and nitrate drip.

Also determine the underlying cause for acute left ventricular failure (such as acute myocardial infarction, severe hypertension, cardiac arrhythmias, thyrotoxicosis).

Pulmonary embolus

This may present in a number of ways. For example:

- Severe dyspnea.
- Cough with hemoptysis.
- Collapse and syncope.
- Hypotension.
- Cardiorespiratory arrest (often with electromechanical dissociation or ventricular fibrillation).

If PE is suspected, anticoagulation should be commenced immediately with an intravenous heparin infusion or subcutaneous low-molecular-weight heparin.

If the patient is hemodynamically unstable (suggesting a massive PE), thrombolysis may be administered or emergency pulmonary angiography carried out in an attempt to disrupt the embolus.

Pneumonia

The patient may be febrile or even show signs of septic shock (e.g., hypotension, renal failure). Blood gases may reveal hypoxia, which may be extremely severe in pneumonia caused by *Pneumocystis carinii*. Patients with PCP have a pulse oximetery (pulse ox) that plummets during ambulation. Suspect this diagnosis if the patient is immunocompromised in some way (via illness or immunosuporessive therapy). Also remember that in severe cases steroids are now being used along with antibiotics to treat this infection.

The chest radiograph may show lobar or patchy consolidation. Radiographic changes may be deceptively mild in *Mycoplasma* or *Legionella* infections.

The most common community-acquired organisms are still pneumococci and atypical organisms such as mycoplasma; thus, appropriate antibiotic therapy should be commenced immediately after blood (and sputum if possible) cultures have been taken.

3. Syncope

Syncope is a loss of conciousness usually due to a reduction in perfusion of the brain.

Differential diagnosis of syncope

Many conditions may give rise to loss of consciousness. They can be divided into cardiac, vasovagal, circulatory, cerebrovascular, neurological, and metabolic (Fig. 3.1).

History in a patient who presents with suspected syncope

The first differentiation to be made is between cardiac and noncardiac (usually neurological) syncope. Differentiation depends upon a detailed history of the syncopal episode with particular emphasis on the features outlined below:

Events preceding the syncope

- Exertion—may precipitate syncope in hypertrophic obstructive cardiomyopathy (HOCM) or aortic stenosis.
- Pain or anxiety—in vasovagal syncope.
- Standing—may precipitate postural hypotension.
- Neck movements—aggravate vertebrobasilar attacks.
- Palpitations—in cardiac arrhythmias, more often in tachyarrhythmias.

Speed of onset of syncope

- Immediate with no warning—classic presentation of Stokes-Adams attacks (arrhythmia). In a patient with coronary artery disease, syncope without warning is ventricular tachycardia (VT) until proved otherwise. In this situation the patient has no prodrome and becomes immediately unconscious.
- Rapid with warning—either preceded by lightheadedness (vasovagal) or by an aura (epilepsy).
- Gradual with warning—hypoglycemia preceded by lightheadedness, nausea, and sweating.

Account of the syncope by a witness

- This is very important—indeed no history is complete without one.
- Patient lies still breathing regularly—Stokes–Adams attack (a prolonged Stokes-Adams attack may cause epileptiform movements secondary to cerebral anoxia).
- Patient shakes limbs or has facial twitching and possibly associated with urinary incontinence and tongue biting—epilepsy.
- Patient becomes very pale and gray immediately before collapsing—vasovagal (patients who have cardiac syncope become very pale after collapse before regaining consciousness).

Recovery of conciousness

- If the patient feels very well soon after episode—a cardiac cause is likely.
- If the patient feels washed out and nauseated and takes a few minutes to return to normal—the cause is probably vasovagal.
- If the patient has a neurological deficit—transient cerebral ischemia (transient ischemic attack, TIA) or epilepsy is likely. (Todd's paralysis is used to describe postictal hemiplegia or hemiparesis or any other focal neurological deficit; the paralysis is usually transient.)
- If the patient is very drowsy and falls asleep soon after regaining consciousness—epilepsy is probable.

Past medical history

As always a thorough history is needed:

- Any cardiac history is important—ischemia may precipitate arrhythmias.
- A history of stroke or TIA may suggest a cerebrovascular cause.
- Diabetes mellitus may cause autonomic neuropathy and postural hypotension, whereas good control of diabetes mellitus puts the patient at risk of hypoglycemia.
- A history of head injury may suggest epilepsy secondary to cortical scarring.
- A history of cancer requires that metastasis to the brain be ruled out.

Differential diagnosis of syncope	
System involved	**Pathology**
Cardiac	Tachyarrhythmia—supraventricular or ventricular Bradyarrhythmia—sinus bradycardia, complete or second-degree heart block, sinus arrest Stokes-Adams attack—syncope due to transient asystole Left ventricular outflow tract obstruction—aortic stenosis, HOCM Right ventricular outflow tract obstruction—pulmonary stenosis Pulmonary hypertension
Vasovagal	After carotid sinus massage and also precipitated by pain (simple faint), micturition, anxiety; these result in hyperstimulation by the vagus nerve, which leads to AV node block (and therefore bradycardia, hypotension, and syncope)
Circulatory	Postural hypotension—usually due to antihypertensive drugs or diuretics; also caused by autonomic neuropathy as in diabetes mellitus Pulmonary embolus—may or may not be preceded by chest pain Septic shock—severe peripheral vasodilatation results in hypotension
Cerebrovascular	Transient ischemic attack Vertebrobasilar attack
Neurological	Epilepsy
Metabolic	Hypoglycemia

Fig. 3.1 Differential diagnosis of syncope. (See also Fig. 9.3.) (AV, atrioventricular; HOCM, hypertrophic obstructive cardiomyopathy.)

Medication history

Important points include the following:

- Antihypertensives and diuretic agents predispose to postural hypotension.
- Class I and class III antiarrhythmics may cause long QT syndrome and predispose to torsades de points—all antiarrhythmic agents may cause bradycardia leading to syncope.
- Some other drugs may also predispose to long QT syndrome (e.g., quinidine, macrolide antibiotics, tricyclic antidepressants; complete list can be found at www.torsades.org)
- Vasodilators precipitate syncope in pulmonary hypertension.

Family history

A family history of sudden death or recurrent syncope may occur in patients who have hypertrophic obstructive cardiomyopathy and also in those rare cases of familial long QT syndrome (Romano-Ward and Jervell-Lange-Nielson syndromes).

A few patients who have epilepsy have a family history.

Social history

Note that:

- Alcohol excess is a risk factor for withdrawal seizures.
- Smoking is a risk factor for ischemic heart disease.
- Recreational drug use could cause syncope.

Examination of patients who present with syncope

The points to note on examination of the patient who has syncope are summarized in Fig. 3.2 and discussed in turn below. On inspection:

- Look for any neurological deficit suggestive of a cerebrovascular cause (e.g., speech deficit or hemiplegia).
- Look for any signs of shock, such as pallor or sweating.

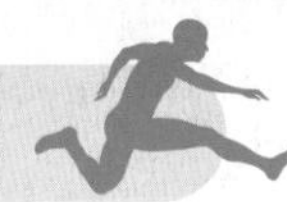

Notes on syncope:

- Cardiovascular syncope is always accompanied by hypotension.
- Syncope with normal blood pressure is likely to have a neurological, cerebrovascular, or metabolic cause.
- Stokes-Adams attacks are episodes of syncope due to cardiac rhythm disturbance.
- Tonic-clonic movements while unconscious are not always caused by epilepsy. They can occur in any patient who has cerebral hypoperfusion or a metabolic disorder (e.g., cardiac syncope or syncope secondary to a pulmonary embolus, cerebrovascular event, hypoglycemia, or alcohol withdrawal).

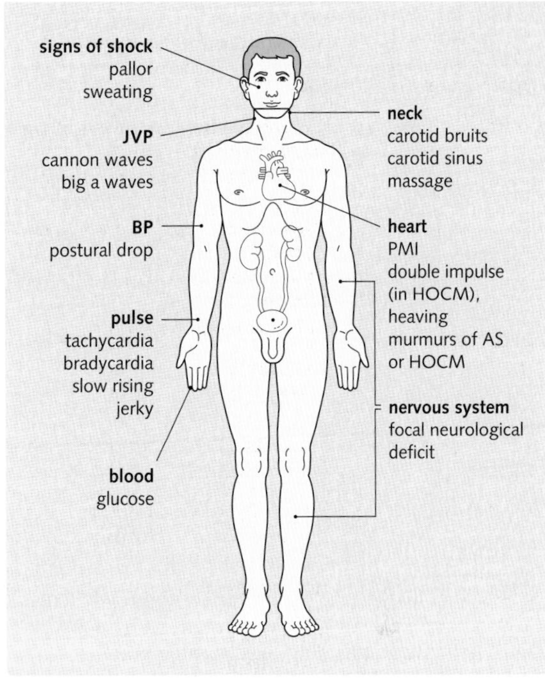

Fig. 3.2 Points to note on examination of a patient presenting with syncope. (AS, aortic stenosis; BP, blood pressure; HOCM, hypertrophic obstructive cardiomyopathy; JVP, jugular venous pressure.)

Always look for trauma secondary to the syncopal episode. The elderly are more at risk for head trauma or other injuries that may occur with lose of consciousness. A patient may present with mental status change not related to a postictal episode but resulting from a subdural hematoma or other traumatic injury. This is especially important in patients on anticoagulation. Always check the international normalized ratio (INR) in anyone who may be on warfarin.

Cardiovascular system

On examination note the following:

- Pulse—any tachy- or bradyarrhythmia and character of pulse (slow rising in aortic stenosis, jerky in HOCM).
- Blood pressure lying and standing to detect orthostatic hypotension (20 mmHg drop in blood pressure from lying to standing or a 10 beat rise in HR).
- Jugular venous pulse—cannon "a" waves in complete heart block (due to the atrium contracting against a closed tricuspid valve); prominent "a" wave in pulmonary hypertension.
- PMI—double impulse (HOCM), heaving (aortic stenosis).
- Any murmurs—crescendo–decrescedo murmur of aortic stenosis.
- Carotid bruits—indicating carotid artery stenosis and cerebrovascular disease.
- Response to carotid sinus massage—apply unilateral firm pressure over the carotid sinus with the patient in bed and attached to a cardiac monitor. Full resuscitative equipment should be easily accessible. Patients who have carotid sinus hypersensitivity will become very bradycardic and may even become asystolic. Do not perform this maneuver on a patient with a carotid bruit.

Neurological system

This system should be fully examined to detect any residual deficit.

Chemstick test for blood glucose

This is an easy test and, if positive, may provide valuable diagnostic information.

First-line tests to exclude an emergency syncope	
Test	**Diagnosis**
EKG	Look for rhythm disturbance or signs of pulmonary embolus
EKG monitoring	If suspected cardiac arrhythmia on CCU
Temperature, Hb, WBC	Look for septic or hemorrhagic cause
Blood sugar	Look for hypoglycemia
Electrolytes	Look for hypokalemia (may precipitate arrhythmias)
Carotid Dopplers	Look for carotid stenosis (TIA)
CT scan	For possible cerebral infarct or TIA or intracranial bleed causing seizures in a patient with a recent head injury

Fig. 3.3 First-line tests to exclude an emergency syncope. (CCU, coronary care unit; CT, computed tomography; CXR, chest radiography; EKG, electrocardiography; Hb, hemoglobin; TIA, transient ischemic attack; WBC, white blood cell count.)

Investigations

First-line tests to exclude emergencies are shown in Fig. 3.3.

Blood tests

The following tests should be performed:

- Complete blood count—anemia may be secondary to hemorrhage, which will cause postural hypotension; leukocytosis in sepsis and in the postictal period.
- Electrolytes and renal function—both hypokalaemia and hyperkalemia predisposes towards arrhythmias, always check magnesium and replace when correcting for hypocalcemia and hypokalemia.
- Calcium—hypocalcemia is a cause of long QT syndrome.
- Cardiac enzymes—a myocardial infarction may cause sudden arrhythmia.
- Blood glucose.

Electrocardiography

This may show:

- A brady- or tachyarrhythmia.
- Heart block.
- A long QT interval.
- Ischemia.
- Evidence of a pulmonary embolus.

Holter monitor

This is used to provide a 24- or 48-hour EKG trace to detect arrhythmias and bradycardias (e.g., sick sinus syndrome, intermittent heart block).

Tilt test

This may aid diagnosis:

- Simple tilt produces hypotension and possibly syncope in autonomic denervation.
- Prolonged tilt may provoke vasovagal syncope with bradycardia and hypotension.

Chest radiography

On the chest radiograph:

- There may be cardiomegaly.
- The lung fields may be oligemic due to a pulmonary embolus.

Echocardiography

This may reveal:

- Aortic stenosis.
- Hypertrophic cardiomyopathy.
- Left atrial enlargement in supraventricular tachycardia.
- Left atrial thrombus in TIA (transthoracic echocardiography cannot reliably diagnose intracardiac thrombus; if this is suspected as a cause of TIA, transesophageal echocardiography is needed). Left atrial thrombus may be seen in atriba fibrillation.
- Left ventricular abnormalities in ventricular tachycardia or ventricular fibrillation.
- Right ventricular abnormalities in pulmonary hypertension.

Carotid duplex ultrasound scan

To detect carotid atheroma as source of emboli in TIA. This should be performed regardless of whether carotid bruits are present in a patient who is strongly suspected of having TIAs. Majority of emboli are from atheromatous plaques involving the carotids.

Computed tomography scan of the brain

This may reveal areas of previous infarction in a patient who has had a TIA or brain metastasis in a patient with cancer.

Electrophysiological study of the heart

Consider this if cardiac arrhythmia is strongly suspected but not revealed by Holter monitor.

Electroencephalography (EEG)

EEG will assist in the diagnosis of epilepsy in selected patients.

Syncope of recent onset

This situation represents a medical emergency requiring rapid diagnosis and treatment. It is necessary in his situation to distinguish among the life-threatening causes:

- Intermittent ventricular tachycardia or fibrillation.
- Third-degree heart block, drug toxicity.
- Intermittent asystole.
- Pulmonary embolus.
- Shock.
- TIA heralding major stroke.
- Hypoglycemia.

Differentiating features of syncope

The method is to differentiate among cardiac, circulatory, and neurological causes.

Cardiac causes

Aortic stenosis (AS)

AS usually presents as effort-induced syncope because the left ventricular output is restricted by the outflow restriction. The diagnosis is made by feeling a slow rising carotid pulse and a heaving cardiac impulse in the precordium. An aortic ejection systolic murmur (cresecendo–decrescendo murmur in right upper sternal border) is present.

Electrocardiography may show left ventricular hypertrophy. Echocardiography reveals the stenotic valve, and assessment by Doppler velocity of change through the valve may give an indication of the severity. Patients who present with syncope secondary to AS have a life expectancy of approximately 3 years. Ask about any signs of CHF secondary to LVH and outflow obstruction, and attempt to elicit any previous episode of angina-type chest pain. Angina is the most foreboding presenting symptom in AS. Survival is only 2 years in patients with angina related to AS without intervention.

Cardiomyopathies

Hypertrophic obstructive cardiomyopathy can give rise to syncope by obstructing left ventricular outflow on exercise or by giving rise to ventricular tachycardia or fibrillation. This arrhythmic "sudden death syndrome" can also occur in patients who have nonhypertrophic myocardial dysplasias and patients who have heart failure (dilated cardiomyopathy).

A wide variety of EKG abnormalities is possible on a resting EKG. Holter monitoring may reveal an intermittent ventricular arrhythmia. Echocardiography reveals hypertrophy, subaortic obstruction, and heart failure (ventricular dilatation). A cardiac electrophysiological study may be necessary in difficult or complex cases.

Long QT syndrome

This may be congenital or drug-induced, usually by psychiatric or class III antiarrhythmic drugs (see Chapter 15). The syncope is caused by a self-limiting ventricular tachycardia characterized by a systematically rotating QRS vector (torsade de pointes). The tachycardia and syncope are relieved by rapid pacing or infusion of magnesium or pharmacological sinus tachycardia (e.g., using isoproterenol). The resting nonarrhythmic EKG shows QT prolongation.

Tachyarrhythmias

Syncope is uncommonly due to a supraventricular tachyarrhythmia unless the heart rate is extremely fast. Ventricular tachycardia is more likely to cause syncope because it is accompanied by asynchronous ventricular contraction. If these arrhythmias are not prominent on Holter monitoring, they may be induced during electrophysiological testing.

Bradyarrhythmias

Syncope may occur secondary to a bradyarrhythmia if cardiac output falls markedly as a consequence of the drop in rate. An ongoing bradyarrhythmia is easily detected using on an EKG (e.g., sinus bradycardia and second degree complete heart block). Some conditions, however, occur intermittently, and the EKG may be normal after the syncopal episode. For example, heart block may occur intermittently with normal sinus rhythm between episodes. Ambulatory EKG monitoring is therefore needed to capture these episodes. This may be difficult if they are separated by long periods of time.

In patients with bradyarrhythmia consider beta-blockers, calcium channel blockers, or digoxin.

Circulatory causes

Hypovolemia

Hypovolemia can present as postural hypotension (i.e., loss of consciousness on standing, relieved by lying flat). This occurs because the blood volume is inadequate, even with an intact baroreflex, to maintain arterial blood pressure in the face of gravity-dependent blood pooling. If it is due to acute hemorrhage, there are usually other obvious manifestations such as trauma or hematemesis and melena. However, internal bleeding can sometimes be difficult to detect. With acute blood loss, the hemoglobin may be normal because there may not have been time for hemodilution to occur.

Septic shock

This causes similar effects by excessive vasodilatation, which prevents baroreflex compensation for postural-dependent blood pooling. However, the patient is usually obviously febrile and septic.

Classical postural hypotension

This is due to inadequate baroreflex control. Along with a drop in blood pressure on standing, there may be very little compensatory tachycardia (part of the baroreflex efferent mechanism is to increase heart rate). This can be formally tested by a simple tilt test, during which there are an excessive blood pressure drop and an inadequate tachycardic response.

Obstruction of pulmonary arteries

Obstruction of pulmonary arteries by embolus enters into the differential diagnosis of all cardiovascular emergencies in which syncope is a feature. Chronic thromboembolism or primary pulmonary hypertension can also lead to postural hypotension because the resistance to right ventricular ejection is too high to allow adequate cardiac output when the filling pressure drops on standing.

Cerebrovascular Causes

Transient cerebral ischemia

This often presents to cardiologists because of the known cardiac or arterial causation. After syncope patients show a neurological deficit that recovers with time. There may be repeated episodes. The etiology of neurological deficit can often be seen on CT or magnetic resonance scans of the brain. When carotid disease is the source of a cerebral embolus, a bruit may be heard over one or the other carotid artery. Even if this is absent, the carotid arteries should be scanned using duplex Doppler to delineate any atheromatous filling defects.

A cardiac source of embolus should be suspected if the patient is in atrial fibrillation.

Left atrial or ventricular thrombus may be difficult to detect by transthoracic echocardiography, in which case a transesophageal echocardiogram should be performed.

Sometimes TIA is due to an embolus from an infective vegetation of the mitral or aortic valve, or very rarely a left atrial myxoma. These conditions are also investigated by transthoracic and transesophageal echocardiography.

Patients who have an atrial septal defect may have TIAs secondary to paradoxical emboli (i.e., emboli arising from the right side of the circulation that pass across to the left).

Vertebrobasilar syndrome

This is caused by obstruction of the arteries to the posterior part of the brain (brainstem and cerebellum). The syncope may be preceded by vertigo or dizziness. Precipitation by neck movement is a classic feature in this syndrome when it is associated with cervical spondylosis because the vertebral arteries course within the cervical vertebrae and can get kinked if there is osteoarthritis.

Other neurological causes

Neurological causes without any cardiac or arterial etiology should be studied in *Crash Course: Neurology*, but epilepsy should always be borne in mind during history taking.

Metabolic Causes

In the common situation of insulin-dependent diabetes mellitus, most patients are inadequately controlled, which leads to more rapid development of heart disease and autonomic neuropathy. Fear of this has driven a few patients to control their diabetes mellitus very obsessively and tightly. These patients tend to experience episodes of loss of consciousness due to hypoglycemia.

However, hypoglycemia can occur in any treated diabetic patient and may be precipitated by exercise or reduction in food intake.

4. Palpitations

Palpitations are an unpleasant awareness of the heart beat. They may be rapid, slow, or just very forceful beats at a normal rate.

Differential diagnosis of palpitations

Palpitations may be caused by any disorder causing a change in cardiac rhythm or rate and any disorder causing increased stroke volume.

Rapid palpitations

These may be regular or irregular. Regular palpitations may be a sign of:

- Sinus tachycardia.
- Atrial flutter.
- Atrial tachycardia.
- Supraventricular re-entry tachycardia.

Irregularly irregular palpitations may indicate:

- Atrial fibrillation.
- Multiple atrial or ventricular ectopic beats.
- Multifocal Atrial Tachycardia (MAT): usually found in patients with lung pathology.

Slow palpitations

Patients often describe these as missed beats or forceful beats (after a pause the next beat is often more forceful due to a long filling time and therefore a higher stroke volume). The following may be causes of slow palpitations:

- Sick sinus syndrome.
- Atrioventricular block.
- Occasional ectopics with compensatory pauses.

Disorders causing increased stroke volume

Increased stroke volume may result from:

- Valvular lesions (e.g., mitral or aortic regurgitation).
- High-output states (e.g., pregnancy, thyrotoxicosis, or anemia).

History to focus on the differential diagnosis of palpitations

When taking a history from a patient complaining of palpitations, aim to find answers to the following three questions:

- What is the nature of the palpitations?
- How severe or life-threatening are they?
- What is the likely underlying cause?

Nature of the palpitations

Ask the patient to describe the palpitation by tapping them out (fast, slow, regular, or irregular). Are the palpitations continuous or intermittent? (Paroxysmal is the term used for intermittent tachycardias.)

Severity of the palpitations

Determine the severity of the palpitations (i.e., are they associated with complications such as cardiac failure, exacerbation of ischemic heart disease, or thromboembolic events?).

Are the palpitations associated with:

- Syncope, dizziness, or shortness of breath—suggesting that cardiac output is compromised.
- Angina—suggesting they are causing or being caused by underlying ischemic heart disease.
- History of structural heart disease—valvular heart disease (severe mitral regurgitation due to mitral valve prolapse), left ventricular aneurysm.
- History of stroke or transient ischemic attack or limb ischemia—suggesting thromboembolic complications of arrhythmia.

Likely underlying causes of palpitation

Are there any features in the history suggestive of the recognized causes of arrhythmias shown in Fig. 4.1.

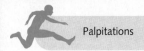

Examination of patients with palpitations

Fig. 4.2 summarizes the important points in the examination of a patient who has palpitations, which are outlined below.

When examining any patient who supposedly has a cardiac problem, you must perform a thorough examination of all systems. Cardiac disease can both cause and be caused by disease in other systems.

General observation

Look for:

- Cyanosis—suggestive of cardiac failure or lung disease (remember that pulmonary embolus is a well-recognized cause of tachyarrhythmia).
- Dyspnea—suggestive of heart failure or lung disease.
- Pallor—suggestive of anemia.
- Thyrotoxic (e.g., exopthalmos) or myxedematous facies.

Features in the history suggesting the cause of an arrhythmia

Features in the history	Cause of arrhythmia
Chest pain, dyspnea on exertion, history of myocardial infarction, history of bypass surgery	Ischemic heart disease
Tremor, excessive sweating, unexplained weight loss, lethargy, obesity, history of thyroid surgery	Thyroid disease
History of rheumatic fever	Heart valve disease
Peptic ulcer disease, menorrhagia, recent surgery	Anemia
Alcohol, caffeine, amphetamine, antiarrhythmic agents	Proarrhythmic drugs
Anxiety	Anxiety

Fig. 4.1 Features in the history that may suggest the cause of an arrhythmia.

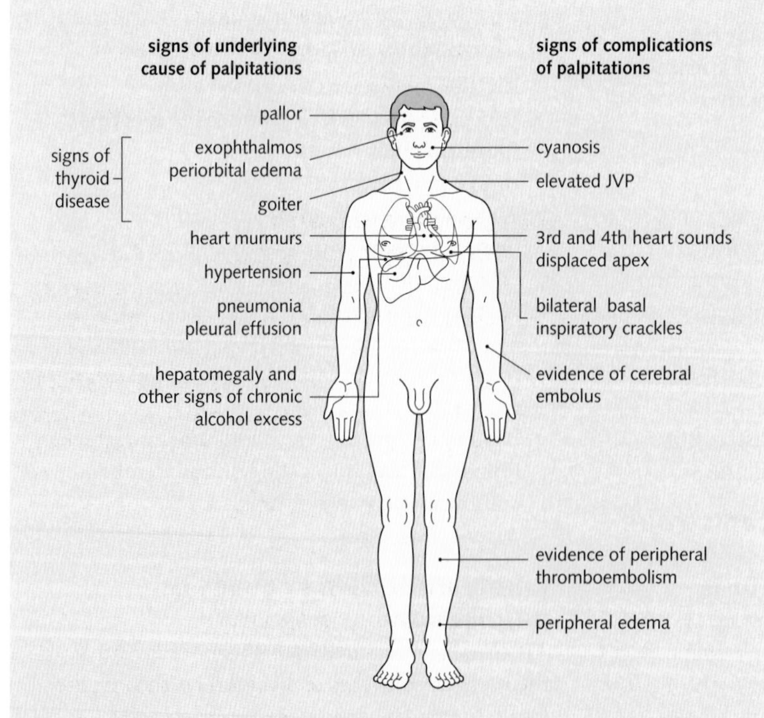

Fig. 4.2 Important points to note when examining a patient who has palpitations. (CVA, cerebrovascular accident; JVP, jugular venous pressure.)

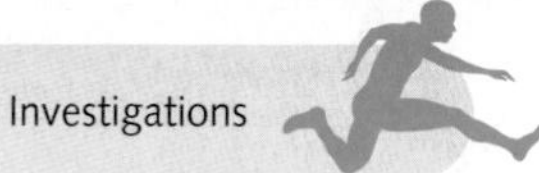

Cardiovascular system

Pulse

Note the rate, rhythm, and character of the pulse at the radial artery (time it for at least 15 s).
Information about the character of the pulse is often more clearly elicited from the carotid pulse, especially features such as:

- A slow rising pulse—due to aortic stenosis.
- A collapsing pulse—due to aortic regurgitation.

A high-volume pulse (due to high-output states and aortic or mitral regurgitation) is often most easily felt at the radial pulse, where it is felt as an abnormally strong pulsation.

Blood pressure

This may be low if the patient has palpitations. Hypertension is a cause of atrial fibrillation. A wide pulse pressure is a sign of aortic regurgitation, whereas a narrow pulse pressure suggests aortic stenosis.

Jugular venous pressure

The jugular venous pressure may be elevated if the patient has congestive heart failure as a consequence of uncontrolled tachycardia or atrial flutter or fibrillation secondary to pulmonary embolism.

Point of maximal impulse

This may be displaced in a patient who has left ventricular failure.

Heart sounds

A third or fourth heart sound may be heard. A third heart sound is heard in patients with mitral regurgitation and heart failure, whereas a fourth heart sound is heard in hypertension and aortic stenosis. Murmurs of mitral or aortic regurgitation are possible causes of high-output state. The murmur of mitral stenosis may be heard in patients who have atrial fibrillation. Of note, you cannot have a fourth heart sound in a patient with atrial fibrillation. There is no atrial kick to precipitate the sound.

Respiratory system

Bilateral basal inspiratory crackles are heard in a patient who has left ventricular failure. There may be signs of an underlying chest infection (consolidation or effusion), a common cause of palpitations.

Gastrointestinal system

Hepatomegaly and ascites may be signs of congestive heart failure or signs of alcoholic liver disease—alcohol is one of the most common causes of tachyarrhythmias. Look for other signs of liver disease if this is suspected.

Limbs

On examining the limbs note the following points:

- Peripheral edema may be a sign of congestive heart failure.
- Tremor may be a sign of thyrotoxicosis or alcohol withdrawal.
- Brisk reflexes seen in thyrotoxicosis.
- Weakness may be a sign of previous cerebral embolus.

Investigations

Blood tests

The following blood tests may aid diagnosis:

- Electrolytes—hypokalemia is an aggravating factor for most tachyarrhythmias. (Hypokalemia, hypocalcemia, and hypomagnesemia all are possible causes of torsades de pointes.)
- Complete blood count—anemia or a leukocytosis suggesting sepsis may be evident.
- Thyroid function tests (TSH will be *low* in thyrotoxicosis).
- Liver function—deranged in congestive heart failure or alcoholic liver disease.

Electrocardiography

12-lead electrocardiography

This may enable the diagnosis to be made instantly. However, if the palpitations are intermittent or paroxysmal, the EKG may be normal.

There may be signs of the cause of the palpitations on the EKG. For example, ischemia, hypertension, or presence of a delta wave or short PR interval as seen in some congenital causes of paroxysmal tachyarrhythmias such as Wolff-Parkinson-White syndrome (pre-excitation).

24-hour electrocardiography

Monitoring of the EKG for 24 hours may reveal paroxysmal arrhythmias. Patients note down the times that palpitations occur, and these can be

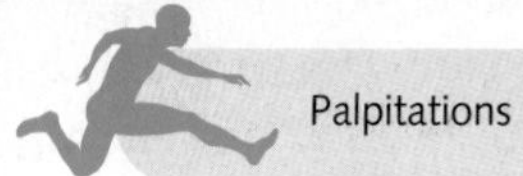

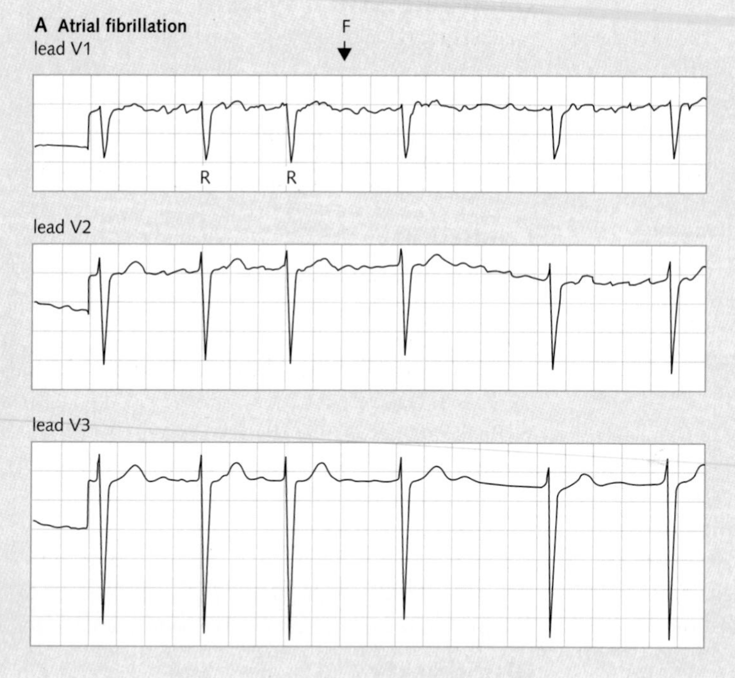

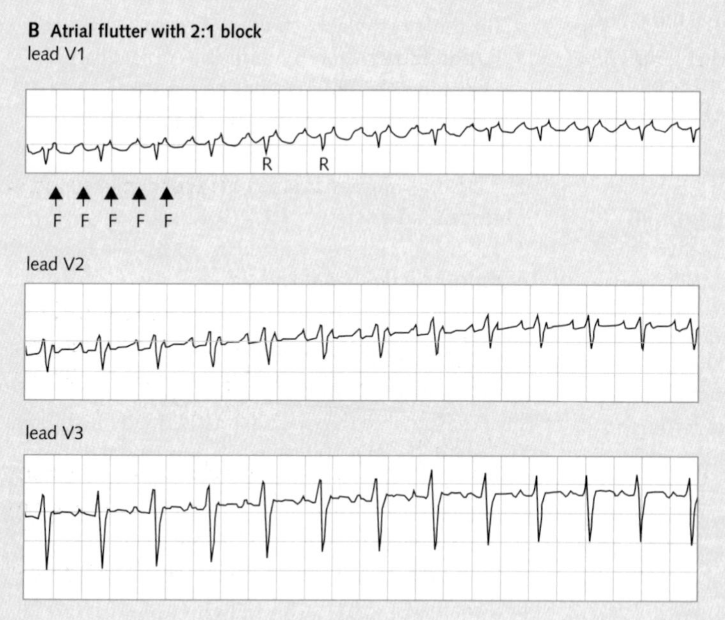

Fig. 4.3 Electrocardiograms illustrating atrial fibrillation, atrial flutter, and supraventricular re-entry tachycardia. (A) Note the narrow QRS complexes. Fibrillation waves (F) can sometimes be seen. Note the irregularly irregular rhythm and the absence of P waves preceding the QRS complexes. The baseline may show an irregular fibrillating pattern. (B) Note the regular rhythm with a rate divisible into 300 (150 beats/min in this case). The P waves are seen in all three leads, but best in V1 at a rate of 300/min. Occasionally the F (flutter) waves form a sawtooth-like pattern (not shown here). Note the F waves at 200-ms intervals (300/min), narrow QRS, and regular RR intervals at 400ms (150/min). (C) The rhythm is regular and fast (usually 140–240 beats/min). P waves may be seen and can occur before or after the QRS. Point X shows reversion back to sinus rhythm—note that the following beat has a normal P wave preceding it.

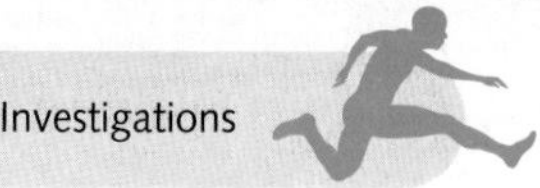

Fig. 4.4 *Continued*

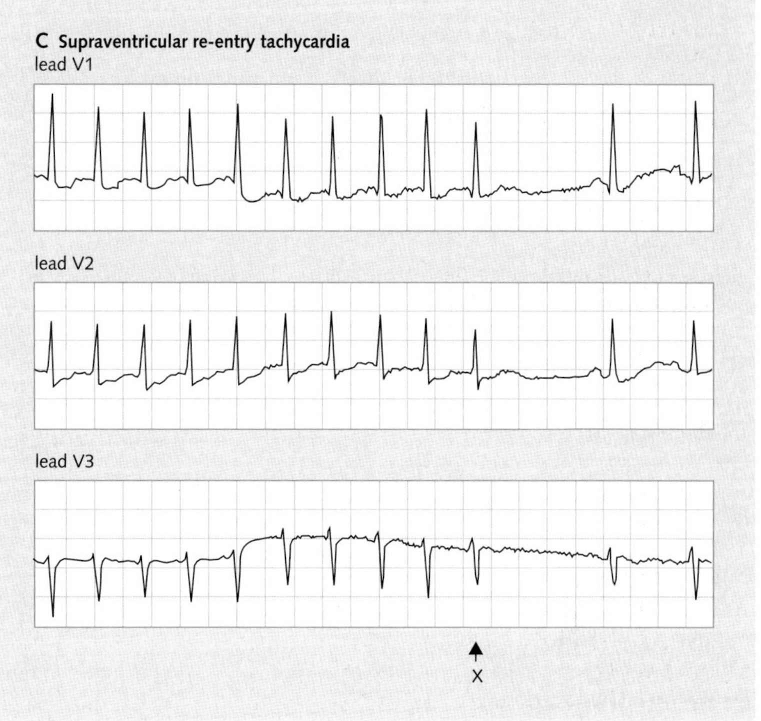

compared with the recorded EKG at that time. Monitors are available that record the EKG for longer periods of time to diagnose more infrequent episodes.

Exercise electrocardiography

This test may be used to reveal exercise-induced arrhythmias. Examples of EKGs illustrating atrial fibrillation, atrial flutter, and supraventricular re-entry tachycardia are shown in Fig. 4.3.

Vagotonic maneuvers

Such maneuvers include:

- Valsalva maneuver.
- Carotid sinus massage.
- Diving reflex: placing the patients face in a bowl of cold water.
- Painful stimuli.

These maneuvers all act by increasing vagal tone, which in turn increases the refractory period of the atrioventricular (AV) node and increases AV node conduction time. By doing this it is possible to differentiate among three common tachyarrhythmias that are sometimes indistinguishable on EKG recording:

- Atrial flutter.
- Atrial fibrillation.
- Supraventricular re-entry tachycardia.

The characteristic features of these tachyarrhythmias are listed in Fig. 4.4.

Adenosine administration

Adenosine is a purine nucleoside that acts to block the AV node. When administered intravenously it will achieve complete AV block. Its half-life is very short, only a few seconds so this effect is very short-lived.

Side effects of adenosine include bronchospasm, so avoid in asthmatics. This medication can actually cause the heart to momentary stop. It is important that you prepare your patients for administration of this drug.

Chest radiography

Look for:

- Evidence of valve disease (e.g., large left atrium and pulmonary vascular congestion in mitral stenosis).
- Evidence of heart failure—enlarged heart shadow, pulmonary edema.

Features of atrial fibrillation, atrial flutter, and supraventricular re-entry tachycardia			
	Atrial fibrillation	**Atrial flutter**	**Supraventricular re-entry tachycardia**
Rate	Any rate; pulse deficit if fast	Atrial flutter rate is 300/min; the ventricular response is therefore divisible into this (usually 100 or 150/min)	140–260 beats/min
Rhythm	Irregularly irregular	Regular	Regular
Response to adenosine or Valsalva maneuver	Slowing of ventricular rate reveals underlying lack of P waves	Slowing of ventricular rate reveals underlying flutter waves	Blocking the AV node may "break" the re-entry circuit and terminate the tachycardia

Fig. 4.4 Characteristic features of atrial fibrillation, atrial flutter, and supraventricular re-entry tachycardia. (AV node, atrioventricular node.)

- Kerley B lines.
- Evidence of pulmonary disease—effusion, collapse, or consolidation.

Echocardiography

This will reveal any valvular pathology. It also enables evaluation of left ventricular function which can be decreased secondary to a previous MI or cardiomyopathy.

Electrophysiological study

This is useful in investigating patients suspected of having tachyarrhythmias due to abnormal re-entry pathways. The technique enables localization of the re-entry circuit, which may then be ablated using a radiofrequency thermal electrode placed inside the heart.

Other investigations

A variety of other investigations may be required to identify a suspected cause of the palpitations. These obviously depend upon the clinical evidence, for example:

- Ventilation/perfusion scan if a pulmonary embolus is likely.
- Coronary angiogram if coronary artery disease is suspected.

Whenever investigating, examining, or taking a history from a patient with palpitations, it is always useful to identify the nature, the severity, and the likely underlying cause of the palpitations. This will enable you to structure your approach and to present your findings in a logical manner.

5. Lower Extremity Edema

Peripheral edema is caused by an increase in extracellular fluid. The fluid will follow gravity; therefore, the ankles are the first part affected in the upright patient. Lower extremity swelling is indicative of edema if there is not a local acute or chronic traumatic cause. Edema may be a feature of generalized fluid retention or obstruction of fluid drainage from the lower limbs.

Differential diagnosis of edema

There are a number of causes of edema; they can be divided into five main groups (Fig. 5.1):

- Cardiac failure—this is due to increased sodium retention secondary to activation of the renin–angiotensin system. In this situation the kidneys do not receive enough blood (e.g., decreased forward flow, which is the hallmark of CHF) and respond as if the intravascular volume were decreased (when the patient is in fact euvolemic or hypervolemic). In an attempt to increase the amount of blood flow, the kidneys react by precipitating a cascade to increase intravascular volume, thereby actually worsening heart failure.
- Hypoalbuminemia—loss of oncotic pressure within the capillaries causes loss of fluid from the intravascular space. This may be secondary to renal loss of protein or decreased liver synthesis of protein. *Note:* To do a quick check of the liver's synthetic function, get a coagulation panel.
- Renal impairment—reduction in sodium excretion results in water retention.
- Hepatic cirrhosis—there are a number of mechanisms involved: hypoalbuminemia (occurs as the hepatic synthetic activity is reduced), peripheral vasodilatation, and activation of the renin–angiotensin system with resulting sodium retention.
- Drugs (e.g., corticosteroids, which act to increase sodium and water retention).

History to focus on the differential diagnosis of edema

The first differentiation to be made is between cardiac and noncardiac edema. The cause of the edema is usually revealed by a detailed systems review because there are often symptoms related to the underlying disorder. Associated dyspnea suggests:

- Pulmonary edema—this can occur due to heart failure or renal failure.
- Chronic lung disease (e.g., chronic obstructive pulmonary disease causes dyspnea).
- Primary and thromboembolic pulmonary hypertension—cause dyspnea and right heart failure.

Other important signs and symptoms include:

- Chest pain and palpitations—suggest underlying cardiac disease (ischemia or arrhythmias, respectively).
- A history of alcohol or drug abuse or of previous liver disease—suggests a hepatic cause for the edema.
- Diarrhea—may be due to a protein-losing enteropathy.

Past medical history

Ask about long-standing history of renal, cardiac, or liver disease.

Drug history

Important points include the following:

- Some drugs may be nephrotoxic (e.g., nonsteroidal anti-inflammatory agents, angiotensin-converting enzyme inhibitors; in patients with renal artery stenosis: cyclosporine, gentamicin, vancomycin, etc).
- Some may be hepatotoxic (e.g., methotrexate, isoniazid).
- Dihydropyridine calcium channel blockers cause ankle edema in some patients.

Differential diagnosis of lower extremity edema	
Pathology	**Cause**
Congestive heart failure	Myocardial infarction, recurrent tachyarrhythmias (particularly artial fibrillation), hypertensive heart disease, myocarditis, cardiomyopathy due to drugs and toxins, mitral, aortic, or pulmonary valve disease
Right heart failure secondary to pulmonary hypertension (cor pulmonale)	Chronic lung disease, primary pulmonary hypertension
Hypoalbuminemia	Excessive protein loss (due to nephritic syndrome, extensive burns, protein-losing enteropathy), reduced protein production (due to liver failure), or inadequate protein intake (due to protein-energy malnutrition)
Renal disease	Any cause of renal impairment (e.g., hypertension, diabetes mellitus, autoimmune disease, infection)
Liver cirrhosis	Alcohol, hepatitis A, B, C, etc., autoimmune chronic active hepatitis, biliary cirrhosis, Wilson's disease, hemachromatosis, drugs
Idiopathic	Premenstrual edema
Arteriolar dilatation (exposing the capillaries to high pressure, thus increasing intravascular hydrostatic pressure)	Dihydropyridine calcium channel blockers (e.g, nifedipine, amlodipine)
Sodium retention	Cushing's disease resulting in excessive mineralocorticoid activity, corticosteroids
Local causes	Cellulitis, venous thrombosis, lympedema

Fig. 5.1 Differential diagnosis of lower extremity edema.

Social history

Important findings may include:

- Smoking—a risk factor for ischemic heart disease.
- Intravenous drug abuse—a risk factor for hepatitis or endocarditis.
- Alcohol use—a risk factor for hepatic cirrhosis.

Causes of localized edema in either the arms or legs include:

- Local venous thrombosis or compression.
- Local cellulitis.
- Local trauma.
- Lymphedema secondary to obstruction of lymphatic drainage (e.g., secondary to malignancy).

Examination of patients with edema

A thorough examination of all systems usually reveals the underlying disease.

Cardiovascular system

Check the pulse and blood pressure:

- The pulse is often fast in the patient who has heart failure.
- Blood pressure may be low.
- Patients who have chronic renal disease are often hypertensive. (They may also be anemic secondary to the kidney's decreased production of erythropoietin. This also may lead to tachycardia.)

Check the jugular venous pressure (JVP). This is elevated in all patients who have generalized fluid overload and is therefore not a specific sign (only an elevated JVP in the absence of edema is specific for right ventricular failure).

On examination of the precordium:

- The PMI may be diffuse and laterally displaced in the patient who has cardiac failure.
- There may be a left parasternal heave suggestive of right ventricular strain.
- There may be added third and fourth heart sounds in heart failure.
- Audible murmurs may be present suggesting a valvular cause for heart failure.

> Remember that left ventricular dilatation causes mitral regurgitation due to stretching of the valve ring. Similarly tricuspid regurgitation is often the result of right ventricular enlargement.

Respiratory system

On inspection, consider the following:

- The patient may be tachypneic and cyanotic—this may be secondary to cardiac or respiratory disease.
- The lungs may be hyperinflated (due to emphysema) or hypoinflated (due to restrictive lung disease).

Expansion is reduced in all causes of lung disease, except perhaps primary pulmonary hypertension.

The lung bases may be stony dull indicating bilateral pleural effusions—these are a sign of generalized fluid retention.

Findings on auscultation of the lungs can include:

- Bilateral basal fine inspiratory crackles suggesting left ventricular failure.
- Coarse crackles or wheeze, which may be heard in bronchitis or emphysema.
- Mid-inspiratory crackles, which may be heard in pulmonary fibrosis.
- Chronic lung disease such as COPD or sleep apnea can predispose patients to pulmonary hypertension. This can eventually cause right heart failure.

Gastrointestinal system

Points to consider on inspection are as follows:

- Does the patient have signs of chronic liver disease such as jaundice, flapping tremor or asterixis, spider nevi, gynecomastia, loss of sexual hair, and testicular atrophy?
- Does the patient have renal failure and look uremic?

Palpation of the abdomen may reveal ascites in patients who have liver, cardiac, or renal disease. A caput medusae may be evident.

Renal system

Dipstick the urine—this is part of every examination of the cardiovascular system. Proteinuria is a feature of nephrotic syndrome and other causes of renal impairment. Hematuria is seen in some diseases causing renal impairment.

Examination of the edema

Edema of generalized fluid retention is pitting in nature. To demonstrate this, the area in question should be pressed firmly for at least 15s—there will be an indent in the edema after this. Be careful: ankle edema is often tender. How far does the swelling extend upward? Is the scrotum involved? The severity of the ankle edema can be roughly gauged by the extent to which the edema can be felt up the leg.

Lymphedema and chronic venous edema do not "pit." Also patients with chronic venous insufficiency frequently have brown discoloration of the skin at the ankles and lower legs from the chronic stasis of blood.

Fig. 5.2 summarizes the findings in patients who have lower extremity edema.

Investigations

Blood tests

The following blood tests should be considered:

- Complete blood count—anemia is common in chronic renal disease and can precipitate heart failure.
- Renal function—this is abnormal in renal disease, but note that patients who have long-standing cardiac or liver disease often have deranged renal function.
- Liver function—this is abnormal in liver disease, but note that hepatic congestion due to heart failure also causes abnormal liver function tests.

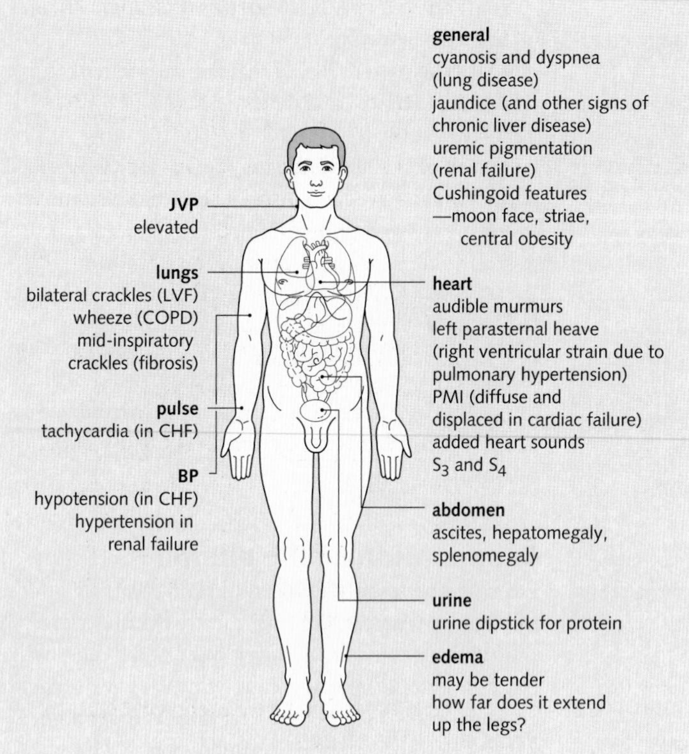

Fig. 5.2 Signs in patients who present with lower extremity edema. (BP, blood pressure; CHF, congestive heart failure; COPD, chronic obstructive pulmonary disease; JVP, jugular venous pressure; PMI, point of maximal impulse; LVF, left ventricular failure.)

- Plasma albumin concentration.
- Thyroid function—hyperthyroidism may precipitate heart failure.
- Coagulation profile—decreased hepatic function can lead to and increase in the PT and INR. Uremia from chronic renal failure can also lead to bleeding secondary to platelet dysfunction.
- BNP—increased in CHF

If Cushing's disease is suspected, the following tests are indicated:

- Random serum cortisol.
- 8 AM serum cortisol.
- Dexamethasone suppression test—low and high dose.
- 24-hour urine cortisol excretion.

Urine tests

With urine tests, note:

- A 24-hour urine protein excretion test is mandatory if there is no evidence of liver disease and the plasma albumin is low.
- Nephrotic syndrome causes loss of at least 3g protein in 24 hours. Nephrotic syndrome is the tetrad of edema, hypoalbuminemia, severe proteinurea, and hyperlipidemia.

Arterial blood gases

These tests may aid diagnosis:

- Hypoxia may be caused by lung or cardiac disease.
- Carbon dioxide retention is a sign of chronic obstructive pulmonary disease.
- Acidosis can occur with normal oxygen and carbon dioxide (metabolic acidosis) in both liver and renal failure.

Electrocardiography

This may show evidence of tachycardia, old myocardial infarction, left or right ventricular enlargement in a patient who has cardiac failure.

Chest radiography

Chest radiography may help diagnose:

- Cardiomegaly.
- Pulmonary edema.
- Pleural effusions.
- Lung overexpansion.

Echocardiography

This may show poor ventricular function or valve lesions. It helps to determine whether the patient has diastolic dysfunction or systolic dysfunction (low ejection fraction in latter).

Ultrasound

Regarding ultrasound:

- In a patient who has no evidence of cardiac, renal, or liver disease and bilateral ankle edema a venous obstruction or external compression must be excluded. Doppler studies of the hepatic/abdominal vasculature should then be performed. If the patient has ascites as well, then this study can also be used to mark for paracentesis.
- Doppler ultrasound to detect venous thrombosis and ultrasound of the pelvis to exclude a mass lesion causing compression are appropriate.

Important aspects

Salt and water retention

It is important to appreciate that edema in heart failure is due to generalized salt and water retention, which results from the neurohumoral response to heart failure. The lack of effective blood flow to the kidneys due to a failing heart activates the renin-angiotensin system and the kidneys act to retain sodium and water. (See Chapter 19). The symptoms and signs, therefore, do not differ from those due to generalized salt and water retention in other conditions with similar neurohumoral response. A similar picture is obtained when the salt and water retention is primarily renal in origin.

Increase in extracellular water and intravascular blood volume

Salt and water retention cause an increase in extracellular water and intravascular blood volume. The increase in volume of blood in the heart and central vessels increases pressures, including right atrial pressure. This is appreciated clinically as raised JVP. It can be observed very simply that the appearance of edema occurs first, and the increase in JVP follows as the central compartment subsequently fills up. When diuretics are administered, the JVP goes down first before the peripheral edema disappears. Therefore, it is incorrect to diagnose right heart failure from a raised JVP in the presence of edema. Right heat failure should be suspected only when the JVP is raised in the absence of edema or despite the removal of edema.

Hypertension treated with calcium channel blockers

Edema commonly appears in patients who have hypertension treated with the dihydropyridine calcium channel blockers (e.g., nifedipine, amlodipine). This is due to disturbance of Starling's forces in the tissue, not to general fluid retention. This type of edema should not be treated with diuretics, which cause electrolyte depletion.

6. Heart Murmur

A heart murmur is caused by turbulence of blood flow, which occurs when the velocity of blood is disproportionate to the size of the orifice it is moving through.

Differential diagnosis of heart murmur

Many conditions can give rise to a murmur:

- Valve lesions—either stenosis or regurgitation of any heart valve.
- Left ventricular outflow obstruction—an example is hypertrophic obstructive cardiomyopathy (HOCM).
- Ventricular septal defect.
- Vascular disorders—coarctation of the aorta, patent ductus arteriosus, arteriovenous malformations (pulmonary or intercostal), venous hum (cervical or hepatic).
- Increased blood flow—normal anatomy, but increased blood flow as in high-output states. Examples of high-output states are anemia, pregnancy, thyrotoxicosis, or childhood.
- Increased flow across a normal pulmonary valve in atrial and ventricular septal defect.

A differential diagnosis of heart murmur is shown in Fig. 6.1.

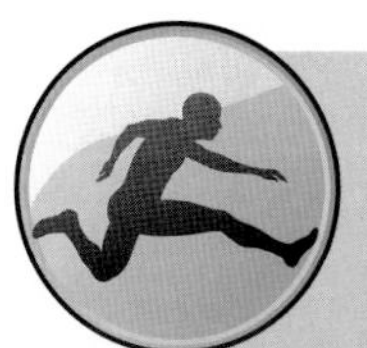

Cardiac sounds may be confused for murmurs; these include:

- Third and fourth heart sounds.
- Mid-systolic clicks, heard in mitral valve prolapse.
- Pericardial friction rub.

History to focus on the differential diagnosis of heart murmur

When taking a history from a patient who has a heart murmur, aim to answer the following questions:

- What is the possible etiology of the murmur (e.g., infective endocarditis, valve lesion secondary to rheumatic heart disease, high-output state)?
- Are there any complications of valve disease (e.g., cardiac failure, exacerbation of ischemic heart disease, arrhythmias, syncope)?

Presenting complaint

Common presenting complaints include:

- Shortness of breath—suggestive of heart failure; also ankle swelling, paroxysmal nocturnal dyspnea, fatigue.
- Chest pain—due to ischemic heart disease, aortic stenosis, or atypical chest pain seen in patients who have mitral valve prolapse.
- Syncope—especially seen in patients who have left ventricular outflow obstruction (e.g., aortic stenosis or HOCM).
- Fever, rigors, and malaise—common presenting complaints in patients who have infective endocarditis.
- Palpitations—for example, mitral valve disease is associated with atrial fibrillation.

Past medical history

Aim to elicit any history of cardiac disease with particular emphasis on possible causes of a murmur:

- History of rheumatic fever in childhood.
- Previous cardiac surgery.
- Myocardial infarction in past—may cause ventricular dilatation and therefore functional regurgitation or rupture or dysfunction of papillary muscle, leading to mitral regurgitation.

Differential diagnosis of heart murmur			
Phase of cardiac cycle	**Nature of murmur**	**Valve lesion**	**Cause of valve lesion**
Systolic	Ejection systolic	Aortic stenosis (AS)	Valvular stenosis, congenital valvular abnormality, rheumatic fever, supravalvular stenosis, subvalvular stenosis, senile valvular calcification
		Aortic sclerosis (murmur that does not radiate to the carotids)	Aortic valve roughening
		HOCM	Left ventricular outflow tract (subaortic) stenosis
		Increased flow across normal valve	High-output states (e.g., anemia, fever, pregnancy, thyrotoxicosis)
	Holosystolic	Mitral regurgitation (MR)	Functional MR due to dilatation of mitral valve annulus Valvular MR: rheumatic fever, infective endocarditis, mitral valve prolapse, chordal rupture, papillary muscle infarct
		Tricuspid regurgitation (TR)	Functional TR Valvular TR: rheumatic fever, infective endocarditis
		VSD with left-to-right shunt	Congenital, septal infarct (acquired)
Diastolic	Early diastolic	Aortic regurgitation (AR)	Functional AR: dilatation of valve ring, aortic dissection, cystic medial necrosis (Marfan syndrome) Valvular AR: rheumatic fever, infective endocarditis, bicuspid aortic valve
		Pulmonary regurgitation (PR)	Functional PR: dilatation of valve ring, Marfan syndrome, pulmonary hypertension Valvular PR: rheumatic fever, carcinoid, Fallot's tetralogy
	Mid-diastolic	Mitral stenosis (MS)	Rheumatic fever, congenital
		Tricuspid stenosis (TS)	Rheumatic fever
		Left and right atrial myxomas	Tumor obstruction of valve orifice in diastole
Continuous		PDA Arteriovenous fistula Cervical venous hum	Congenital

Fig. 6.1 Differential diagnosis of heart murmur. (HOCM, hypertrophic obstructive cardiomyopathy; PDA, patent ductus arteriosus; VSD, ventricular septal defect.)

- Family history of cardiac problems or sudden death—as may occur for patients who have HOCM.
- Recent dental procedures or operations—may be a cause of infective endocarditis.
- Anemia—ask about menorrhagia, liver disease, kidney disease, whether the patient is on iron therapy.

Social history

Ask in particular about:

- Smoking—an important risk factor for coronary artery disease.
- Alcohol intake—excessive intake may result in dilated cardiomyopathy.
- History of intravenous drug abuse—increases the risk of right sided endocarditis.

Examination of patients with heart murmur

General observation

Look for signs of cardiac failure (i.e., dyspnea, cyanosis, or edema). Look also for clues indicating the cause of the murmur:

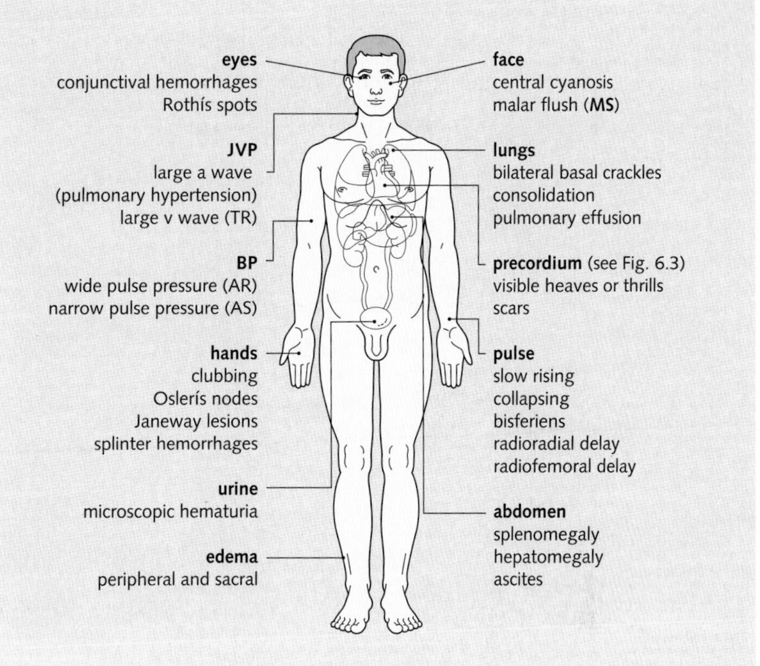

Fig. 6.2 Possible findings in a patient who has a heart murmur. (AS, aortic stenosis; AR, aortic regurgitation; MS, mitral stenosis; TR, tricuspid regurgitation.)

- Anemia—may cause a high-output state or be caused by infective endocarditis.
- Scars of previous cardiac surgery—median sternotomy, thoracotomy scars.

Examine the eyes for retinal hemorrhages (Roth's spots) and conjunctival hemorrhages. These are signs of infective endocarditis.

Fig. 6.2 gives a summary of the findings on examination of a patient who has a heart murmur.

Hands

Look for peripheral stigmas of infective endocarditis:

- Splinter hemorrhages—more than five is pathological. Splinter hemorrhages are proximal in the nail bed and do not appear until 2 weeks after the start of infectious endocarditis. Distal splinter hemorrhages are either really old or the result of trauma.
- Osler's nodes (painful, purplish, raised papules on finger pulps).
- Janeway lesions (erythematous nontender lesions on the thenar eminence).
- Finger clubbing.

Cardiovascular system

Pulse

Examine the pulse both at the radial site and the carotid artery. Examples of abnormal pulse due to valvular disease include:

- Slow rising or plateau pulse in aortic stenosis.
- Collapsing or waterhammer pulse in aortic regurgitation or patent ductus arteriosus.
- Birefringent pulse in mixed aortic valve disease.
- A jerky pulse in HOCM.

Blood pressure

This may also give important clues:

- A narrow pulse pressure associated with hypotension is a sign of severe aortic stenosis.
- A wide pulse pressure may be seen in aortic regurgitation or high-output states.

Jugular venous pressure

Remember that he patient must be at 45 degrees with the neck muscles relaxed (e.g., the patient facing forward). Since we all remember from anatomy that the sternocleidomastoid muscle (SCM) pulls the head to the opposite side, if we tilt the patients head away from us, the SCM will

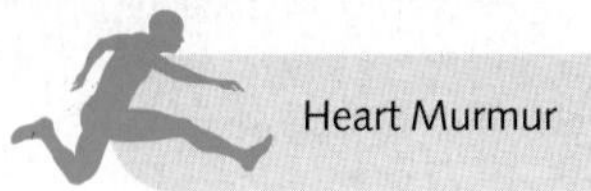

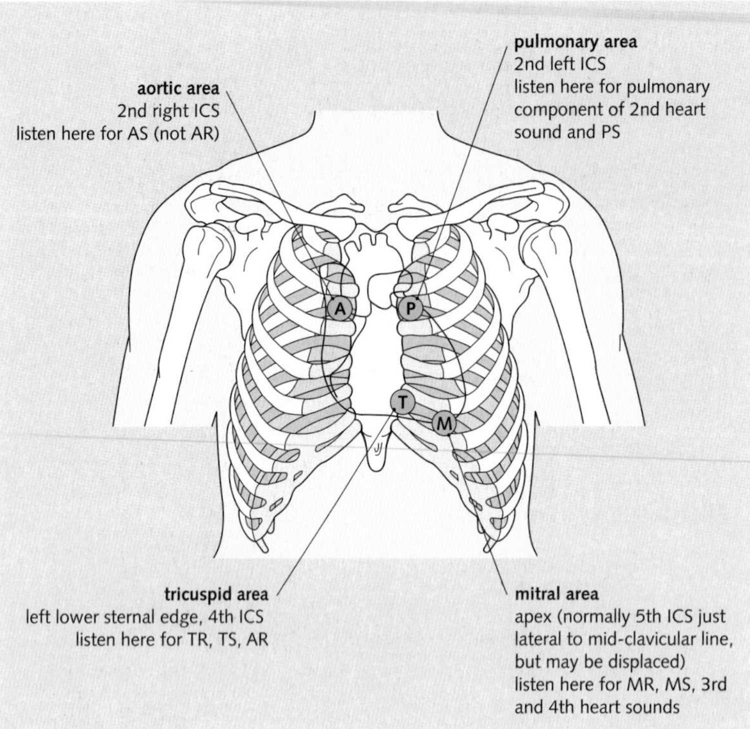

Fig. 6.3 Precordium, illustrating the position of valve areas. AR, aortic regurgitation; AS, aortic stenosis; ICS, intercostal space; MR, mitral regurgitation; MS, mitral stenosis; PS, pulmonary stenosis; TR, tricuspid regurgitation; TS, tricuspid stenosis.

contract over the vein we are attempting to observe. The jugular venous pressure is measured as the height of the visible pulsation vertically from the sternal angle. Possible findings include:

- An elevated jugular venous pressure in congestive heart failure.
- Large a waves in pulmonary stenosis and pulmonary hypertension.
- Large v waves—a sign of tricuspid regurgitation.
- Cannon A waves—the atria contracting against a closed tricuspid valve in AV disassociation.

Precordium

Remember to look for scars of previous surgery. On palpation the PMI (point of maximal impulse) is the point at which the impulse is the strongest. Possible abnormalities in a patient who has a murmur include:

- Displaced PMI—due to mitral regurgitation and aortic regurgitation.
- Double apical impulse—due to HOCM, also left ventricular aneurysm.
- Tapping PMI—due to mitral stenosis.
- Heaving PMI—due to aortic stenosis.
- Thrusting PMI—due to aortic or mitral regurgitation or any high-output state.

Right ventricular heave is a sign of right ventricular strain and may be felt in patients who have right ventricular failure due to mitral valve disease.

Thrills (or palpable murmurs) may be felt in any of the cardiac areas where the corresponding murmurs are best heard). The position of valve areas is shown in Fig. 6.3.

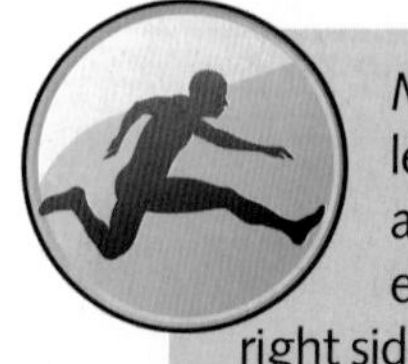

Murmurs from valves on the left side of the heart (mitral and aortic) are heard best in expiration. Those from the right side of the heart (pulmonary and tricuspid) are heard best in inspiration.

Maneuvers—straining or performing a Valsalva maneuver will increase the sound of a systolic

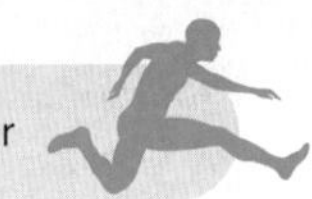

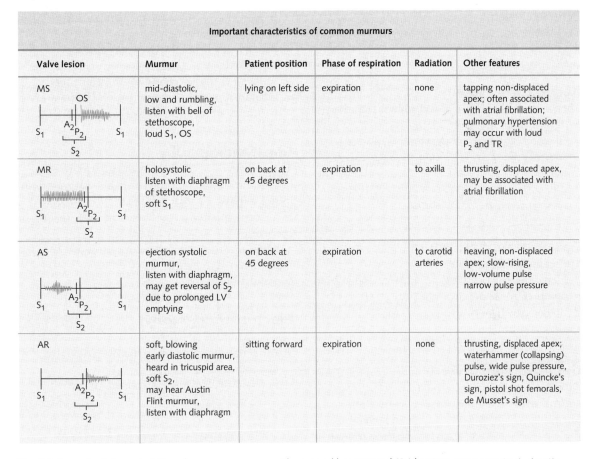

Valve lesion	Murmur	Patient position	Phase of respiration	Radiation	Other features
MS (diagram: S_1, OS, A_2, P_2, S_2, S_1)	mid-diastolic, low and rumbling, listen with bell of stethoscope, loud S_1, OS	lying on left side	expiration	none	tapping non-displaced apex; often associated with atrial fibrillation; pulmonary hypertension may occur with loud P_2 and TR
MR (diagram: S_1, A_2, P_2, S_2, S_1)	holosystolic listen with diaphragm of stethoscope, soft S_1	on back at 45 degrees	expiration	to axilla	thrusting, displaced apex, may be associated with atrial fibrillation
AS (diagram: S_1, A_2, P_2, S_2, S_1)	ejection systolic murmur, listen with diaphragm, may get reversal of S_2 due to prolonged LV emptying	on back at 45 degrees	expiration	to carotid arteries	heaving, non-displaced apex; slow-rising, low-volume pulse narrow pulse pressure
AR (diagram: S_1, A_2, P_2, S_2, S_1)	soft, blowing early diastolic murmur, heard in tricuspid area, soft S_2, may hear Austin Flint murmur, listen with diaphragm	sitting forward	expiration	none	thrusting, displaced apex; waterhammer (collapsing) pulse, wide pulse pressure, Duroziez's sign, Quincke's sign, pistol shot femorals, de Musset's sign

Fig. 6.4 Important characteristics of common murmurs. The second heart sound (S_2) has two components: A_2 (aortic valve closure) and P_2 (pulmonary valve closure). Duroziez's sign = a double murmur over the femoral or other large artery due to aortic insufficiency. Quincke's sign = alternating blanching and flushing of the skin that may be elicited in several ways, such as observing the nail bed or skin at the root of the nail while pressing on the end of the nail. De Musset's sign = rhythmic jerking movement of the head seen in cases of aortic aneurysm and aortic insufficiency. (AS, aortic stenosis; AR, aortic regurgitation; MR, mitral regurgitation; MS, mitral stenosis; OS, opening snap; S_1, first heart sound; TR, tricuspid regurgitation.)

murmur caused by HOCM. Also, an AR murmur is more easily heard with the patient leaning forward and holding his/her breath.

Characteristics of common murmurs are listed in Fig. 6.4.

Peripheral vascular system

All peripheral pulses should be palpated. Radioradial delay and radiofemoral delay may be found with coarctation of the aorta. Also seen in this condition is discrepancy in the blood pressure taken in each arm. It is important to look for these signs as part of the cardiovascular examination.

It is important to know these important characteristics for each of the common murmurs:

- Location at which to listen for the murmur.
- Position of the patient for each murmur.
- Phase of respiration during which each murmur is best heard.
- Nature of the murmur and where it radiates.

Peripheral edema

This may be elicited by applying firm pressure for at least 15 seconds.

Respiratory system

The chest should be carefully examined. Possible findings include:

- Bilateral basal fine end-inspiratory crackles—suggest pulmonary edema due to heart failure.
- Evidence of respiratory tract infection—sepsis may cause a high-output state.

Gastrointestinal system

Important findings include:

- Hepatomegaly or ascites, seen in right-sided heart failure or congestive heart failure.
- Splenomegaly, a feature of infective endocarditis.

Genitourinary system

Dipstick test of the urine should always be performed as part of the bedside examination. Microscopic hematuria (secondary to hemolysis caused by the growing vegetation on the heart valve) is a common finding in patients who have infective endocarditis.

Investigations

Blood tests

These include:

- Complete blood count—anemia may be seen as a sign of chronic disease in a patient who has infective endocarditis and is also a cause of hyperdynamic state; leukocytosis is also a feature of infective endocarditis.
- Urea and creatinine—may be elevated in patients who have heart failure as a result of poor renal perfusion or diuretic therapy.
- Electrolytes—may be deranged in patients who have heart failure as a result of diuretic therapy.
- Liver function tests—may be abnormal in patients who have hepatic congestion secondary to cardiac failure.
- Blood cultures—at least three sets should be taken before commencement of antibiotic therapy in all patients in whom infective endocarditis is suspected.
- ESR and C-reactive protein—these markers of inflammation or infection are useful in monitoring treatment of infective endocarditis.

Chest radiography

This may reveal an abnormal cardiac shadow (e.g., large left atrium and prominent pulmonary vessels in mitral stenosis, enlarged left ventricle in mitral or aortic regurgitation, or the abnormal aortic shadow in coarctation).

Abnormality in the lung fields may also be seen (e.g., pulmonary edema, pleural effusion, consolidation).

Electrocardiography

The 12-lead EKG may give useful information:

- Atrial fibrillation may be a sign of mitral valve disease.
- Left ventricular strain pattern may be seen in aortic stenosis.
- P mitrale may be seen in the ECG if there is pulmonary hypertension secondary to valve disease (as occurs in severe mitral stenosis).

Echocardiography

Transthoracic (or surface) echocardiography

Transthoracic echocardiography enables visualization of the valves and assessment of pressure gradients across valves. Left ventricular function and pulmonary artery pressure can be estimated. The presence of ventricular septal defect or patent ductus arteriosus may be more accurately assessed by cardiac catheterization, but they may be visualized using echocardiography.

Transesophageal echocardiography

Transesophageal echocardiography is very useful because it gives highly detailed information about structures that are difficult to see using transthoracic echocardiography. Examples of its uses include:

- Assessment of prosthetic valves.
- Detailed evaluation of the mitral valve before mitral valve repair.

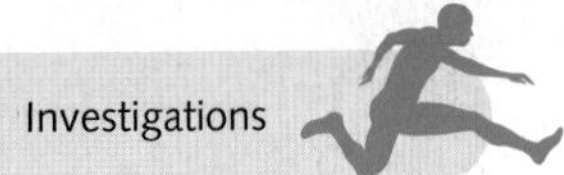

Cardiac catheterization

Before valve replacement this is performed to obtain information about the:

- Presence of coexisting coronary artery disease.
- Degree of pulmonary hypertension in patients who have mitral valve disease.

This investigation can also be used to assess the severity of the left-to-right shunt in patients who have ventricular or atrial septal defects.

7. Hypertension

A person has stage 1 hypertension if blood pressure measurements taken on the average of 2 or more properly measured, seated BP readings on each of 2 or more office visits are higher than 140/90mmHg (or above 130/80mmHg if they are diabetic). If the blood pressure is found to be very high, however (e.g., over 160 systolic), three such measurements may not be required to make the diagnosis. The stages of hypertension are listed in Fig. 7.1

Differential diagnosis of hypertension

Systemic hypertension may be classified as:

- Primary (essential) hypertension, for which there is no identified cause. This accounts for 95% of cases.
- Secondary hypertension, for which there is a clear cause (Fig. 7.2).

History to focus on the differential diagnosis of hypertension

Presenting complaint

Hypertensive patients are often asymptomatic. Occasionally they complain of headaches, tinnitus, recurrent epistaxis, or dizziness. In this situation a detailed systems review may reveal clues to a possible cause of hypertension:

- Weight loss or gain, tremor, hair loss, heat intolerance, or feeling cold may suggest the presence of thyroid disease.
- Paroxysmal palpitations, sweating, headaches, or collapse may indicate the possibility of a pheochromocytoma.

Ask the patient about symptoms that may indicate the presence of complications of hypertension such as:

- Dyspnea, orthopnea, or ankle edema suggesting heart failure.
- Chest pain indicating ischemic heart disease.
- Unilateral weakness or visual disturbance (either persistent or transient) suggesting cerebrovascular disease.

Past medical history

To gain information about a condition that has so many varied causes it is crucial to ask about all previous illnesses and operations. Examples include:

- Recurrent urinary tract infections, especially in childhood, may lead to chronic pyelonephritis, a common cause of renal failure.
- A history of asthma/COPD may reveal chronic corticosteroid intake, leading to Cushing's syndrome.
- Thyroid surgery in the past.
- Evidence of peripheral vascular disease (e.g., leg claudication or previous vascular surgery may suggest the possibility of underlying renovascular disease).

Drug history

A careful history of all drugs being taken regularly is needed, including use of over-the-counter analgesics (e.g., aspirin, nonsteroidal anti-inflammatory drugs), which are a possible cause of renal disease, as well as prednisone and cyclosporine. Remember that steroids use can lead to hypertension.

Family history

Essential hypertension is a multifactorial disease requiring both genetic and environmental inputs. A family history of hypertension is therefore not an uncommon finding. Some secondary causes of hypertension have a genetic component:

- Adult polycystic kidney disease is an autosomal dominant condition associated with hypertension, renal failure, and cerebral artery aneurysms.
- Pheochromocytoma may occur as part of a multiple endocrine neoplasia syndrome associated with medullary carcinoma of the thyroid and hyperparathyroidism (MEN 2, autosomal dominant).

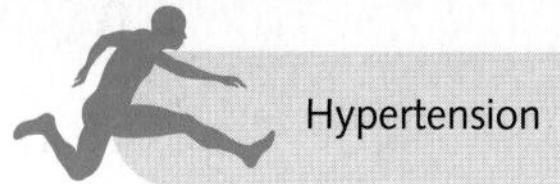

Stages of hypertension				
BP classification	**Systolic BP (mmHg)**		**Diastolic BP (mmHg)**
Normal	<120	*and*	<80
Prehypertension	120–39	*or*	80–9
Stage 1 hypertension	140–59	*or*	90–9
Stage 2 hypertension	≥160	*or*	≥100

Fig. 7.1 The stages of hypertension.

Social history

Smoking, like hypertension, is a risk factor for ischemic heart disease. Excessive alcohol intake may cause hypertension. Recreational drugs like cocaine and amphetamines can also can an increase in blood pressure by acting on adrenergic receptors.

Examination of patients with hypertension

When performing the examination, look for:

- Signs of end-organ damage (i.e. heart failure, ischemic heart disease, peripheral artery disease, cerebrovascular disease, and renal impairment).
- Signs of an underlying cause of hypertension: renal artery bruit (renal artery stenosis), radiofemoral delay (coarctation of aorta).

Blood pressure

Important points to note are:

- Patient should be seated comfortably—preferably for 5 minutes before measurement of blood pressure in a quiet, warm setting.
- Correct cuff size should be used—if the cuff is too small, a spuriously high reading will result; if the cuff is too large, a falsely low measurement will result.
- The manometer should be correctly calibrated.
- The bladder should be inflated to 20mmHg above systolic blood pressure.
- Systolic blood pressure is recorded as the point during bladder deflation where regular sounds can be heard. Systolic blood pressure can also be measured as the pressure at which the palpated distal pulse disappears.

Cause of secondary hypertension	
Mechanism	**Pathology**
Renal	Renal parenchymal disease (e.g., chronic atrophic pyelonephritis, chronic glomerulonephritis), renal artery stenosis, renin-producing tumors, primary sodium retention
Endocrine	Acromegaly, hypo- and hyperthyroidism, hypercalcemia, adrenal cortex disorders (e.g., Cushing's disease, Conn's syndrome, congenital adrenal hyperplasia), adrenal medulla disorders (e.g., pheochromocytoma)
Vascular disease	Coarctation of the aorta
Other	Hypertension of pregnancy, carcinoid syndrome
Increased intravascular volume	Polycythemia (primary or secondary)
Drugs	Alcohol, oral contraceptives, monoamine oxidase inhibitors, glucocorticoids
Psychogenic	Stress
Neurological	Increased intracranial pressure

Fig. 7.2 Causes of secondary hypertension.

- Diastolic blood pressure is recorded as the point at which the sounds disappear (Korotkoff phase V). In children and pregnant women, muffling of the sounds is used as the diastolic blood pressure (Korotkoff phase IV).
- If BP is monitored at home, have the patient bring in the BP cuff so that a staff member make sure that it is calibrated and used correctly. It is pointless to have a patient record home BPs if you cannot rely on their accuracy.

When performing the initial blood pressure measurements, measure blood pressure in both arms. A marked difference suggests coarctation of the aorta.

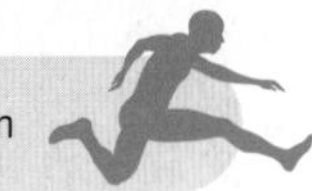

The blood pressure in some patients goes up when they see a doctor—this is "white coat hypertension."

Cardiovascular examination

Examine the pulses, considering the following:

- Rate—tachycardia or bradycardia may indicate underlying thyroid disease.
- Rhythm—atrial fibrillation may result from hypertensive heart disease.
- Symmetry—compare the pulses. Radioradial delay is a sign of coarctation (common in Turner's syndrome), as is the finding of abnormally weak foot pulses.

Keep in mind:

- Weak or absent peripheral pulses along with cold extremities suggest peripheral vascular disease.
- Jugular venous pressure may be elevated in congestive heart failure, a complication of hypertension.
- A displaced PMI is seen in left ventricular failure due to dilatation of the left ventricle. An extra heart sound that precedes the closure of the mitral and tricuspid valvues, an S4, is suggestive of left ventricle hypertrophy.
- Mitral regurgitation may occur secondary to dilatation of the valve ring during left ventricular dilatation.
- In patients who have coarctation, bruits may be heard over the scapulas and a systolic murmur may be heard below the left clavicle.

Respiratory system

Bilateral basal crackles of pulmonary edema may be heard on examination of the respiratory system.

Gastrointestinal system

Hepatomegaly and ascites may be seen in cases with congestive heart failure. The patient must be examined for an abdominal aortic aneurysm because it is a manifestation of generalized atherosclerosis. Palpable kidneys may be evident in patients who have polycystic kidney disease. A renal artery bruit may be heard in patients with renal artery stenosis.

Limbs

Peripheral edema is a sign of congestive heart failure or underlying renal disease.

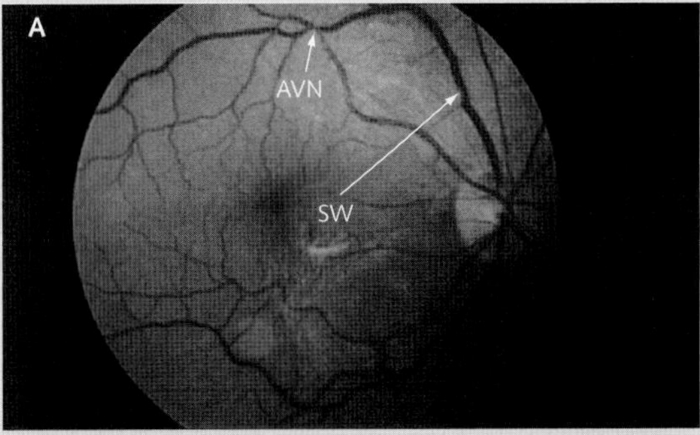

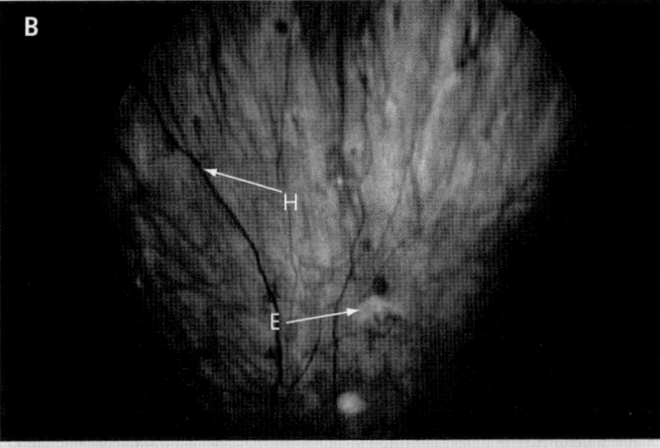

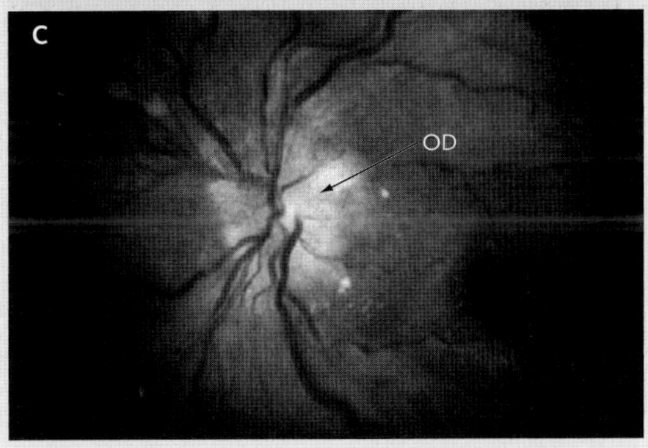

Fig. 7.3 Stages of hypertensive retinopathy. (A) Grade II, showing silver wiring (SW) and arteriovenous nicking (AVN) where an artery crossing above a vein causes apparent compression of the underlying vein. (B) Grade III, showing evidence of hemorrhages (H) and exudates (E). (C) Papilledema—the optic disc (OD) is swollen and edematous—a sign of malignant hypertension.

Eyes

Hypertensive retinopathy

A detailed examination of the fundi is crucial in all patients who have hypertension because it provides valuable information about the severity of the hypertension (Fig. 7.3). Patients exhibiting grade III or IV hypertensive retinopathy have accelerated or malignant hypertension and need urgent treatment.

Features of hypertensive retinopathy on ophthalmoscopy	
Grade	**Features**
I	Narrowing of the arteriolar lumen occurs, giving the classical "silver wiring" effect
II	Sclerosis of the adventitia and thickening of the muscular wall of the arteries lead to compression of underlying veins and arteriovenous "nicking"
III	Rupture of small vessels, leading to hemorrhages and exudates
IV	Papilledema (plus signs of grades I–IV)

Fig. 7.4 Features of hypertensive retinopathy on ophthalmoscopy.

Fig. 7.4 highlights the features of the different grades of hypertensive retinopathy.

Other findings on examination

In examining a patient with a disorder that has many possible causes, a thorough examination of all systems is vital. Remember to look out for signs of thyroid disease, Cushing's disease, acromegaly, renal impairment, etc.

Investigations

Look for evidence of end-organ damage and possible underlying causes.

Blood tests

The following blood tests may help in the diagnosis:

- Electrolytes and renal function—many patients who have hypertension may be treated with diuretics and therefore may have hypokalemia or hyponatremia as a result. Renal impairment as a result of either hypertension or its treatment must be excluded.
- Complete blood count—polycythemia may be present. Macrocytosis may be seen in hypothyroidism; anemia may be a result of chronic renal failure.
- Blood glucose—elevated blood glucose may be seen in diabetes mellitus or Cushing's disease.
- Thyroid function.
- Blood lipid profile—like hypertension, an important risk factor for ischemic heart disease.

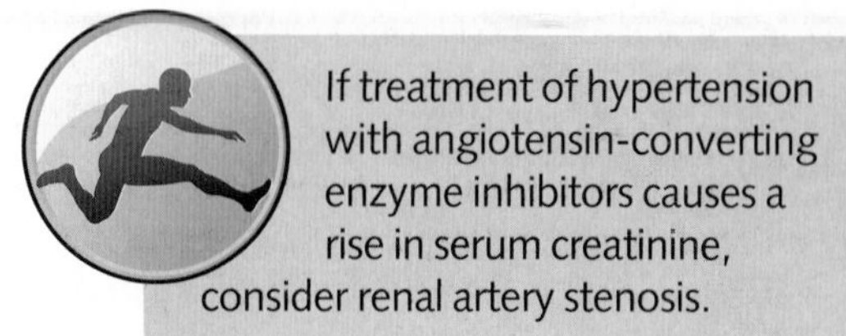

If treatment of hypertension with angiotensin-converting enzyme inhibitors causes a rise in serum creatinine, consider renal artery stenosis.

Urinalysis

Look for protein casts or red blood cells—a sign of underlying renal disease.

Electrocardiography

There may be evidence of left ventricular hypertrophy. Features of left ventricular hypertrophy, shown in Fig. 7.5, are:

- Tall R waves in lead V6 (25mm).
- R wave in V5 plus S wave in V2 greater than 35mm.
- Deep S wave in lead V2.
- Inverted T waves in lateral leads (i.e., I, AVL, V5, and V6).

There may be evidence of an old myocardial infarction or of rhythm disturbance, especially atrial fibrillation.

Chest radiography

Look for:

- An enlarged left ventricle—seen on the chest radiograph as an enlarged cardiac shadow. The normal ratio of cardiac width to thoracic width is 1:2.
- Evidence of coarctation of the aorta—this is seen as poststenotic dilatation of the aorta with an indentation above producing the reversed figure three, along with rib notching due to dilatation of the posterior intercostal arteries.

Echocardiography

This investigation is used to:

- Reveal left ventricular hypertrophy.
- Reveal poor left ventricular function.
- Show any areas of left ventricular hypokinesia suggestive of old myocardial infarction.

Investigations to exclude secondary hypertension

The above investigations may point to possible underlying causes of secondary hypertension but are

Fig. 7.5 Electrocardiographic features of left ventricular hypertrophy (LVH). Note the three cardinal features indicating LVH—R wave in V5 plus S wave in V2 exceeds 7 large squares; the R wave in V6 and S wave in V2 are greater than 5 large squares; T wave inversion in lateral leads V4–V6.

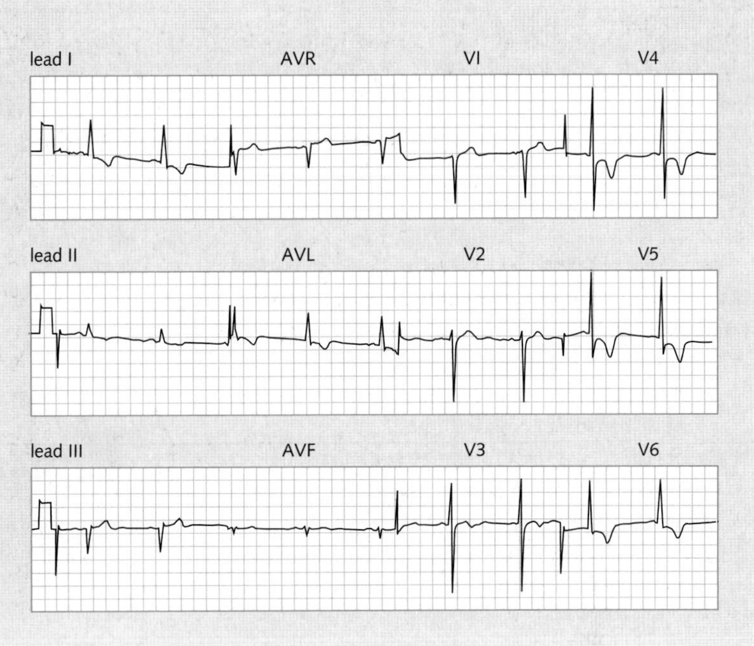

Investigation of secondary hypertension		
Underlying cause	**Investigation**	**Notes/result**
Renal parenchymal disease	24-hour creatinine clearance 24-hour protein excretion Renal ultrasound Renal biopsy	↓ ↑ Bilateral small kidneys In some cases
Renal artery stenosis	Renal ultrasound Radionucleotide studies using DTPA Renal angiography or MRI angiography	Often asymmetrical kidneys Decreased uptake on affected side; this effect is highlighted by administration of an ACE inhibitor
Pheochromocytoma	24-hour urine catecholamines CT scan of abdomen MIBG scan	↑, VMA measurements now rarely used Tumor is often large To identify extra-adrenal tumors (seen in 10% cases)
Cushing's disease	24-hour urinary free cortisol Dexamethasone suppression test 0800 blood cortisol Adrenal CT scan Pituitary MRI scan Chest X-ray	↑ Low-dose 48-hour test initially, high-dose test to rule out ectopic source of ACTH Reveals loss of circadian rhythm in Cushing's disease May show adrenal tumor May show enlarged pituitary May show oat cell carcinoma of bronchus (ectopic ACTH)

Fig. 7.6 Investigation of secondary hypertension. (ACE, angiotensin converting enzyme; ACTH, adrenocorticotrophic hormone; CT, computed tomography; MIBG, meta-iodobenzylguanidine; MRI, magnetic resonance imaging; VMA, vanillylmandelic acid.)

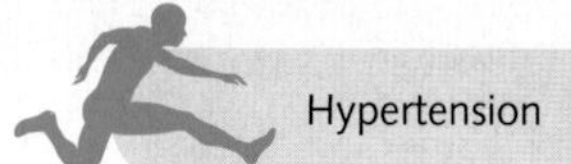

not exhaustive. It would not, however, be cost-effective to investigate all hypertensive patients for these disorders because over 95% of cases of hypertension are primary.

Careful selection of patients who are more likely to have secondary hypertension is therefore needed before embarking on more detailed and invasive investigations.

Secondary hypertension is more likely in patients who are under 35 years of age and also in patients who have:

- Symptoms of malignant hypertension (i.e., severe headaches, nausea and vomiting, blood pressure >180/100 mmHg, papilledema).
- Evidence of end-organ damage (i.e., grade III or IV retinopathy, raised serum creatinine, heart failure).
- Signs of secondary causes (e.g., hypokalemia in the absence of diuretics, signs of coarctation, abdominal bruit, symptoms of pheochromocytoma, family history of renal disease or stroke at a young age).
- Poorly controlled blood pressure despite medical therapy.

Investigations for secondary hypertension are listed in Fig. 7.6.

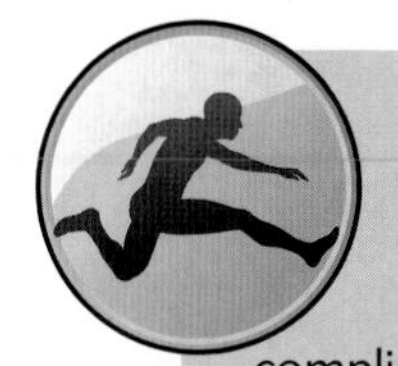

Failure of hypertension to respond to treatment may be due to an underlying secondary cause or lack of compliance with therapy.

8. Fever Associated with a Cardiac Symptom or Sign

Differential diagnosis

Some very serious and potentially fatal cardiac conditions are accompanied by fever. It is therefore important to have at hand a working list of differential diagnoses when presented with such a case.

The differential diagnosis includes:

- Infective endocarditis (bacterial or fungal infection within the heart).
- Myocarditis (involvement of the myocardium in an inflammatory process, which is usually viral).
- Pericarditis (inflammation of the pericardium, which may be infective, postmyocardial infarction, or autoimmune).
- Other rare conditions, such as cardiac myxoma.

The fever may be of noncardiac origin.

Rare conditions

Cardiac myxomas:

- Are benign primary tumors of the heart.
- Are most often located in the atria.
- May present with a wide variety of symptoms (e.g., dyspnea, fever, weight loss).
- Can cause complications such as thromboembolic phenomena or sudden death.
- Are diagnosed by echocardiography.
- Are treated with anticoagulation to prevent thromboembolic phenomena and resection (they may recur if incompletely resected).

On the wards a well-presented list of differential diagnoses implies that you can think laterally and adapt your knowledge of cardiac conditions to fit a clinical scenario.

Whenever presenting a list of differential diagnoses, start with either the most dangerous or the most common disorder first. Leave the rare conditions to the end (even though they are invariably the ones that immediately spring to mind.)

History to focus on the differential diagnosis of fever

When presented with a set of symptoms that cover a potentially huge set of differential diagnoses, it is important to be systematic. Remember that sepsis is a common cause of atrial fibrillation and flutter. Patients who have sepsis may therefore present with fever and palpitations.

Presenting complaint

Common presenting complaints include:

- Fever—ask when it started and whether the patient can think of any precipitating factors (e.g., an operation or dental work, IV drug use).
- Chest pain—to differentiate between, for example, ischemic and pericarditic pain, establish the exact nature of the pain, where it radiates, duration, and exacerbating factors (Fig. 8.1).
- Palpitations—ask about rate and rhythm to obtain information about the likely nature of the palpitations. Also ask about the possible complications of palpitations (e.g., dyspnea, angina, dizziness).
- Malaise—ask about generalized malaise, fatigue, or weight loss.

Past medical history

It is crucial to obtain a detailed past medical history. In particular, the following aspects of the past medical history are important in these patients:

- Recent dental work—this is a common source of bacteremia and cause of infective endocarditis.

Important features of ischemic and pericarditic pain		
Condition	Pericarditis	Ischemia
Location	Precordium	Retrosternal with or without radiation to left arm, throat, or jaw
Quality	Sharp, pleuritic (may be dull)	Pressure pain (usually builds up)
Duration	Hours to days	Minutes, usually resolving (occasionally lasts hours)
Relationship to exercise	No	Yes, unless unstable angina or myocardial infarction
Relationship to posture	Worse when recumbent, relieved when sitting forward	Usually no effect

Fig. 8.1 Important features of ischemic and pericarditic pain.

- Recent operations—these may also cause transient bacteremia (e.g., gastrointestinal surgery, genitourinary surgery, or even endoscopic investigations).
- History of rheumatic fever—although rare in the developed world now, this condition was common in the early twentieth century and is the cause of valve damage in many elderly patients. Such abnormal valves are vulnerable to colonization by bacteria.
- Previous myocardial infarction—a possible cause of pericarditis and Dressler's syndrome (a nonspecific, possibly autoimmune inflammatory response to cardiac necrosis in surgery, post MI or PE. It usually presents between a few weeks to months after the initial event).
- Recent viral infection (e.g., a sore throat or a cold)—myocarditis and pericarditis are commonly caused by viral infection.
- Past history of endocarditis.
- Past history of heart valve replacement.

Drug history

Ask about any recent antibiotics taken—obtain exact details of drugs and doses. Remember that some drugs may cause pericarditis. Examples include penicillin (associated with hypereosinophilia), hydralazine, procainamide, and isoniazid.

Social history

Ask about:

- History of intravenous drug abuse, which is a risk factor for infective endocarditis (especially right sided).
- Risk factors for human immunodeficiency virus infection, which may be associated with infection due to unusual organisms (i.e., the HACEK organisms: *Hemophilus*, *Actinobacillus*, *Cardiobacterium*, *Eikenella*, and *Kingella*). These are gram-negative organisms that grow slowly over many weeks.
- Smoking—a common cause for recurrent chest infection or myocardial infarction.

Examination of patients with fever associated with a cardiac symptom or sign

Fig. 8.2 highlights the important features on examination of a patient who has fever and a cardiac sign or symptom.

Temperature

If using a mercury thermometer, shake it well before use and leave it in the mouth for 3 full minutes.

Hands

Look for signs of infective endocarditis:

- Clubbing.
- Osler's nodes (tender purplish nodules on the finger pulps).
- Janeway lesions (erythematous areas on palms).
- Splinter hemorrhages—up to four can be considered normal. The most common cause for a lesion that has the same appearance as a splinter hemorrhage is trauma, so they are common in gardeners.

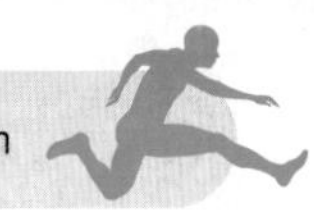

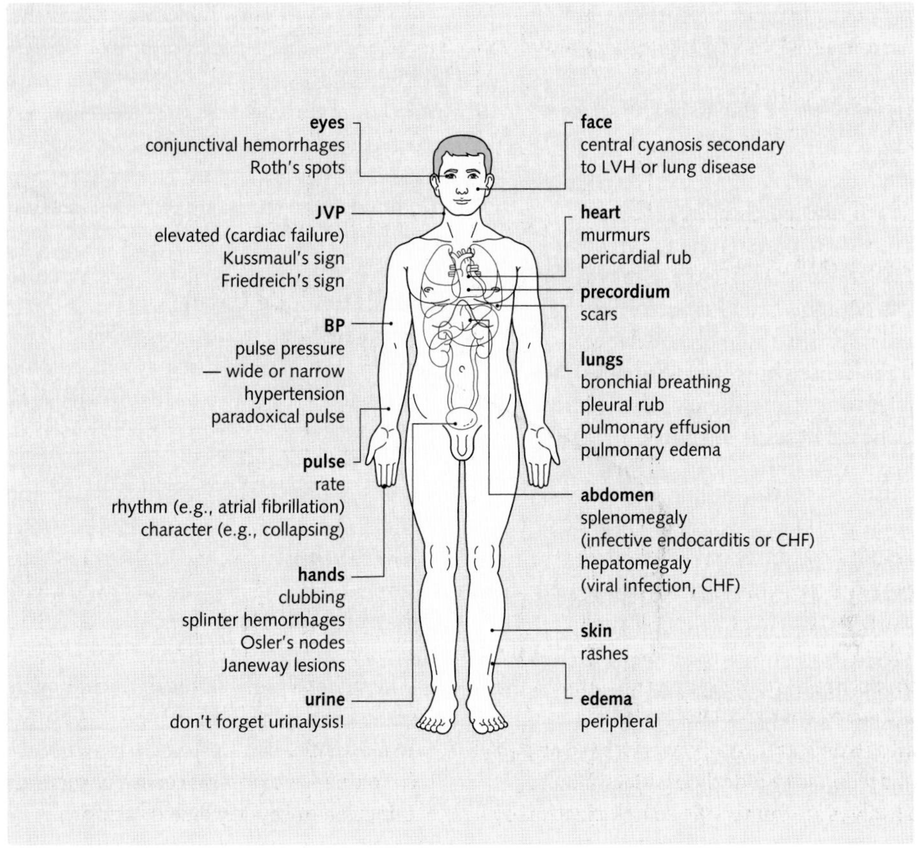

Fig. 8.2 Important signs in a patient who has fever and a cardiac symptom or sign. (CHF, congestive heart failure; JVP, jugular venous pressure.)

All these are signs of vasculitis and may be found in other conditions causing vasculitis (e.g., autoimmune disease).

Facies

Look for:

- Conjunctival hemorrhages and Roth's spots (retinal hemorrhages)—both signs of infective endocarditis.
- Central cyanosis—this may be a sign of a chest infection or cardiac failure.
- A vasculitic rash (e.g., the butterfly rash of systemic lupus erythematosus).

Cardiovascular system

Pulse

Check the:

- Rate and rhythm—may reveal underlying tachyarrhythmia (e.g., atrial fibrillation or, more commonly, sinus tachycardia—a common finding in a patient who is febrile.
- Quality of pulse—may reveal an underlying valve abnormality (e.g., waterhammer or collapsing pulse suggesting aortic regurgitation caused by endocarditis affecting the aortic valve).

Blood pressure

Hypotension may be found, suggesting septic shock or heart failure.

A large pericardial effusion causing tamponade may result in pulsus paradoxus, which is an exaggeration of the normal variation of the blood pressure during respiration (i.e., the blood pressure falls during inspiration; a fall greater than 10mmHg is abnormal).

Jugular venous pressure

Look for:

- Kussmaul's sign—jugular venous pressure (JVP) increases with inspiration (normally, it falls), as seen in cases where pericardial effusion leads to cardiac tamponade.

- Friedreich's sign—a rapid collapse of the JVP during diastole seen in aortic regurgitation.

The JVP may be elevated due to heart failure.

Precordium

Look for scars of previous valve replacement (prosthetic valves are more prone to infective endocarditis). The scar used in these operations is the median sternotomy scar. Listen for:

- Murmurs, especially those of valvular regurgitation caused by infective endocarditis. (Remember to ask the patient about the murmur. Patients whose history is unknown in your hospital may have a long-standing heart murmur of which they are well aware. Simply ask patients if they have ever been told that they have a murmur.)
- Prosthetic valve sounds.
- Pericardial rub—this may be heard in patients who have pericarditis and has been described as the squeak of new leather. It is best heard with the diaphragm of the stethoscope and can be distinguished from a heart murmur because its timing with the heart cycle often varies from beat to beat and may appear and disappear from one day to the next.

Respiratory system

Examine carefully for signs of infection such as bronchial breathing, a pleural rub, or pleural effusion.

Gastrointestinal system

Possible findings include:

- Splenomegaly, which is an important finding because it is a sign of infective endocarditis.
- Hepatomegaly, which may be found as a consequence of heart failure or of viral infection (e.g., infectious mononucleosis).

Skin

Infective endocarditis and many viral infections may be associated with a rash.

Investigations

Blood tests

Blood cultures

This is the most important diagnostic test in infective endocarditis.

At least three sets of blood cultures should be taken, if possible 1 hour apart, from different sites before commencing antibiotics. This enables isolation of the causative organism in over 98% of cases of bacterial endocarditis. Therapy is often started immediately after this and can then be modified when the blood culture results are available.

Complete blood count

A complete blood count may reveal:

- Anemia of chronic disease, which is commonly seen in patients who have infective endocarditis.
- A leukocytosis, which is an indicator of infection or inflammation.
- Thrombocytopenia, which may accompany disseminated intravascular coagulation in cases of severe sepsis.

Other blood tests

These include:

- Antistreptolysin O titers, which may be useful in cases of rheumatic fever.
- Monospot test if Epstein-Barr virus infection is suspected as a possible cause of viral myocarditis.
- Clotting screen because clotting may be deranged in cases of sepsis associated with disseminated intravascular coagulation.
- Renal function tests, which may be abnormal in infective endocarditis because the associated vasculitis may involve the kidneys causing glomerulonephritis. Autoimmune disease may also cause renal dysfunction and is a cause of pericarditis and myocarditis.
- Liver function tests, which are abnormal in many viral infections.
- Erythrocyte sedimentation rate and C-reactive protein measurements because these inflammatory markers are a sensitive indicator of the presence of infection or inflammation. They are also invaluable as markers of the response to treatment. Because C-reactive protein has a short half-life (approximately 8 hours), it is often a more sensitive marker of disease activity than the erythrocyte sedimentation rate.
- Viral titers, which are taken in the acute and convalescent phase of the illness and may reveal the cause of pericarditis or myocarditis. If viral illness is suspected, throat swabs and fecal culture are also appropriate investigations to isolate the organism.

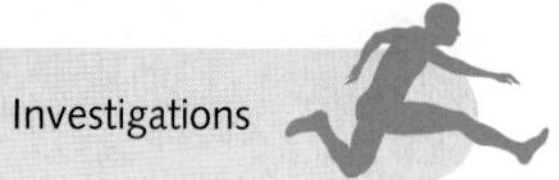

Urinalysis

No examination of a cardiovascular patient is complete without dipstick of the urine to look for microscopic hematuria. This is an extremely sensitive test for infective endocarditis and must not be forgotten. Urine microscopy almost always reveals red blood cells in infective endocarditis. Bacterial endocarditis can lead to immune complex deposition within the kidney that can lead to glomerulonephrits. The kidney can also be showed with septic emboli, which can progress to a renal abscess or infarction. Proteinuria may also be a finding.

Electrocardiography

In patients who have pericarditis, the EKG may show characteristic ST segment elevation. This differs from that seen in myocardial infarction because it is:

- Concave.
- Present in all leads.
- Associated with upright T waves.

Eventually with time the ST segments may flatten or invert, but unlike infarction, there is no loss of R wave height.

Myocarditis may be associated with atrial arrhythmias or interventricular conduction defects. Rarely complete heart block may occur.

Chest radiography

This may reveal an underlying cause of cardiac disease:

- Pneumonia—a possible cause of atrial fibrillation.
- Lung tumor—may invade the pericardium causing pericardial effusion.
- Cardiac failure—an enlarged cardiac shadow and pulmonary edema may be seen in patients who have valve disease or myocarditis.
- A globular heart shadow—characteristic of a pericardial effusion.
- Calcified heart valves—may be visible in a patient who has a history of rheumatic fever.

Transthoracic echocardiography (TTE or surface echocardiography)

TTE is a very useful investigation in the patient who has fever and a cardiac symptom or sign:

- Left ventricular function can be accurately assessed—in myocarditis this is found to be globally reduced (in patients who have left ventricular failure due to ischemic heart disease, the left ventricle often shows regional dysfunction according to the site of the vascular lesion).
- Valve lesions may be identified, and in cases of infective endocarditis the vegetations may be visualized on the valve leaflets. It is important to remember, however, that infective endocarditis cannot be excluded by the absence of vegetations on echocardiography. This investigation is by no means 100% sensitive, and blood cultures remain the most important investigation for this condition.

Transesophageal echocardiography (TEE)

TEE is more sensitive than transthoracic echocardiography because the resolution is much better. It allows a more detailed examination to be made and is especially useful in cases where TTE does not provide adequate imaging. For example:

- Prosthetic heart valves—the acoustic shadows cast by these make imaging with TTE very difficult.
- Localization of vegetations—TEE will visualize vegetations in many cases of infective endocarditis.

Pericardiocentesis

This may be appropriate if a pericardial effusion is found at echocardiography. The procedure is performed by an experienced operator and uses echocardiography as a guide for positioning of a catheter in the pericardial space. An EKG lead is often attached to the needle when attempting to enter the pericardium and will show an injury current (with ST elevation) if the myocardium is touched, thus enabling myocardial puncture to be avoided.

Pericardiocentesis may be:

- Therapeutic—if it relieves cardiac tamponade.
- Diagnostic—if the pericardial fluid can be cultured to reveal an infective organism.

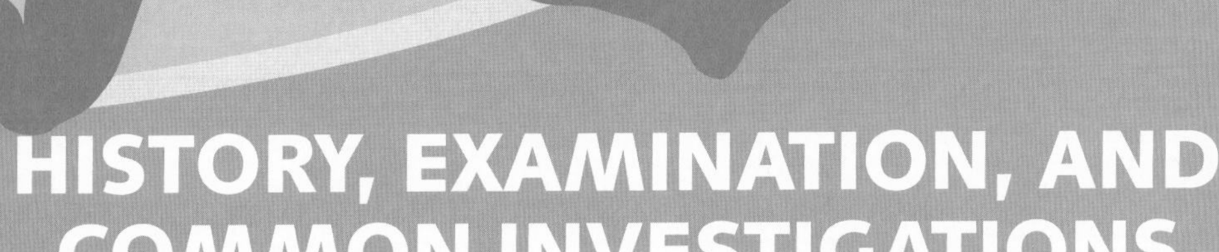

HISTORY, EXAMINATION, AND COMMON INVESTIGATIONS

9. History

Aim of history-taking

The aim of history-taking is to observe the following points:

- Highlight important symptoms and present them in a clear and logical manner.
- Obtain information about the severity of the symptoms and therefore of the underlying disease.
- Ask questions relevant to suspected diseases and so narrow the list of suspected differential diagnoses.
- Evaluate to what extent the individual's lifestyle has been affected by or has contributed to the underlying disease.

Always remember to find out the reason the patient decided to seek medical treatment. Determine what was the inciting factor that brought the patient to the hospital. For example, if the patient has had pain for one week, why did he or she decide to present to you now?

Presenting complaint

The presenting complaint will usually be one of the following:

- Chest pain.
- Dyspnea, including paroxysmal nocturnal dyspnea (PND), orthopnea.
- Syncope or dizziness.
- Palpitations.
- Lower extremity edema.

It may be an incidental finding of a murmur or hypertension.

Chest pain

Ascertain the following points as you would for any type of pain:

- Nature of the pain (e.g., sharp, dull, heavy, burning). If the patient makes a well-clenched fist to describe the pain, then the pain is more likely to be of cardiac origin—known as Levine's sign (after Samuel Levine, MD, the professor at Harvard Medical School who described it).
- Site and radiation of the pain (have the patient point with a finger to the site of the pain).
- Exacerbating and relieving factors.
- Duration of the problem—is it getting worse? Is it not going away as it used to? Is it brought on by activities that used to be performed pain-free?
- Severity of the pain or "quantity of the pain" (how would you rate your pain on a ten-point scale? (e.g., 7/10).
- Determine Canadian Cardiovascular Society Angina Class—there are four functional classes:
  1. Class I: Angina occurs only with strenous or rapid or prolonged exertion.
  2. Class II: There is slight limitation of ordinary activity (e.g., climbing more than one flight of ordinary stairs at a normal pace and in normal conditions).
  3. Class III: There is marked limitation of ordinary activity (e.g., climbing more than one flight in normal conditions).
  4. Class IV: Inability to carry out any physical activity without discomfort. Anginal syndrome may be present at rest.
- Associated features (Fig. 9.1).

Paroxysmal nocturnal dyspnea may be the first feature of pulmonary edema. This occurs when fluid accumulates in the lungs when the patient lies flat during sleep. When awake, the respiratory centers are very sensitive and register edema early with dyspnea; during sleep sensory awareness is depressed, allowing pulmonary edema to accumulate. The patient is therefore woken by a severe sensation of breathlessness, which is extremely frightening and is relieved by sitting or standing up.

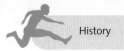

Features of different types of chest pain					
	Angina pectoris	**Pericarditis**	**Pulmonary embolus or pneumonia**	**Esophagitis or esophageal spasm**	**Cervical spondylosis**
Location	Retrosternal	Central or left-sided	Anywhere in chest	Epigastric or retrosternal	Central or lateral
Nature	Pressure or dull ache	Sharp	Sharp	Dull or burning	Aching or sharp
Radiation	Left arm, neck, or jaw	No	No	Neck	Arms
Exacerbating factors	Exertion, cold weather, stress	Recumbent position, deep inspiration	Deep inspiration, coughing	Recumbent position, presence or lack of food	Movement
Relieving factors	Rest, sublingual NTG, oxygen mask	Sitting forward	Stopping breathing	Food or antacids, NTG spray	Weather, position in bed
Associated features	Shortness of, breath, sweating, nausea, palpitations	Shortness of breath, sweating, palpitations, fever	Shortness of breath, hemoptysis, cough, fever	Sweating, nausea	Dizziness, pain in neck or shoulder

Fig. 9.1 Features of different types of chest pain. (NTG, nitroglycerin.)

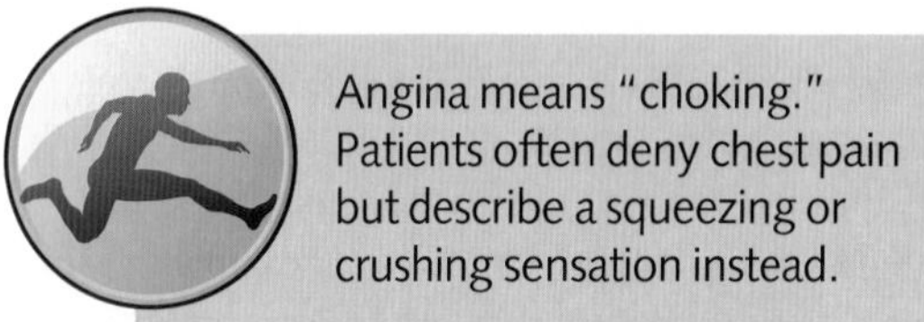

Angina means "choking." Patients often deny chest pain but describe a squeezing or crushing sensation instead.

Dyspnea

This is an uncomfortable awareness of one's breathing. Ascertain the following:

- Precipitating factors.
- Duration of the problem—is it getting worse?
- Determine New York Heart Association Class—there are four classes:
  1. Class I: Dyspnea that occurs on unaccustomed exertion
  2. Class II: Dyspnea on accustomed exertion
  3. Class III: Dyspnea with activities of daily living (such as washing, bathing, etc.).
  4. Class IV: Dyspnea at rest.
- Associated features such as chest pain, palpitations, sweating, cough, or hemoptysis (Fig. 9.2)
- Ask what the patient was doing when the pain started.
- Determine whether there are any recent risk factors for pulmonary embolism (PE).

Syncope

This is a loss of consciousness due to inadequate perfusion of the brain. The differential diagnosis is given in Fig. 9.3.

Cardiac syncope often occurs with no warning and is associated with rapid and complete recovery. Be careful, therefore, because the patient will usually be well when you take the history despite having a potentially life-threatening condition.

Ask about the following:

- Speed of onset.
- Precipitating events.
- Nature of the recovery period.
- Determine whether there was loss of continence.

Features of the conditions causing dyspnea		
System involved	**Disease**	**Features of dyspnea**
Cardiovascular	Pulmonary edema	May be acute or chronic, exacerbated by exertion or lying flat (orthopnea and PND), associated with sweating (and cough) with pink, frothy sputum)
	Ischemic heart disease	Exacerbated by exertion or stress, relieved by rest, associated with sweating and angina
Respiratory	COPD	Chronic onset, exacerbated by exertion and respiratory infections, may be associated with cough and sputum, always associated with history of smoking
	Interstitial lung disease	Chronic onset, no real exacerbating or relieving factors, may have history of exposure to occupational dusts or allergens
	Pulmonary embolus	Acute onset, associated with pleuritic chest pain and hemoptysis
	Pneumothorax	Acute onset, pleuritic chest pain
	Pneumonia and neoplasms of the lung	Associated with pleuritic pain
Other	Pregnancy	Gradual progression due to splinting of diaphragm or anemia
	Obesity	Gradual progression due to effort of moving and chest wall restriction
	Sleep apnea	Increased somnolence, snoring, and obesity
	Anemia	History of blood loss, peptic ulcer, operations, etc.

Fig. 9.2 Features of conditions causing dyspnea. (COPD, chronic obstructive pulmonary disease; PND, paroxysmal nocturnal dyspnea.)

- Remember to ask about trauma from the syncopal episode. The fall may have lead to head injury, etc.

Palpitations

Ask the following questions:

- Can you describe the palpitations? Ask the patient to tap them out.
- Are there any precipitating or relieving factors?
- How long do they last and how frequent are they?
- Are there any associated features (e.g., shortness of breath, chest pain, or loss of consciousness? (Fig. 9.4).

Commonly used vagotonic maneuvers include:

- Valsalva maneuver (bearing down against a closed glottis).
- Carotid sinus massage—remember only one side at a time! And listen for carotid bruits beforehand.
- Painful stimuli (e.g., immersing the hands into iced water or ocular pressure).
- Diving reflex (i.e., immersing the face in water).

Lower extremity edema

Cardiac causes of lower extremity edema include congestive heart failure (fluid retention caused by heart failure). There are many causes of cardiac failure.

Causes of left heart failure include:

- Ischemic heart disease.
- Hypertension.
- Mitral and aortic valve disease.
- Cardiomyopathies (e.g., dilated cardiomyopathy from viral infection, cocaine use, chemotherapy, postpartum cardiomyopathy).

Causes of right heart failure include:

- Left heart failure (the number one cause of right heart failure).
- Chronic lung disease (e.g., COPD (cor pulmonale)).
- Pulmonary embolism.
- Tricuspid and pulmonary valve disease.
- Mitral valve disease with pulmonary hypertension.
- Right ventricular infarct.
- Primary pulmonary hypertension.

From the above list it can be seen that a history encompassing all aspects of cardiac disease needs to be taken to identify the possible causes of lower extremity edema.

Differential diagnosis of syncope			
Cause	**Speed of onset**	**Precipitating events**	**Nature of recovery**
Stokes–Adams attack (transient asystole; results from cerebral hypoxia occurring during prolonged asystole)	Sudden—patient feels entirely well immediately before syncope	Often none	Rapid, often with no sequelae
Tachycardia—VT or very rapid SVT	Sudden	Often none	Rapid
AS and HOCM	Sudden	Exertion, sometimes no warning	Rapid
Vasovagal syncope	Preceded by dizziness, patient often feels nauseated or vomits	Sudden pain, emotion, micturition	Rapid
Orthostatic hypotension	Rapid onset after standing	Standing up suddenly, prolonged standing, use of antihypertensive or antianginal agents	May feel nauseated
Carotid sinus hypersensitivity	Dizziness or no warning	Movement of the head	May feel nauseated
Neurological (may be associated with convulsions during the period of unconsciousness)—epileptiform seizure or cerebrovascular event	May have classical aura or focal neurological signs, rapid onset	Often none (certain types of flashing lights or alcohol withdrawal may precipitate epilepsy)	Often drowsy, may have residual neurological deficit
Pulmonary embolus	Chest pain, dyspnea, or no warning	None (but ask about recent travel, hospitalization, etc.)	May have dyspnea or pleuritic chest pain
Hypoglycemia (may be associated with convulsions during the period of unconsciousness)	Slower onset, nausea, sweating, tremor	Exercise, insulin therapy, missing meals	Often drowsy

Fig. 9.3 Differential diagnosis of syncope. (AS, aortic stenosis; HOCM, hypertrophic obstructive cardiomyopathy; SVT, supraventricular tachycardia; VT, ventricular tachycardia.)

Ankle swelling secondary to cardiac causes is classically worse later in the day after the patient has been walking around. The hydrostatic pressure in the small blood vessels is greater when the legs are held vertical, thus increasing the accumulation of fluid in the interstitial spaces. At night, however, the legs are raised, reducing intravascular pressure and allowing flow of fluid back into the venules with reduction of the edema by morning.

Noncardiac causes of lower extremity edema include:

- Renal—due to proteinuria.
- Hepatic—due to low serum albumin (remember to do a quick check of liver function; just look at the PT/INR).
- Protein malnutrition—due to low serum albumin.
- Pulmonary due to hypercapnia and hypoxia in COPD.

Review of systems

It is very important to learn the skill of taking a rapid but detailed systems review. This part of the history consists of direct questions covering the important symptoms of disease affecting systems other than the one covered in the presenting complaint. Learn the questions by heart so that you automatically ask them every time you take a history (note that this is time-consuming only if the doctor has trouble remembering the questions to ask).

Respiratory system

Cough

Cough may suggest the presence of infection, a common cause of arrhythmias. Cough is also a symptom of heart failure.

Causes of palpitations		
Rhythm	**Precipitating factors**	**Relieving factors**
Sinus tachycardia	Anxiety, exertion, thyrotoxicosis, anemia	Rest or specific treatment of underlying condition
Atrial fibrillation	Ischemia, thyrotoxicosis, hypertensive heart disease, mitral valve disease, alcoholic heart disease, pulmonary sepsis or embolism, idiopathic	Anti-arrhythmic agents or treatment of the underlying disorder
Atrial flutter	Thyrotoxicosis, sepsis, alcohol, caffeine, pulmonary embolus, idiopathic	Anti-arrhythmic agents or treatment of the underlying cause
AV and AV nodal re-entry tachycardias	Caffeine, emotion, alcohol, or no obvious cause	Vasovagal stimulation, ablation of re-entry pathways, or anti-arrhythmic drugs
VT	Ischemia, ventricular dysplasia	Anti-arrhythmic agents, treatment of the underlying cause, or ablation of focus of arrhythmia
Bradyarrhythmias (AV nodal block or sinus node disease)	Often none (overtreatment of tachycardia with anti-arrhythmic agents)	Stop anti-arrhythmic agent or insert permanent pacemaker

Fig. 9.4 Causes of palpitations. (AV, atrioventricular; VT, ventricular tachycardia.)

Hemoptysis

Hemoptysis is a feature of pulmonary embolism, pulmonary edema (sputum may be pink and frothy), pulmonary hypertension secondary to mitral valve disease, and pulmonary infection.

Wheeze

Wheeze is classically seen in asthmatics (remember that some asthmatics cannot take beta blockers), but it is also a feature of cardiac asthma as a sign of pulmonary edema. Patients who have chronic obstructive airways disease may complain of wheeze; these patients have often been heavy smokers and are therefore at risk of cardiac disease.

Gastrointestinal system

Appetite

Appetite is often reduced in cardiac failure because patients are too breathless to eat; this and other factors lead to cardiac cachexia. Do not forget about mesenteric ischemia. Cardiac patients are at risk for build-up of athlerosclerotic deposits in the mesenteric blood vessels, which may lead to intestinal angina with eating and food fear.

Weight loss or gain

Edema can cause marked weight gain. Severe heart failure or infective endocarditis can cause weight loss.

Nausea and vomiting

Nausea and vomiting often complicate an acute myocardial infarction, vasovagal syncope, and drug toxicity (e.g., digoxin toxicity).

Indigestion

This may be confused with ischemic cardiac pain and vice versa. Remember, just because you give someone nitrates and the pain goes away, it does not mean that the pain was of cardiac origin. Esophageal spasms may be stopped by nitrate administration. Conversely, if a patient's pain dissipates after receiving viscous lidocaine and antacids, it may still be cardiac in nature because the time waited may have relieved the pain rather than the medication administered.

Diarrhea and constipation

Diarrhea may lead to electrolyte imbalance affecting cardiac rhythm or may be a sign of viral illness leading to myocarditis or pericarditis.

Central nervous system

Headache

Headache may be a side effect of cardiac drugs (e.g., nitrates, calcium channel blockers).

Weakness, sensory loss, visual or speech disturbance
These signs may suggest thromboembolic disease, which may complicate atrial fibrillation or may alter the decision to give thrombolysis to a patient who has acute myocardial infarction.

Skin and joints
Rashes
Rashes are an important sign in the patient who has infective endocarditis or a possible drug side effect. They are also seen in many viral illnesses and autoimmune disease.

Joint pain
Joint pain can occur in infective endocarditis, viral disease, rheumatic fever, and autoimmune disease. A history of arthritis will affect the decision to undertake an exercise tolerance test to diagnose angina.

Genitourinary system
Proteinuria
This suggests a renal cause of edema.

Hematuria
Macroscopic hematuria is sometimes seen in infective endocarditis.

Frequency, hesitancy, nocturia, and terminal dribbling
Symptoms of prostatism are common in middle-aged male patients who have heart disease and may affect their compliance with diuretic therapy.

Impotence and failure of ejaculation
These symptoms can be caused by beta blockers and are also quite common in diabetics and patients with arterial disease.

Past medical history

For any patient the past medical history should include all previous illnesses and operations and the dates when they occurred. In particular, in cardiac patients emphasis should be placed on the following aspects of the past medical history:

- Risk factors for ischemic heart disease—male sex, age over 55, smoking, diabetes mellitus, hypercholesterolemia, hypertension, or family history. It may be easier to ask about this along with the other risk factors rather than in the family history section of the history.
- Past history of cardiac catheterization, PTCA/stent (does the patient have a pocket card with type of stent?), coronary artery bypass grafting (does the patient have a "diagram" outlining the location of grafts?), valve replacement, implantation of pacemaker (does the patient have a pocket card with details of type and settings of pacemaker?)
- History of rheumatic fever.
- History of recent dental work—an important cause of infective endocarditis (others include recent invasive procedures such as upper gastrointestinal endoscopy, colonoscopy, or bladder catheterization).

Drug history

For all patients this should include all regular medications with details of doses and times. In addition, in the cardiac patient, attention should be paid to the following features:

- Nitrates should be taken in such a way as to allow for a drug-free period; therefore, if a twice-daily nitrate is being used it is important to establish that it is not being taken at 12-hour intervals. For example, isosorbide mononitrate should be taken at 8 AM and 2 PM so that drug levels fall to very low levels overnight.
- Remember to ask about sildenafil (Viagra) and related drugs. Patients who have taken the drug within the past 24 hours should be given nitrates with caution.
- Pay particular attention to drugs that have cardiac effects (e.g., antidepressants, antiasthmatics).

Allergies
All drug allergies should be carefully documented with information about the precise effects noted. In particular, inquire about allergies to IV contrast dye, cough with angiotensin coverting enzyme (ACE) inhibitors.

Fig. 9.5 Heart conditions that have a genetic component. (AD, autosomal dominant; AR, autosomal recessive; HOCM, hypertrophic obstructive cardiomyopathy.)

Heart conditions that have a genetic component		
Disorder	**Inheritance**	**Cardiac complications**
Familial hypercholesterolemia	AR	Premature ischemic heart disease
HOCM	AD	Sudden death, arrhythmias
Marfan syndrome	AD	Aortic dissection, mitral valve prolapse or incompetence
Hemochromatosis	AR	Cardiomyopathy
Romano-Ward, Jervell, Lange-Nielsen syndromes	AR	Long QT syndrome, may lead to sudden death due to ventricular arrhythmias
Homocystinuria	AR	Premature ischemic heart disease, recurrent venous thrombosis

Cardiovascular effects of heavy alcohol consumption	
Cardiovascular effect	**Comments**
Cardiomyopathy	Alcohol is the second most common cause of dilated cardiomyopathy in developed countries (the most common is IHD due to a direct toxic effect of alcohol on the myocardium and also due to a nutritional deficiency of thiamine, which often accompanies alcohol excess and may lead to beriberi; dilated cardiomyopathy is most commonly seen in men aged 35–55 years of who have been drinking heavily for over 10 years
Arrhythmias	Most commonly atrial arrhythmias (e.g., atrial fibrillation, but also ventricular arrhythmias)
Sudden death	Due to ventricular arrhythmias
Hypertension	Alcohol is an independent risk factor for hypertension, possibly due to stimulation of the sympathetic nervous system
Coronary artery disease	In small quantities alcohol has a protective effect on IHD, but heavy alcohol intake is associated with an increased risk of IHD

Fig. 9.6 Cardiovascular effects of heavy alcohol consumption. (IHD, ischemic heart disease.)

Family history

Ischemic heart disease is recognized as having a genetic component, and this should have been ascertained earlier in the history. Also determine at what the age of relatives at the onset of disease (e.g., premature coronary artery disease). In addition, other cardiac conditions have a genetic component (Fig. 9.5).

Laboratory tests

Many patients are able to give history regarding laboratory tests:

- Lipid profile, blood sugar, and glycosylated hemoglobin levels.
- Serum electrolyte, BUN, and creatinine levels in patients with CHF.
- Serum levels of drugs: many patients are able to

tell about serum digoxin levels, and heart transplant patients are able to give history of serum cyclosporine levels, etc.

Social history

The social history aims to identify any areas in the patient's lifestyle that may contribute to or be affected by his or her disease:

- Occupation—always ask about the patient's occupation. In cardiac patients this is particularly important because a history of ischemic heart disease, for example, may result in the loss of a heavy machinery driver's licence. There are many other similar situations where a patient may not be able to continue work, and these need to be identified.
- Smoking—a recognized risk factor in cardiovascular disease.
- Use of illegal drugs—intravenous drug abuse is associated with a high risk of infective endocarditis. The organisms involved are unusual (e.g., *Staphylococcus aureus*, *Candida albicans*, Gram-negative organisms, and anerobes). Cocaine abuse is associated with coronary artery spasm and increased myocardial oxygen demand, resulting in some cases in myocardial ischemia and infarction. Long-term use of cocaine may result in dilated cardiomyopathy. Do not give beta-blockers to patients presenting with cocaine-induced chest pain. It is believed that the beta blocker effect will unmask the alpha receptors to the cocaine, resulting in more constriction of blood vessels.
- Alcohol intake—heavy alcohol consumption has many cardiac effects (Fig. 9.6). Alcohol is a potent myocardial depressant when taken in excess over a long period.
- Obtain contact address and details of primary care physician and other health care providers and next of kin.

10. Examination

This chapter provides information about how to examine the cardiovascular system. Remember that cardiovascular cases are among the most popular used in examinations.

How to begin the examination

Always start by introducing yourself and gently shaking hands (many elderly patients have painful arthritic joints—never make the patient wince when you shake hands). Ask the patient if you can examine his or her chest and heart.

Position the patient correctly. The patient should remove all clothing from the waist upward. It is acceptable for a female patient to cover her breasts when you are not observing or examining the precordium.

The patient should be sitting comfortably against the pillows with his or her back at 45 degrees with the head supported so that the neck muscles are relaxed. The only two circumstances when you may deviate from this position are:

- If the patient has such bad pulmonary edema that he or she needs to sit bolt upright.
- If the jugular venous pressure (JVP) is not raised, a more recumbent position will fill the jugular vein and allow examination of the venous pressure waveform.

Observation

As soon as you see the patient and during your introductions, you should be observing the patient and his or her surroundings. Once the patient has been positioned expose the chest, step to the end of the bed, and observe for a few seconds.

Observation is an art, and you will be surprised how much information you can obtain and remember after only a few seconds. In many cases this part of the examination provides valuable clues about the diagnosis. The secret is knowing what to look for.

Look at the patient's face for the following signs:

- Breathlessness, central cyanosis.
- Malar flush of mitral stenosis.
- Corneal arcus or xanthelasma—suggestive of hypercholesterolemia.
- Any signs of congenital abnormality such as the classical appearance of Down syndrome (endocardial cushion defects) or Turner's syndrome (coarctation and aortic stenosis).

Look at the neck and precordium:

- Visible pulsation in the neck may be due to a high-volume carotid pulse or giant "v" waves in the JVP (the JVP usually has a double pulsation).
- Scars—it is important to have a working knowledge of the common scars seen (Fig. 10.1).
- Visible pulsation on the chest: the PMI may be visible.

Look for peripheral edema if the patient's feet are visible.

Examination of the hands

Pick up the patient's right hand gently (alternatively you can ask the patient to lift both hands and look at them one after the other, thus avoiding the risk of causing any pain). Look for the following:

- Peripheral cyanosis and cold peripheries—suggests peripheral vascular disease or poor cardiac output.
- Nail changes such as clubbing (Fig. 10.2), splinter hemorrhages, nicotine staining.
- Janeway lesions on the finger pulps and Osler's nodes on the palm of the hand—suggest infective endocarditis.

Examination of the pulse

After examining the pulse you should be able to comment on three things: rate, rhythm, and character.

Feel for the radial pulse and time it against your watch for 15–30 seconds. At the same time make note of whether it is:

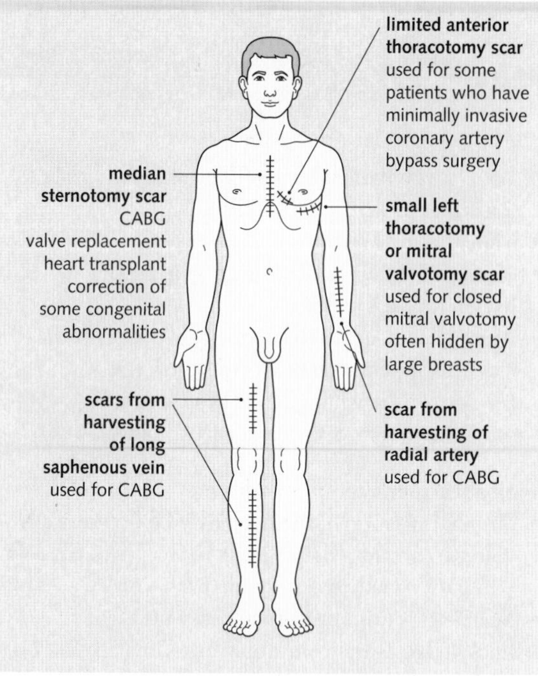

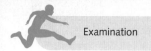

Fig. 10.1 Common scars related to cardiac surgery. Note that a larger left lateral thoracotomy is used for correction of coarction and patent ductus arteriosus. (CABG, coronary artery bypass grafting.)

Don't get confused by occasional ectopic beats, which make the pulse seem irregularly irregular for a short time. In these patients it is important to feel the pulse for at least 15 seconds because you will notice that the basic rhythm is sinus.

- Regular and sinus rhythm or atrial flutter/re-entry tachycardia if rapid—note that atrial flutter may be slow.
- Irregularly irregular—atrial fibrillation.
- Regularly irregular—Wenckebach heart block gives this rhythm because the PR interval progressively lengthens and finally a beat is dropped—you are very unlikely to be asked to diagnose Wenckebach rhythm by feeling the pulse.

Causes of clubbing	
System involved	**Pathology**
Respiratory	Carcinoma of the lung (especially squamous cell), suppurative lung conditions (e.g., lung abscess, empyema, bronchiectasis), fibrosing alveolitis
Cardiovascular	Cyanotic heart disease, infective endocarditis (takes several weeks for clubbing to develop)
Gastrointestinal	Inflammatory bowel disease, cirrhosis

Fig. 10.2 Causes of clubbing.

The character of the pulse is usually best assessed at the carotid pulse, but you may notice a slow rising pulse at the radial pulse (Fig. 10.3).

A collapsing pulse can usually be felt by gently lifting the patient's arm and feeling the pulse with the fingers laid across it. The impulse is felt as it hits the examiner's finger and then rapidly declines.

Finally, check briefly for radioradial delay by feeling both radial pulses together. This may result from coarctation of the aorta (proximal to the left subclavian artery) or unilateral subclavian artery stenosis.

Pulsus paradoxus describes an exaggeration of the normal (not actually a paradox) blood pressure on inspiration (>10 mmHg less than on expiration). Causes are cardiac tamponade, constrictive pericarditis, and severe asthma.

Measurement of blood pressure

Always ask whether you can take the blood pressure yourself and be sure that you know how to do so properly. The blood pressure should be measured in both arms, if the radial pulses are unequal (suggesting coarctation of the aorta).

of cardiac dullness is affected by lung conditions (e.g., emphysema). However, an increased area of dullness indicates cardiac enlargement or pericardial effusion. This is useful if the PMI is not palpable.

Causes of different types of apex beat	
Character	**Causes**
Tapping	MS
Thrusting	MR, AR
Heaving	AS
Diffuse (the normal apex beat should be discrete and localized to an area no bigger than a penny)	Left ventricular failure, cardiomyopathy
Double	HOCM, left ventricular aneurysm

Fig. 10.6 Causes of different types of apex beat. (AR, aortic regurgitation; AS, aortic stenosis; HOCM, hypertrophic obstructive cardiomyopathy; MR, mitral regurgitation; MS, mitral stenosis.)

This is still important in trauma situations when pneumomediastinum is a possibility.

Auscultation

When listening to the heart, every murmur should be systematically excluded. You should at all times be able to explain exactly which sounds you are expecting to hear at any stage during auscultation.

Learn a systematic approach, not necessarily the one described in this chapter, but always listen to the heart in the same way.

Knowing when systole and diastole occur is fundamental. Know this at all times during auscultation by keeping a finger or thumb on the carotid pulse.

The order for auscultation is as follows:

- Using the diaphragm of the stethoscope, listen quickly at the mitral, tricuspid, pulmonary, and aortic areas in that order. You should already know where these are; if not then learn their location now (Fig 10.7). This enables you to hear any loud murmurs and possibly begin to approach the diagnosis.

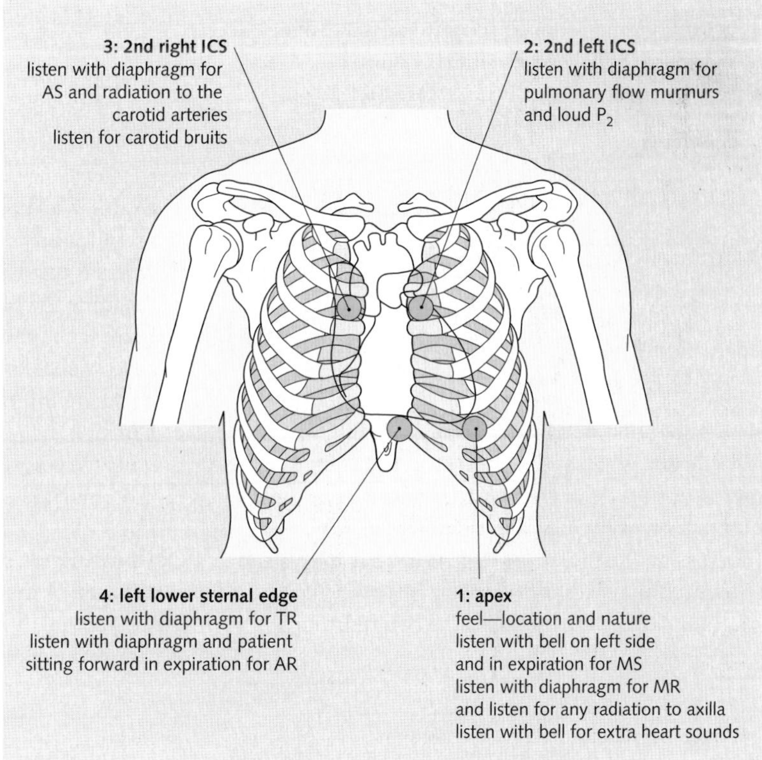
3: 2nd right ICS
listen with diaphragm for AS and radiation to the carotid arteries
listen for carotid bruits
2: 2nd left ICS
listen with diaphragm for pulmonary flow murmurs and loud P_2
4: left lower sternal edge
listen with diaphragm for TR
listen with diaphragm and patient sitting forward in expiration for AR
1: apex
feel—location and nature
listen with bell on left side and in expiration for MS
listen with diaphragm for MR and listen for any radiation to axilla
listen with bell for extra heart sounds

Fig. 10.7 Sequence of auscultation of the heart. (AR, aortic regurgitation; AS, aortic stenosis; ICS, intercostal space; MR, mitral regurgitation; MS, mitral stenosis; TR, tricuspid regurgitation.)

- Listen at the apex: first with the bell of the stethoscope to hear any extra heart sounds (i.e., third and fourth heart sounds); listen for mitral stenosis by asking the patient to lie on his or her left side and breathe out fully. Again the bell of the stethoscope should be used for this. Listen for mitral regurgitation at the apex with the diaphragm of the stethoscope. If a holosystolic murmur is heard, listen at the axilla for radiation of the murmur.
- Listen at the pulmonary area—using the diaphragm to hear a pulmonary flow murmur and loud P_2 if present. Both are accentuated in inspiration.
- Listen in the aortic area for the ejection systolic murmur of aortic stenosis using the diaphragm. This murmur is usually loud, but if there is any doubt, ask the patient to exhale, because left-sided murmurs are loudest in expiration. Take this opportunity to listen over the carotid arteries for radiation of an aortic stenotic murmur if one is present or for evidence of carotid artery stenosis.
- Finally, listen over the tricuspid area for a holosystolic murmur of tricuspid regurgitation or the murmur of HOCM. Then ask the patient to sit forward and listen in expiration for the murmur of aortic regurgitation (this murmur is often soft and requires accentuation by asking the patient to exhale). Both murmurs are heard best with the diaphragm of the stethoscope.

> You cannot say that mitral stenosis has been excluded unless you have listened with the bell of the stethoscope at the apex with the patient lying on his or her left side in full expiration.

Remember that both the murmurs of HOCM and MVP lessen when a patient squats. Squatting increases the size of the ventricle and lessens the obstruction of HOCM and tightens the MV (decreasing the prolapse). Also note that the Valsalva maneuver increases the intensity of a HOCM murmur and decreases the sound of a murmur caused by AS.

Rest of the examination

The rest of the examination must be completed efficiently and thoroughly with just as much care as the first part of the cardiovascular examination. The aim of this part of the examination is to look for signs of heart failure and for any peripheral signs to confirm the diagnosis, which by now you may suspect:

- At this stage the patient is sitting forward. Start with auscultation of the lung bases. Listen for fine end-inspiratory crackles and assess how far up the chest these extend (an evaluation of the severity of pulmonary edema).
- Pleural effusions occur in heart failure and are detected by finding dullness to percussion at one or both lung bases.
- With the patient still sitting forward, check for sacral edema by gently pressing over the sacrum for at least 10 seconds. Then ask the patient to sit back against the pillows. Water follows Newton's laws. Therefore, if the patient has been standing, check the feet/LE; if the patient has been lying, check the sacrum.
- Look for swelling of the lower legs, again very gently, and assess how far up the leg the edema extends (a guide to its severity). Remember that edema is often tender.
- Examine the abdomen for tender hepatomegaly (in CHF), splenomegaly (in infective endocarditis), ascites (in CHF), and palpable aortic aneurysm.
- Examine all peripheral pulses by palpation, and listen for bruits to look for evidence of peripheral vascular disease.
- Examine the fundi.
- Look at the temperature chart for all patients who have a valve lesion to look for a fever, which may be due to infective endocarditis.
- Dipstick the patient's urine. Hematuria is a very sensitive test for infective endocarditis, and proteinuria is associated with renal edema.

Obviously if you suspect that the patient has coarctation of the aorta, it is mandatory to examine the peripheral pulses and look for radiofemoral delay as part of the examination.

11. How to Write a History and Physical (H and P)

There is no single correct way to write an H and P, but there are several incorrect ways! Remember that doctors, nurses, physiotherapists, and many other health professionals use the medical notes during the course of a patient's medical care. The notes need to last for years, and your entries may provide valuable information to doctors looking after the patient in several years time. It is also worth remembering that the medical notes are legal documents that may one day be used as evidence in a court of law.

The basic principles when making entries into the notes are as follows

- Always write legibly—this sounds obvious, but notes are often illegible. Remember if no one else can read your entry, you may as well not write anything.
- A date and time should precede every entry, no matter how brief. At the end of the entry you should sign your name and, if your signature does not clearly show your name, your surname and initials should be written in capitals below it. There are no exceptions to this rule ever!
- Always be courteous to your patients and colleagues when writing in the notes. Rude or angry entries may give a certain degree of satisfaction when they are made but only serve to make you look unprofessional when read at a later date.
- Write everything down. Every time you see a patient an entry should be made in the notes, stating accurately the content and outcome of the consultation. This may sometimes seem pedantic, but most qualified doctors will be able to recall situations when careful documentation has resolved difficult situations.

History

The history should always have the following information at the top of the first page:

- Name of patient in full plus at least one other unique identifier (e.g., date of birth or hospital number). Because loose sheets often fall out of the notes, all pages of the history should have this information so they are not replaced in the notes of another patient with the same name.
- Date and time of entry.
- Route of admission. If the patient is being admitted to the hospital, it is useful to state the route by which the admission came about (i.e., via general practitioner or ED).

Remember, the main headings of the history are:

- Chief complaint (CC)
- History of presenting illness (HPI)
- Review of systems (ROS)
- Past medical history (PMH)
- Medications
- Allergies
- Family history (FH)
- Social history (SH)

Chief complaint

This should be a short list of the presenting complaint(s). There is no place in this section for any descriptions. The purpose of the presenting complaint section is to state clearly the patient's main symptoms so that an initial differential diagnosis can be formulated. It is important that at this stage the list of differential diagnoses is large.

Examples of presenting complaints are shown in the chapter titles in the first half of this book:

- Shortness of breath.
- Palpitations (see Chapter 4).
- Collapse.
- Lower extremity edema (see Chapter 5).
- Chest pain (see Chapter 1).

History of the present illness (HPI)

It is here that information about the presenting complaint is expanded. A full description of the presenting complaint(s) in turn should be noted.

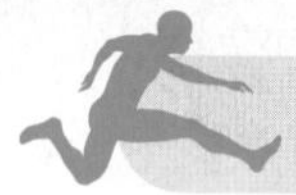

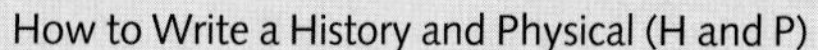

Important questions to ask during the review of systems	
System	**Symptoms and signs to ask about**
Cardiovascular (CVS)	Chest pain, shortness of breath, orthopnea, paroxysmal nocturnal dyspnea, lower extremity swelling, palpitations, syncope
Respiratory (RS)	Cough, sputum, hemoptysis, shortness of breath, wheeze
Gastrointestinal (GI)	Appetite, vomiting, hematemesis, weight loss, indigestion, abdominal pain, change in bowel habit, description and frequency of stools, blood and/or mucus per rectum
Genitourinary (GU)	Frequency, dysuria, hesitancy, urgency, poor stream, terminal dribbling, impotence, hematuria, menstrual cycle, menorrhagia, oligomenorrhea, dyspareunia
Neurological (CNS)	Headache, photophobia, neck stiffness, visual problems, any other focal symptoms (e.g., weakness, numbness; don't forget olfactory problems), tremor, memory, loss of consciousness
Other	For example, muscle pain, joint pain, rashes, depression

Fig. 11.1 Important questions to ask during the review of systems.

It is also important in this section to ask other relevant questions pertaining to the likely organ system(s) involved. For example:

- A patient presenting with chest pain should be asked fully about the nature of the pain and should also be asked about all relevant cardiovascular and respiratory symptoms.
- For a patient who has abdominal pain, a full gastrointestinal and genitourinary systems review should be included in the HPI.

Review of systems

A full systems review of the other organ systems should be entered here (Fig. 11.1).

It is not necessary to document negatives unless they are particularly relevant.

Once you have memorized the questions, they will become second nature and the review of systems will be very quick to do. It is worth the initial time-consuming effort to do this properly; after all, you will be taking histories for the rest of your career.

Past medical history

All previous illnesses and operations should be noted, along with details of when they happened and whether there were any complications.

Patients may be very vague about these details, and you may need to speak to the relatives or the primary care physician for more information.

Medications

All drugs taken should be documented. Remember to ask about over-the-counter medications and herbal remedies/supplements.

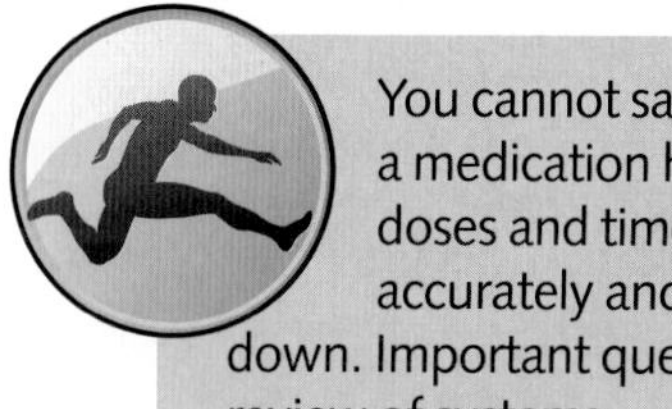

You cannot say that you have a medication history unless the doses and times of all drugs are accurately and legibly written down. Important questions to ask on review of systems.

Allergies

Not only should the drugs that the patient is allergic to be documented, but the type of reaction and when it occurred should be stated.

Many patients say they are allergic to penicillin when they have only experienced some gastric discomfort while taking it. In the situation when the patient is readmitted with for example suspected meningitis this may influence whether or not a potentially life-saving dose of penicillin can be given safely.

Family history

Any diseases that have a potential genetic causation should be documented. The family member who had

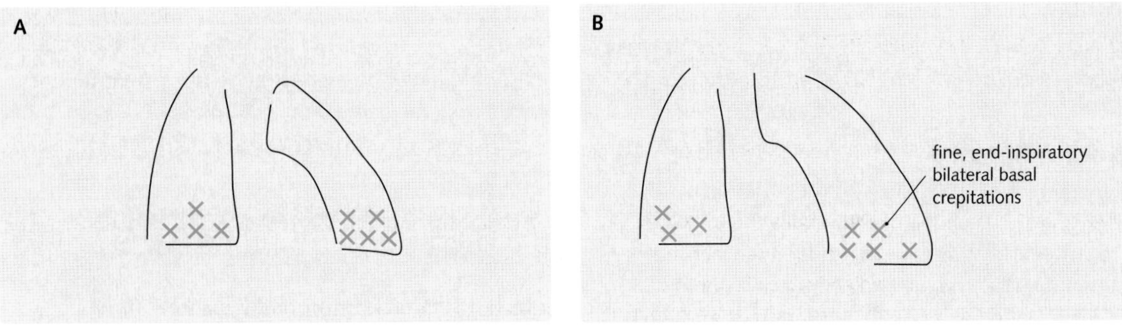

Fig. 11.2 Potential confusion caused by lack of annotation. (A) This diagram is usually used to represent bilateral basal crackles secondary to pulmonary edema. The same diagram, however, may be used to represent coarse inspiratory crackles due to bronchiectasis. (B) This diagram is unequivocal and confirms the finding of pulmonary edema.

Sample notes for an H and P

Mr. John Smith
D.O.B. 11/06/35
Hosp. No. 345678
63-yr-old man
CC: shortness of breath
HPI: gradual onset of shortness of breath approximately 6 months ago. Initially only on exertion, but breathlessness has deteriorated and now patient is breathless on minimal exertion (e.g., when dressing in the morning)
Associated features
Orthopnea
Lower extremity swelling
Cough with clear sputum and occasional flecks of blood
Palpitations—feels heart beating rapidly and irregularly from time to time with no obvious precipitating factors
No chest pain
No known risk factors for coronary artery disease
NB: patient unaware of his cholesterol level
Review of systems
GI
Recent loss of appetite
No weight loss or vomiting
No abdominal pain
No change in bowel habit
CNS: no abnormalities on questioning
GU: no abnormalities on questioning
PMH
Rheumatic fever when 10 years old
Cholecystectomy 1989 no complications
Meds: furosemide 40 mg—started by PCP last week
Allergies: none known
FH
Mother died aged 68—stroke
Father still alive—hypertensive
SH
Never smoked
Alcohol—approx. 10 units a week
Retired accountant
Married with 2 children (family healthy)

PE
General: looks short of breath at rest
No central or peripheral cyanosis
VS: 36.5°C Pulse 80, regular BP 120/80 mmHg Respiratory rate 30 breaths/min
Head, eyes, ears, nose, and throat (HEENT): pupils equal round and reactive to light and accommodation (PERRLA)
CVS
JVP—elevated 6 cm
Apex not displaced
Marked right ventricular heave and loud P_2
Lower extremity edema to knees
RS
Percussion and expansion normal
GI
2 cm hepatomegaly
Ascites detected
No palpable kidneys or spleen
CNS: no abnormalities detected on full neurological examination
Assessment and plan: progressive dyspnea in a man who has a history of rheumatic fever and clinical signs of mitral stenosis
Diagnosis: pulmonary edema and congestive cardiac failure secondary to rheumatic mitral stenosis
Differential diagnosis
Mitral stenosis of another etiology
Paroxysmal atrial fibrillation leading to congestive cardiac failure
Treatment plan
Blood tests: CBC, U +E, LFT, TFT
Chest radiography
EKG and 24-hour EKG to rule out paroxysmal atrial fibrillation
Echocardiography
Intravenous diuretics, initially furosemide 80 mg bid.
Daily U + E to check effect of diuretics on electrolytes and renal function
Daily weights and fluid input and output chart
Fluid restriction to 1500 ml/24 hours
Referral to consultant cardiologist

Fig. 11.3 Sample notes for an H and P. Abbreviations: D.O.B., date of birth; Hosp. No., hospital number; CC, chief complaint; HPI, history of presenting illness GI, gastrointestinal; CNS, central nervous system; GU, genitourinary; PMH, past medical history; Meds, medications; PCP, primary care practitioner; FH, family history; SH, social history; PE, physical exam; CVS, cardiovascular system; BP, blood pressure; JVP, jugular venous pressure; HS, heart sounds; S_1, first heart sound; S_2, second heart sound; P_2, pulmonary component of second heart sound; RS, respiratory system; CBC, complete blood count; U+E, urea and electrolytes; LFT, liver function tests; TFT, thyroid function tests; bid., twice daily.

the disease and whether it was the cause of death should be stated. Specifically ask for family history of diabetes mellitus, CVA, CAD, and sudden death.

Social history

This should include notes on the following:

- Accurate alcohol and drug intake history.
- Smoking—should be carefully documented (i.e., what is smoked, how many, for how long).
- Occupation and possible exposure to industrial dusts or chemicals.
- If HIV infection is a possible differential diagnosis, get a thorough history of possible risk factors. This may be embarrassing both for you and for the patient, but it is important not to miss a diagnosis as serious as this.

Physical examination

There are many ways of documenting the findings on examination, and it does not really matter how you do this provided a few rules are obeyed:

- The patient's name and another unique identifier are written on every sheet of paper—this should come as second nature to you.
- Any positive findings are represented in writing—diagrams can be used to aid the description but should never be used alone to document findings because they are likely to be interpreted differently by different people (Fig. 11.2).

Assessment and plan

The last section is important because it brings together all the information from the notes. The following should be seen at the end of every H and P:

- A list of differential diagnoses with the most likely diagnosis at the top of the list.
- A list of investigations performed and to be performed—it is good practice to tag those tests that have been done already.
- A plan of action, including initial drugs to be given, any intravenous fluids, specific observations needed (e.g., fluid balance chart or daily weights and any consultant referrals to be made).

This reads like a long list, but you do not need to learn it. The only thing you need to remember is that if you do something that concerns a patient, then write it down. Fig. 11.3 shows sample notes for an H and P.

12. Common Investigations

Electrocardiography (EKG)

This investigation records the electrical activity of the heart.

Lead placement

Limb leads

There are six limb leads, one attached to each extremity (Fig. 12.1):

- Bipolar limb lead: I, II, III.
- Unipolar limb leads: aVL, aVR, aVF.

Chest leads

There are six chest leads (Fig. 12.1):

- V1—4th right intercostal space.
- V2—4th left intercostal space.
- V3—between V2 and V4.
- V4—cardiac apex—you need to feel for it before placing the lead.
- V5—anterior axillary line at same level as V4.
- V6—midaxillary line at same level.

12-lead EKG

The standard 12-lead EKG is derived from information given by the ten EKG electrodes placed on the patient.

It is important to know how this information is obtained when interpreting EKG findings and also when the lead positioning is incorrect.

Leads I, II, and III

These are bipolar leads and were first used by Einthoven. They record the differences in potential between pairs of limb leads:

- I records the difference in potential between LA and RA.
- II records the difference in potential between LF and RA.
- III records the difference in potential between LF and LA.

These three leads form Einthoven's triangle (Fig. 12.2).

AVR, AVL, and AVF

With regard to these leads:

- The letter V indicates that the lead is unipolar.
- The information is obtained by connecting the electrode to a central point, which is said to have zero voltage (the reference electrode).
- AVR records the difference between RA and zero.
- AVL records the difference between LA and zero.
- AVF records the difference between LF and zero.

Chest leads

The chest leads:

- Are the precordial leads V1 to V6 and are unipolar (as seen by the prefix V).
- They each record the difference between the voltage at their location and zero.

QRS axis

The normal axis is between –30 and +90 degrees (Fig. 12.3). A positive, or an upward spike on the EKG is when the depolarization of the myocardium in going toward that lead or in that direction. A negative wave is myocardial depolarization that is going away from the lead.

The most accurate way to calculate the axis (Fig. 12.4) is to take the lead in which the complex is isoelectric (i.e., the complex with equal magnitude in the positive and negative direction). Once this lead has been identified, the QRS axis can be found because it is at right angles to this.

Causes of right and left axis deviation are given in Fig. 12.5.

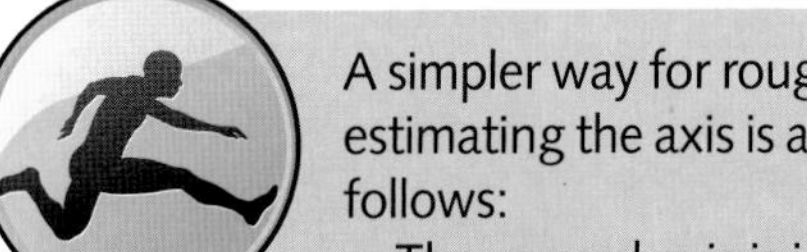

A simpler way for roughly estimating the axis is as follows:

- The normal axis is in the same direction as I and II; therefore, both should be positive.
- In right axis deviation the axis swings to the right and lead I becomes negative and III more positive.
- In left axis deviation the axis swings to the left so lead III and lead II become negative and lead I remains positive.

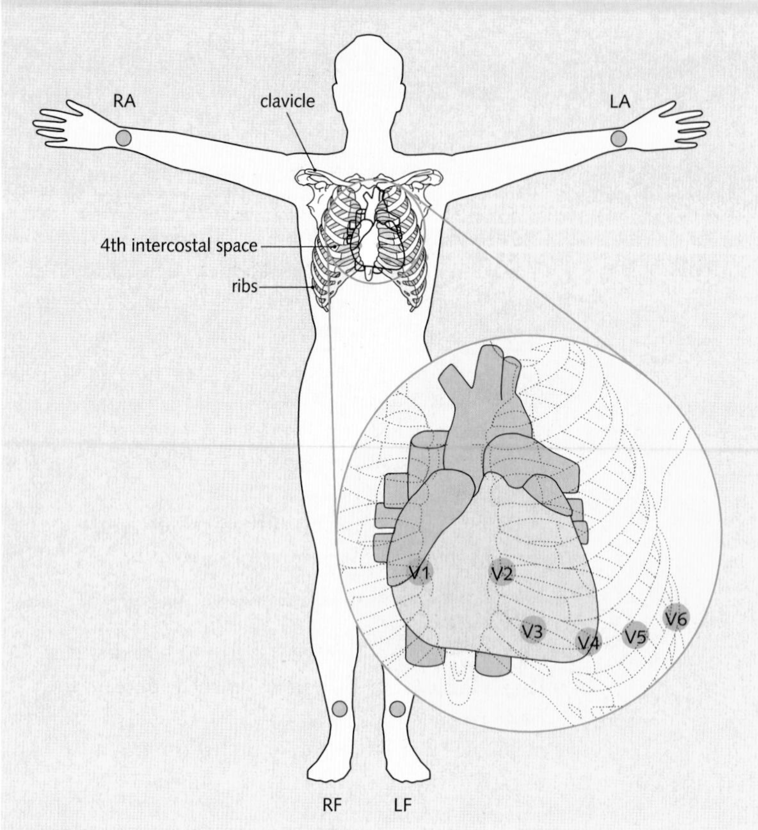

Fig. 12.1 Lead positions for electrocardiography. (LA, left arm; LF, left foot; RA, right arm; RF, right foot.)

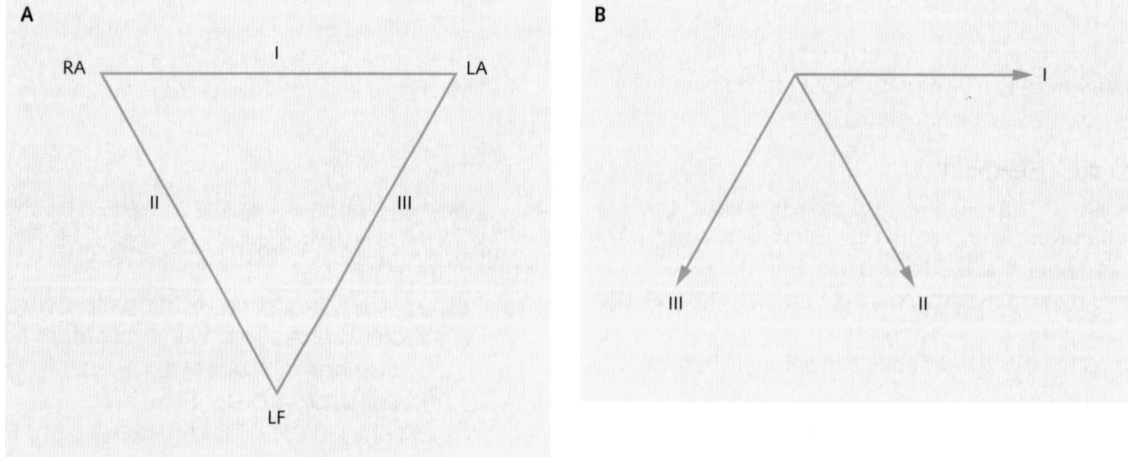

Fig. 12.2 Leads I, II, and III. (A) Lead I is 0 degrees to the horizontal, II is +60 degrees to the horizontal, and lead III is +120 degrees to the horizontal—Einthoven's triangle. (B) Leads I, II, and III are often drawn as shown here.

Fig. 12.3 Hexaxial reference system.

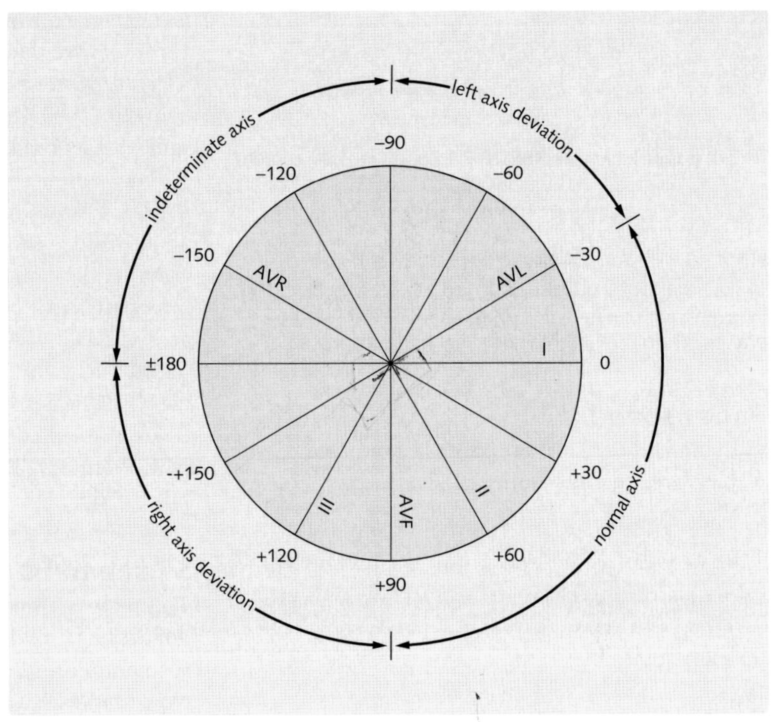

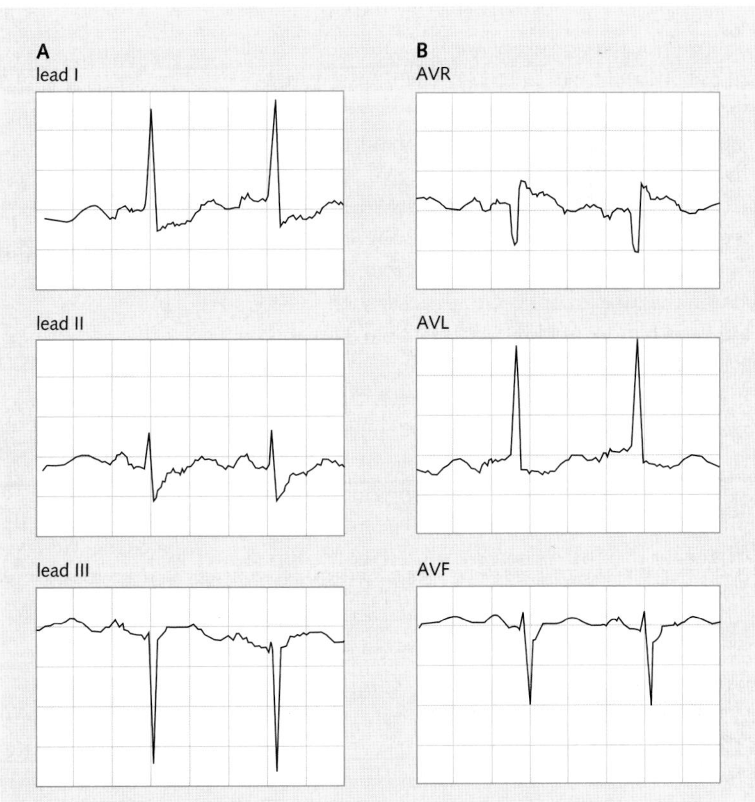

Fig. 12.4 Calculation of the axis. The QRS complex that is almost isoelectric is in lead II. Using the hexaxial reference system the two leads`at right angles are –30 and +150 degrees. The axis is –30 degrees because the positive lead I excludes +150 degrees.

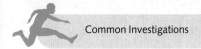

Causes of right and left axis deviation	
Left axis deviation	LBBB, left anterior hemiblock, LVH, septum primum ASD
Right axis deviation	RBBB, RVH, cor pulmonale, septum secundum ASD

Fig. 12.5 Causes of right and left axis deviation. (ASD, atrial septal defect; LBBB, left bundle branch block; LVH, left ventricular hypertrophy; RBBB, right bundle branch block; RVH, right ventricular hypertrophy.)

Paper speed

The standard EKG paper speed is 25mm/sec:

- One large square (5mm) is 0.2sec.
- One small square (1mm) is 0.04sec.

The rate is calculated by counting the number of large squares between each QRS and dividing into 300 (e.g., if there are five large squares, the rate is 60 beats/min)

P wave

The P wave represents atrial depolarization, which originates in the SA node on the right atrium and spreads across the right and then the left atria.

The duration of the P wave is normally less than 0.12sec (three small squares). The P wave is usually upright in leads I and II and has the same interval, size, and shape for the heart to be in normal sinus rhythm. If the P waves are of different shape and sizes, this can represent ectopic atrial beats or atrial depolarization not occurring at the SA node.

The PR interval represents the time taken for conduction of the impulse to pass through the AV node and bundle of His. This is normally no greater than five small squares (0.2sec). This interval represents the pause between when the atria contract and the ventricles contract. This allows the blood to adequately fill the ventricles. When this pause is greater than 0.2sec and still followed by a QRS complex, it is called first-degree heart block. Whenever the QRS is not conducted, or "dropped," this is called second-degree heart block. Variations in second-degree heart block are covered in Chapter 18. Third-degree heart block is complete dissociation between the P waves and the QRS complex.

QRS complex

The QRS represents the depolarization of the ventricles, which begins at the septum. The septum is depolarized from left to right, and the left and right ventricles are then depolarized. The left ventricle has a larger muscle mass; therefore, more current flows across it. The left ventricle thus exerts more influence on the EKG pattern than the right.

The maximum normal duration of the QRS is 0.12sec (three small squares) and the QRS is abnormally wide in bundle-branch block (left and right bundle-branch block (Chapter 18), interventricular conduction delay, and ventricular arrhythmias). It is also wide when the ventricles are paced (Fig. 12.6). Wide complex tachycardia is usually considered to be ventricular tachycardia unless proved otherwise. Other causes include SVT with aberrancy, hyperkalemia, paced rhythym, or false reading.

ST segment

This segment is normally isoelectric (i.e., it shows no deflection from the baseline). Elevations in the ST segment represent myocardial ischemia or lack of oxygen and are usually concerning for a MI. This would be called an ST elevation MI (STEMI). Depending on the pattern of ST segment changes, sometimes the blocked vessel can be predicted. For instance II, III, aVF pattern suggests inferior MI or involvement of the RCA. ST segment depressions also represent myocardial ischemia, but usually it is an incomplete blockage of the artery. This is referred to as a non-ST elevation MI (NSTEMI) or unstable angina (USA). Of note, digoxin may cause down-sloping of the ST segment in some patients. If you see a down-sloping ST segment on an EKG, the first thing to do is to check the medication list.

T wave

The T wave represents ventricular repolarization. Normally the only leads that show negative T waves are AVR and V1; the rest are positive. (A negative QRS should, however, be accompanied by a negative T wave.) Certain T wave abnormalities suggest particular noncardiac disorders (Fig. 12.7). T waves that are flipped, or inverted, can be caused by myocardial ischemia.

QT interval

The QT interval extends from the beginning of the QRS complex to the end of the T wave and therefore represents time from depolarization to repolarization of the ventricles.

Fig. 12.6 Ventricular pacing. The sharp spikes are the artificial stimuli from the pacemaker. Each is followed by a wide QRS complex indicating the left ventricular response. Whenever the impulse is generated in one ventricle either due to a pacing wire or a ventricular ectopic focus, the QRS is widened. This mimics the electrical disturbances seen in bundle-branch block because the two ventricles are not depolarized in the normal sequence.

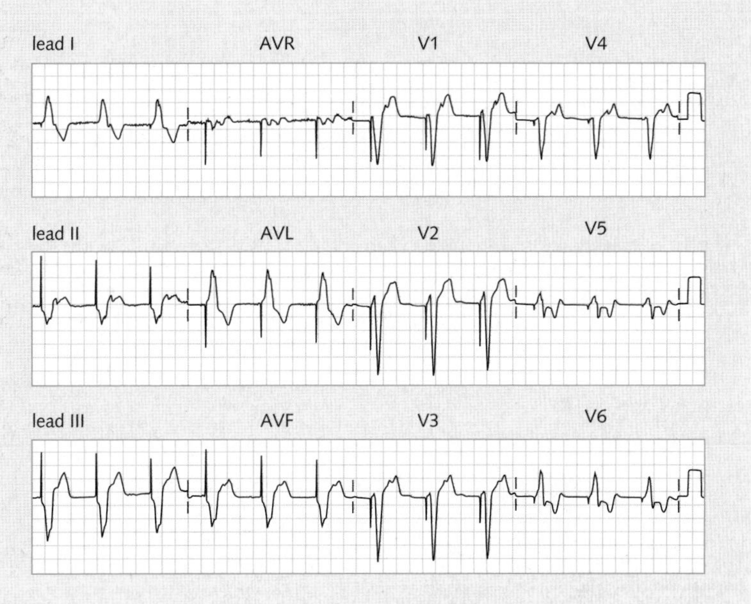

EKG abnormalities in noncardiac disease	
Cause	**EKG abnormalities**
Hypothermia	J waves, baseline shiver artifact, bradycardia; watch out for arrhythmias as the patient is warmed up
Hyperkalemia	Tall peaked T waves, small P wave, gradual widening of the QRS; if serum potassium is very high—ventricular fibrillation
Hypokalemia	Decreased T wave amplitude, long QT interval, U waves
Hypocalcemia	Long QT interval, U waves
Hypercalcemia	Short QT interval, ST segment depression
Digoxin	Downsloping ST segment (reverse tick shape), T wave inversion
Digoxin toxicity	AV block, atrial tachycardia with block, ventricular arrhythmias

Fig. 12.7 Electrocardiographic abnormalities in noncardiac disease. (AV, atrioventricular.)

The duration of the QT interval is dependent upon cycle length, and the corrected QT interval (QTc) is normalized (QTc = QT/square root of RR in sec). The upper limit of normal is 0.39 in women and 0.44 in men. A prolonged QT interval can be caused by some drugs and may predispose to dangerous arrhythmias like torsades de pointes.

Q waves

A Q wave is a negative deflection at the beginning of the ventricular depolarization. Small, nonsignificant Q waves are often seen in the left-sided leads due to the depolarization of the septum from left to right. Significant Q waves:

- Are more than 0.04sec (one small square) in duration and more than 2mm in depth.
- Occur after transmural myocardial infarction where the myocardium on one side of the heart dies. This myocardium has no electrical activity; therefore, the leads facing it are able to pick up the electrical activity from the opposite side of the heart. (The myocardium depolarizes from the inside out; therefore, the opposite side of the heart depolarizes away from these leads, resulting in a negative deflection or Q wave.)

U wave

This is an abnormal wave in some patients but can appear in the chest leads of normal EKGs. It is an upright wave that appears after the T wave (Fig. 12.8). Causes include:

- Hypokalemia.
- Hypocalcemia.

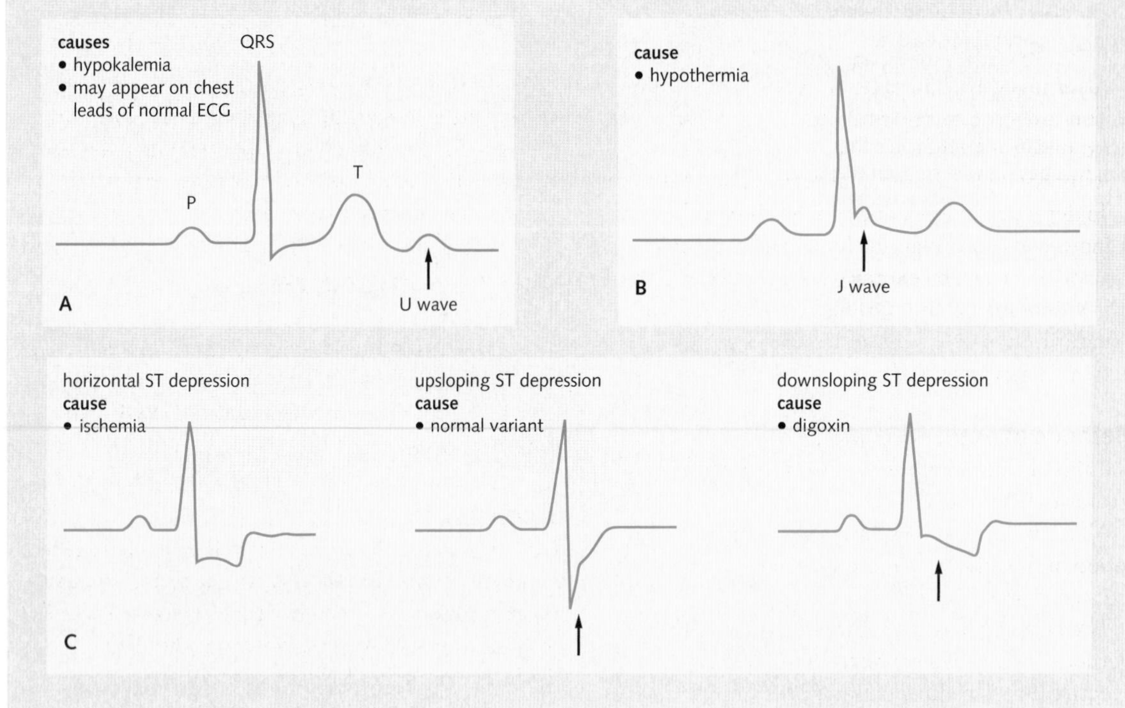

Fig. 12.8 U waves, J waves, and ST segment depression.

Reporting an EKG

You will often be asked to comment on an EKG, and it is difficult to remember to include everything. This exercise should be treated like the history or the examination in that you should always follow a strict routine. After a short time this will become second nature to you.

The order of examination of an EKG is as follows:

- Name of the patient and date of the EKG.
- Check whether the calibration tracing is 2 large squares vertically.
- Rate (i.e., the number of large squares between the QRS complexes divided into 300).
- Rhythm (e.g., regular, irregular, irregularly irregular).

Axis intervals

- Look at each part of the complex P waves, QRS complexes, T waves, PR interval, and QRS duration—and comment on these either out loud when you are starting to do this or in your head when you are more experienced. Also comment on any abnormalities, and remember to look for q waves.

If there are abnormalities look to see whether they are global or territorial. Remember the territories:

- Anterior—V1–V4.
- Inferior—II, III, and AVF.
- Lateral—I, AVL, V4–V6.

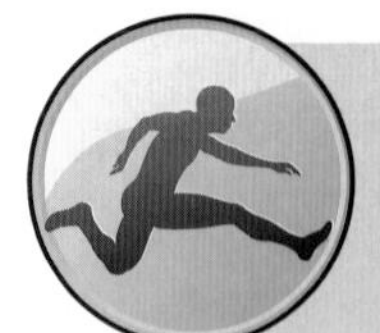

When reporting an EKG:

- Note the patient's name and date.
- Look at the rate and rhythm.
- Comment on P, QRS, and T waves (note shape and duration).
- Look at the distribution of changes—is it global or regional?

Exercise electrocardiography

This investigation is important in the diagnosis of ischemic heart disease. In addition, it provides prognostic information.

Indications for exercise testing

The most common indication for exercise testing is to establish the diagnosis of ischemic heart disease in a symptomatic patient. Other indications are as follows

- After myocardial infarction to evaluate prognosis.
- After myocardial infarction to aid rehabilitation. This gives the patient and doctor an idea of exercise capabilities.
- After angioplasty to evaluate results of treatment.
- To detect exercise-induced arrhythmias. The increased catecholamine levels and metabolic acidosis caused by exercise potentiate arrhythmias in vulnerable patients vulnerable. This gives an indication of prognosis and whether or not treatment is required.

Methods of exercise

The aim of the exercise test is to stress the cardiovascular system.

All exercise protocols have a warm-up period, a period of exercise with increasing grades of intensity, and a cool-down period.

The best method is treadmill exercise. Other methods such as bicycle testing are often less effective because many patients are not used to the cycling action and therefore leg fatigue often sets in before cardiovascular fatigue, resulting in early termination of the test. However, bicycle testing has the advantage that the workload can be controlled and recorded in watts.

The Bruce protocol is often used in conjunction with treadmill testing. This involves 3-min stages starting with 3min at a speed of 1.7 miles/hour and a slope of 10 degrees. Subsequent stages are at incrementally higher speeds and steeper gradients. The final stage (stage 6) is at a rate of 5.5 miles/hour and a gradient of 20 degrees.

The modified Bruce protocol is sometimes used for patients likely to have poor exercise tolerance. An additional two stages are added to the beginning of the standard Bruce protocol. Again, they are 3min in duration and at a speed of 1.7 miles/hour, but the gradient starts at 0 and increases to 5 degrees in the first and second stage, respectively. Of note: women tend to have nondiagnostic exercise stress tests. In light of this, consider a stress echocardiogram or another cardiac imaging study in female patients.

Patient preparation

The following should be completed before testing:

- All patients should have been seen and examined by a physician to ensure that there are no contraindications to testing.
- The test and its indications and risks should have been fully explained to the patient.

Certain patients are advised to stop all antihypertensive and antianginal medication before the test. The operator should be aware of patients who are still taking their medication because it affects the response to exercise.

Variables measured

12-lead EKG

The patient is fitted with the standard 12-lead EKG equipment. Poor electrode contact is avoided by shaving hair and gently abrading the skin with sandpaper or gauze.

Blood pressure

Normal response to exercise involves an increase in blood pressure, sometimes with the systolic pressure rising to 200mmHg. An inadequate response or a fall in blood pressure with exercise indicates the likelihood of the following disorders:

- Coronary artery disease—the most common cause.
- Cardiomyopathy.
- Left ventricular outflow tract obstruction.
- Hypotensive medication.

Heart rate response

Heart rate normally increases with exercise. If the increase is inadequate, ischemic heart disease or sinus node disease must be suspected (also ingestion of beta blockers and calcium channel blockers).

An excessive increase in heart rate indicates reduced cardiac reserve as in left ventricular failure or anemia.

These variables are measured before, during, and after exercise. Measurements are stopped once all variables have returned to their pre-exercise levels.

Test end-points

The following are appropriate indications for terminating an exercise test:

- Attainment of maximal heart rate (in a modified Bruce protocol the submaximal heart rate is used, which is 85% of maximal heart rate. Maximal heart rate is 220–age in years).
- Completion of all stages of the test with no untoward symptoms and without attaining maximum heart rate.

Premature termination of the exercise test is indicated if any of the following occur:

- Excessive dyspnea or fatigue.
- Chest pain.
- Dizziness or faintness.
- Any form of arrhythmia.
- Failure of blood pressure to increase or an excessive increase in blood pressure (e.g., systolic >220mmHg).
- Failure of heart rate to increase.
- ST segment depression greater than 1mm.
- ST segment elevation.
- Ventricular arrhythmias.
- Abnormal blood pressure response.

Causes of ST segment depression are listed in Fig. 12.10.

Positive exercise test

The following are indications of a positive exercise test (i.e., highly suggestive of coronary artery disease):

- ST segment depression of more than 1mm. This should occur in more than one lead, and the ST segments should preferably not be upsloping (Fig. 12.9).
- ST segment elevation.
- Chest pain—provided that the pain has the characteristics of angina pain.

Contraindications to exercise testing

This list includes conditions in which additional stress on the heart may be very hazardous:

- Marked aortic stenosis—gradient greater than 50mmHg with normal left ventricular function.
- Acute febrile or flu-like illness.
- Cardiac failure.
- Unstable angina.
- Second- or third-degree atrioventricular (AV) block.
- Patients unable to walk effectively (e.g., due to severe arthritis or peripheral vascular disease).

Despite adhering to these rules exercise testing does have a mortality rate of approximately 0.5–1/10000. In all cases, a defibrillator and all the necessary equipment for advanced cardiopulmonary resuscitation should be at hand.

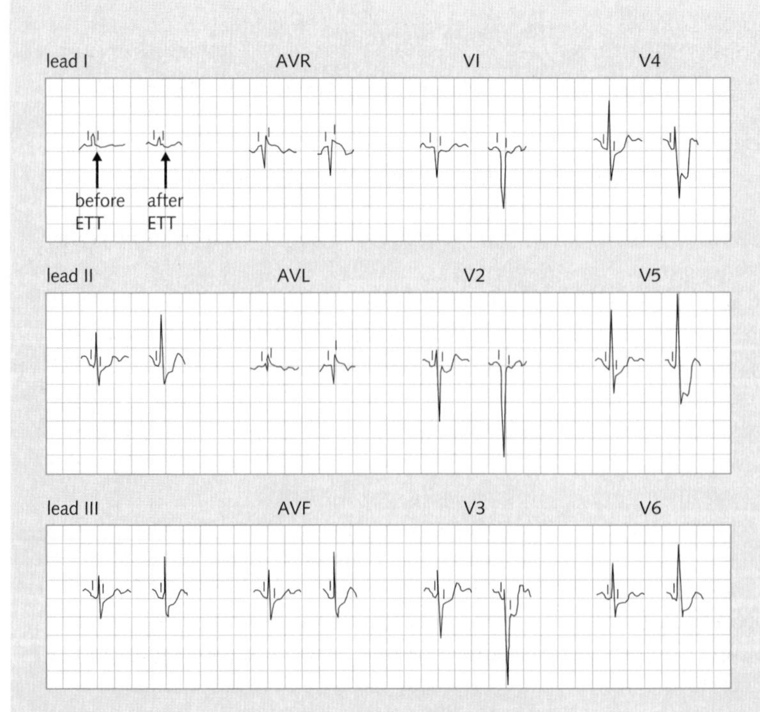

Fig. 12.9 Computer-averaged exercise EKG report showing ST depression after exercise (right-hand trace) compared with resting EKG (left-hand trace) in each of the EKG leads. There is a good tachycardia in response to exercise and the blood pressure rises to 166/84mmHg. The ST depression is in the lateral leads V3–V6 and the inferior leads II, III, and AVF. (ETT, exercise tolerance test.)

Causes of ST segment depression	
Source	**Pathology**
Cardiac	Ischemia, AS, LVH, intraventricular conduction defect (e.g., LBBB)
Noncardiac	Hypokalemia, digoxin, hypertension

Fig. 12.10 Causes of ST segment depression. (AS, aortic stenosis; LBBB, left bundle-branch block; LVH, left ventricular hypertrophy.)

Echocardiography

Echocardiography is the use of ultrasound to investigate the structure and function of the heart.

The frequency of the waves used is between 1 and 10MHz (1MHz = 1000000Hz). The upper limit of audible sound is 20kHz (1kHz = 1000Hz).

The ultrasound waves are generated by a piezoelectric element within the transducer. They travel through certain structures (e.g., blood) and are reflected off others (e.g., muscle and bone). The reflected waves are picked up by the transducer, and by knowing the time taken for the sound to return and the speed of the waves through the medium, the distance of the reflecting object from the transducer can be calculated.

By rapidly generating waves and detecting reflected waves a picture of the heart can be built up.

M-mode echocardiography

The transducer is stationary and records only a single cut through the heart, producing an image on a moving page. The result is the activity along that line seen changing with time. This mode of echocardiography is useful for:

- Visualizing the movement of the mitral and aortic valve leaflets.
- Assessing left ventricular dimensions and function.
- Assessing aortic root size.
- Assessing left atrial size.

Two-dimensional echocardiography

The ultrasound generator moves from side to side so that a sector of the heart is visualized. In the echocardiographic examination standard views of the heart are taken (Fig. 12.11) to provide information about:

- Valve structure and function.
- Left ventricular contractility.
- Size of the chambers.
- Congenital cardiac malformations.
- Pericardial disease.

The inadequacies of this approach are:

- The presence of lung between the heart and chest wall precludes ultrasound travel—"poor windows."
- The posterior part of the heart is farthest from the transducer and may not be viewed adequately, particularly when searching for thrombi and vegetations.

Doppler echocardiography

This uses the principle of the Doppler effect to record blood flow within the heart and great vessels. Doppler effect is the phenomenon in which the frequency of ultrasound reflected off moving objects (e.g., blood cells) varies according to the speed and direction of movement. Color Doppler echocardiography uses different colors, depending upon the direction of blood flow, thus enabling the operator to assess both the speed and the direction of blood flow.

Doppler echocardiography is used for:

- Assessment of valve stenosis and regurgitation.
- Assessment of atrial and ventricular septal defects, patent ductus arteriosus, and other congenital anomalies.
- Assessment of pulmonary hypertension.

Transesophageal echocardiography

Transesophageal echocardiography (TEE) uses a flexible endoscope with a two-dimensional transducer incorporated into the tip. Images are obtained by introducing the transducer into the distal esophagus. The advantage of TEE is that images are much clearer because the transducer is in close apposition to the heart. Because of this TEE is the investigation of choice for:

- Assessment of intracardiac thrombus—transthoracic echocardiography (TTE) is unreliable.
- Assessment of prosthetic valve function—the planes used in TTE result in a great deal of artifact generated by the prosthesis.
- Assessment of valve vegetations.

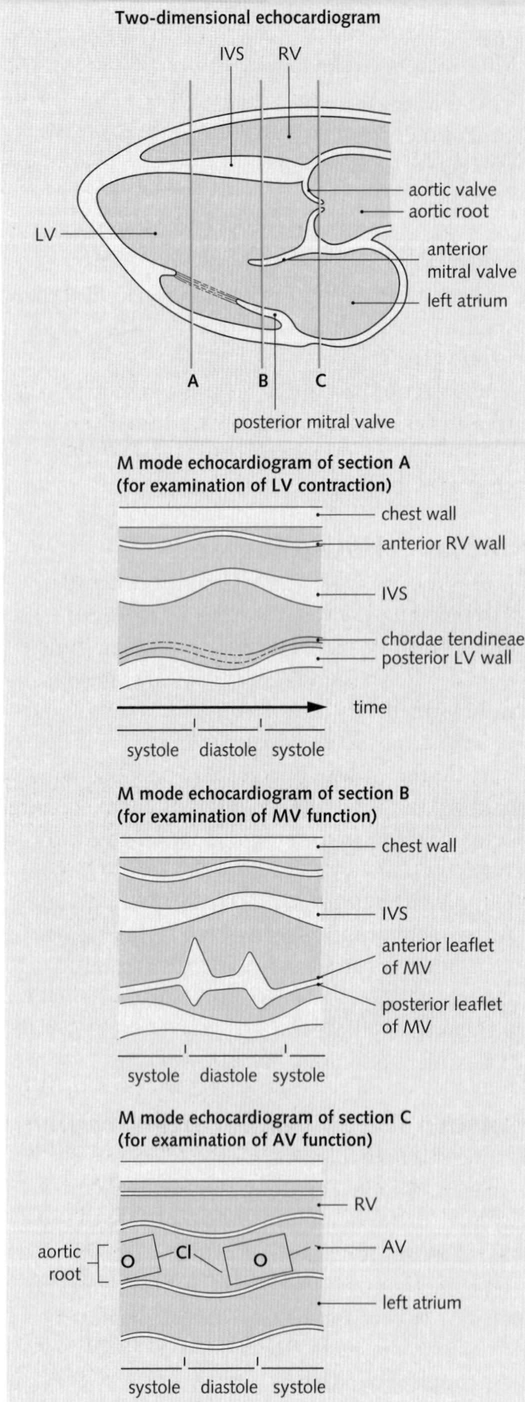

Fig. 12.11 Two-dimensional and M-mode echocardiography. The top illustration shows a long axis view of the heart taken from the left parasternal position with the transducer placed at the left lower sternal edge. The B view shows the opening and closing of the mitral valve (MV). The normal valve gives an M shape when opening and closing with time. Left and right ventricular diameters are also measured with this view. The C view shows the aortic valve (AV) leaflets, which make a box shape when opening and closing with time. Left atrial and aortic root measurements can be made here. (Cl, closed; IVS, interventricular septum; LV, left ventricle; O, open; RV, right ventricle.)

- Assessment of congenital heart lesions (e.g., atrial and ventricular septal defects).
- Imaging can be performed in multiple planes, whereas TTE is restricted to a few planes.
- TEE can be used intraoperatively during cardiac surgery to provide information about valve function and left ventricular function.

Stress echocardiography

When myocardium is ischemic, it contracts less strongly and efficiently.

The patient's heart is stressed with a drug such as dobutamine, which increases the rate and force of contraction and causes peripheral vasodilatation, thus mimicking exercise. With a skilled operator echocardiography images are obtained before, during, and after dobutamine, and areas of ischemia are seen as areas of dyskinesia (or regional wall motion abnormalities), which recover at rest.

Myocardial perfusion imaging

This investigation uses radiolabeled agents, which are taken up by the myocardium proportional to local myocardial blood flow. It is more sensitive and specific than exercise testing alone but much more expensive.

A number of radiolabeled agents are used:

- Technetium-99m labelled agents (e.g., ^{99m}T–sestamibi). This agent has a half-life of 6 hours and is taken up by perfused myocardium. It remains in the myocardium for several hours and imaging of the heart provides an accurate picture of regional myocardial perfusion. Because of this phenomenon resting and exercise images are obtained on two different days with an injection of ^{99m}Tc–sestamibi for each day.
- Thallium-201 is also taken up by the myocardium only in perfused areas. Unlike ^{99m}Tc–sestamibi, thallium is continually passed across the cell membrane (i.e., it is extruded by one cell and

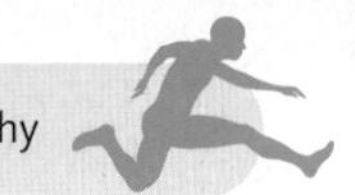

taken up by another). This redistribution allows for early and late images to be taken after exercise using only a single injection. The image early after exercise (or drug stimulation) shows any areas of reduced uptake, and the second image a few hours later will show whether these areas have normal uptake, suggesting the presence of reversible ischemia.

Myocardial perfusion imaging is used in the following situations:

- If the exercise EKG is equivocal and confirmation of reversible ischemia is required before coronary angiography.
- If the patient cannot perform an exercise EKG due to poor mobility—in this situation a perfusion scan is performed using drugs to stress the heart.

In all other situations an exercise EKG is the first investigation.

Methods of stressing the heart

There are a number of ways for stressing the heart. Wherever possible physical exercise should be used because this is actual physiological stress.

For those patients who are unable to exercise due to poor mobility, peripheral vascular disease, or respiratory disease, pharmacological stress may be used. (Patients who have aortic stenosis or heart failure should not have any sort of stress testing.)

The following are commonly used agents for pharmacological stress:

- Dipyridamole—this blocks the reabsorption of adenosine into the cells, so increasing intravascular adenosine concentrations. Adenosine is a powerful vasodilator and vasodilates normal coronary arteries but not diseased coronary arteries. It therefore redistributes blood flow away from diseased vessels. This relative hypoperfusion of diseased areas is picked up by radionucleotide myocardial imaging.
- Adenosine—a direct infusion of adenosine may be used.
- Dobutamine infusion—this drug mimics exercise by increasing myocardial rate and contractility.

Note that both dipyridimole and adenosine are contraindicated in patients who have bronchospasm. Patients that are undergoing adenosine stress testing should not be consuming any products with caffeine within 12 hours of the test. This includes coffee, tea, chocolate, etc.

Multigated acquisition scanning

Multigated acquisition (MUGA) scanning is a radionucleotide technique for evaluating cardiac function.

Technetium-99m label is used to label the patient's red blood cells. The amount of radioactivity detected within the left ventricle is proportional to its volume, and its degree of contraction during systole will affect this finding.

The imaging of the cardiac blood pool is synchronized to the EKG trace, and each image is identified by its position within the cardiac cycle. Hundreds of cycles are recorded, and an overall assessment of the left ventricular ejection fraction can be made using the averaged values for end-systolic and end-diastolic volume.

Magnetic resonance imaging

Magnetic resonance imaging (MRI) will soon be widely used in cardiology. It has a number of advantages:

- It is noninvasive.
- It can be gated by an EKG trace, thus producing still images from each stage of the cardiac cycle.

Depending upon which imaging mode is used, MRI has a number of uses:

- In ischemic heart disease myocardial perfusion can be assessed using contrast techniques. The coronary arteries can be directly visualized, and this has good correlation with conventional angiography. Also myocardial function before and after pharmacological stress can be assessed.
- In structural heart disease MRI can provide a very wide range of soft tissue contrast and detailed structural information.

Positron emission tomography

Positron emission tomography (PET) scanning provides images of the metabolic processes of the myocardium. It is used to assess myocardial viability in patients when conventional techniques (radionucleotide perfusion scanning and coronary angiography) have given equivocal results.

Cardiac catheterization

This invasive investigation is used when noninvasive techniques are unable to give adequately detailed information on a cardiac lesion. In addition, it allows an intervention to take place such as balloon angioplasty with possible stent placement.

> Cardiac catheterization and coronary angiography are mandatory before a patient can undergo a coronary artery bypass operation. It provides detailed information about the severity and location of coronary atherosclerotic lesions, without which surgery cannot be undertaken.

Technique

Before the procedure it is important to determine serum electrolytes, BUN, creatinine, and INR (if the patient is on oral anticoagulants).

Access to the right side of the heart (right heart catheter) is gained by one of the great veins (e.g., femoral, subclavian, or internal jugular vein). Access to the left side of the heart is gained by a peripheral artery (e.g., femoral, brachial, or radial artery).

In either case the vessel is punctured using a Seldinger needle (a large hollow needle), and a guide wire is passed through the center of the needle and into the heart using x-ray guidance. Hollow catheters can then be passed over the wire into the great vessels or the desired chamber, where a number of investigations may be carried out:

- The pressure in the chamber or vessel can be recorded.
- Oxygen saturation of the blood at that location can be measured.
- Radiopaque dye can be injected via the catheter to provide information depending upon the location of the catheter. If in the ostia of the coronary arteries, the anatomy and patency of the coronary arteries can be assessed (coronary angiography); if in the left ventricle, the contractility of the ventricle can be assessed by visualizing the manner in which the dye is expelled from the ventricular cavity; if in the aortic root, the size and tortuosity of the aortic root can be seen by the outline of the dye within it.

Left heart catheterization and coronary angiography

Indications

This is indicated for patients who:

- Have a positive exercise test or myocardial perfusion scan.
- Give a good history of and have multiple risk factors for ischemic heart disease.
- Have had a cardiac arrest.
- Have had a cardiac transplantation. There is a high incidence of atherosclerosis after transplant, and yearly angiograms are performed.
- Occupational reasons—for patients who have chest pain even if noninvasive tests are negative (e.g., airline pilots).

> Older patients undergoing valve replacement surgery also have coronary angiography before surgery to exclude coexistent coronary artery disease. If this is found, coronary artery bypass may be undertaken at the same time as valve replacement.

Note that the list of indications is much more complicated than this, but you only need to have a general idea of the common indications.

Patient preparation

The following must be completed before the procedure:

- A detailed history to ensure that the indications are appropriate and that the patient has no other serious diseases that may affect the decision to proceed. Any history of allergy to iodine must be noted.

- Examination of the patient to ensure that he or she is well. Peripheral pulses must all be palpated and their absence or presence noted. If the femoral approach is to be used, the groin area will need to be shaved just before the procedure.
- Patients with a creatinine of 1.3 or greater are at risk for renal failure secondary to the contrast dye. In this situation they should be pretreated with intravenous fluid (although be careful about giving fluid to a patient with CHF) and acetylcysteine. This will help to protect renal function.
- The INR should be checked in patients on warfarin or with liver failure. An INR >1.5 is associated with increased risk of bleeding.
- The procedure must be carefully explained to the patient.
- The risks must be explained.
- Informed consent is obtained.

Left ventriculogram

This is performed to assess left ventricular function. Dye is injected rapidly to fill the left ventricle and X-ray images are obtained of ventricular contraction.

Coronary angiography

The left and right coronary ostia are located in turn, and dye is gently injected into the arteries. Several images are obtained of each artery from different angles so that a detailed picture of the anatomy of the arteries can be obtained. Images are recorded using X-ray video recording or cine camera.

Complications of coronary angiography

The average mortality and serious complication rate of coronary angiography is 1/1000 cases. The following complications may occur:

- Hemorrhage from the arterial puncture site. This is more common at the femoral site, where percutaneous puncture is used. At the brachial site the artery is dissected out and surgically incised, and after the procedure the incision is sutured. Firm pressure should be applied to the site of bleeding and a clotting screen performed; rarely operative repair is necessary.
- Formation of a pseudoaneurysm. This results from weakening of the femoral artery wall and may require surgical repair.
- Infection of the puncture site or rarely septicemia may occur. Blood cultures and intravenous antibiotics may be required.
- Dye reaction—which may range from mild urticaria and a febrile to full-blown anaphylactic shock. This can be avoided by pretreating the patients with steroids and antihistamines.
- Thrombosis of the artery used. This results in a cold blue foot or hand and necessitates peripheral angiography and a referral to the vascular surgeons.
- Arrhythmias. These may occur during the angiogram due to coronary arterial spasm or occlusion by the catheter. Any form of arrhythmia may occur (ventricular arrhythmias are more common).
- Pericardial tamponade. This is rare and occurs as a result of coronary artery tear or left ventricular tear. The patient becomes acutely cyanosed and hypotensive. Pericardial aspiration is required urgently.
- Displacement of atherosclerotic fragments, which then embolize more distally, resulting in myocardial infarction, cerebrovascular emboli, ischemic toes, etc.
- Renal failure.

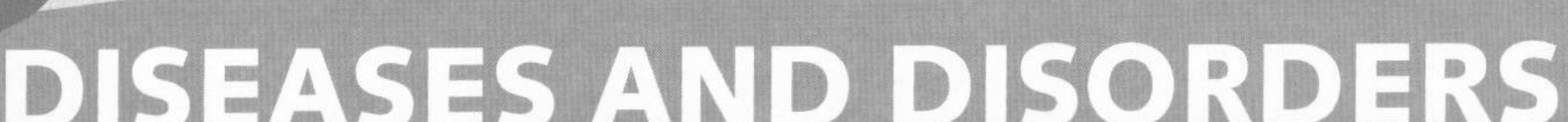

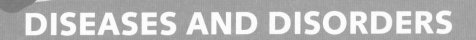

DISEASES AND DISORDERS

13. Angina Pectoris

Definition of angina pectoris

Angina pectoris is characterized by coronary arterial insufficiency leading to intermittent myocardial ischemia. (Ischemia refers to the effect of reduced delivery of oxygen and nutrients to an organ or cell.)

Pathophysiology of angina pectoris

Myocardial ischemia occurs when oxygen demand exceeds supply (Fig. 13.1).

Supply may be reduced for a number of reasons:

- Stenotic atheromatous disease of epicardial coronary arteries—the most common cause of angina.
- Thrombosis within the arteries.
- Spasm of normal coronary arteries as in Prinzmetal's angina or cocaine abuse.
- Inflammation—arteritis (this can occur in polyarteritis nodosa).

Demand may be increased for a number of reasons:

- In conditions requiring increased cardiac output—exercise, stress, thyrotoxicosis.
- In conditions necessitating greater cardiac work to maintain an adequate output—aortic stenosis.
- In conditions where peripheral vascular resistance is increased—hypertension.

The rest of this chapter discusses angina due to atherosclerotic narrowing of the coronary arteries because this is the most common cause of angina.

Risk factors for coronary artery disease

Any modifiable risk factors should be sought and treated to reduce the risk of disease progression and eventual myocardial infarction (Fig. 13.2).

Clinical features of angina pectoris

Symptoms

These include:

- Chest pain—classically a tight, crushing, bandlike pain across the center of the chest. The pain may radiate to the left arm, throat, neck, or jaw. Precipitating factors include exercise, anxiety, and cold air. As the coronary artery narrowing worsens, the amount of stress required to produce angina reduces and the pain may occur even at rest or on minimal exertion. Relieving factors include rest and nitrates.
- Dyspnea—often experienced. This occurs when the ischemic myocardium becomes dysfunctional with an increase in left ventricular filling pressure and, if severe, progression to pulmonary edema.
- Fatigue—may be a manifestation of angina, which should be suspected if it occurs abnormally early into exercise and resolves rapidly at rest or with nitrates.

Most patients have no obvious signs on examination. The patient may be breathless or sweaty. There may be a tachycardia due to anxiety. Be aware of "angina equivalents," which are symptoms other than the classical chest pain that patients may exhibit during episodes of myocardial ischemia. Indigestion, jaw numbness, or arm heaviness/numbness are only a few of such symptoms. These presenting complaints may occur more in diabetics, because their neuropathy may make them unable to feel the typical chest pain of angina, and in the elderly.

There may also be evidence of an underlying cause:

- Hypertension.
- Corneal arcus or xanthelasma—suggesting hypercholesterolemia.
- Nicotine staining of the fingers.
- Aortic stenosis.
- Abnormal tachyarrhythmia.
- Anemia.

Factors involved in the development of ischemia	
Supply factor	**Comments**
Coronary blood flow	Decreased by fixed stenosis (e.g., atheroma, thrombus); vascular tone—depends upon a number of factors, including endothelium-dependent relaxing factor (nitric oxide), prostaglandins, and autonomic nervous system input
Oxygen-carrying capacity	Reduced in anemia and carboxyhemaglobinemia
Demand factor	**Comments**
Heart rate	Increased by exercise, emotion, tachyarrhythmias, outflow obstruction, hypertension, etc.
Contractility	Decreased by rest and negatively inotropic and chronotropic agents (e.g., beta blockers); increased by exertion and positive inotropes (e.g., adrenaline)
Wall tension	Increased by left ventricular dilation (e.g., nocturnal angina)

Fig. 13.1 Factors involved in the development of ischemia.

Risk factors for coronary artery disease
Nonmodifiable risk factors Age—risk increases with age; older patients have a higher risk and therefore a potentially greater risk reduction if modifiable risk factors are treated Sex—men > women (incidence in women increases rapidly after menopause) Family history—this is a strong risk factor even when known genetic diseases (e.g., familial hypercholesterolemia) are excluded
Modifiable risk factors Hypertension Diabetes mellitus Smoking Hypercholesterolemia—important studies include MRFIT, Helsinki Heart Study (*N Engl J Med* 317), SSSS (*Lancet* 344), WOSCOPS (*N Engl J Med* 333), CARE (*N Engl J Med* 335), and LIPID (*N Engl J Med* 339), HPS (*Lancet* 2002 36:7–22)
Other risk factors currently being researched Fibrinogen Homocysteine Low levels of antioxidants Insulin resistance short of overt diabetes mellitus

Fig. 13.2 Risk factors for coronary artery disease. (CARE, Cholesterol and Recurrent Events Trial; LIPID, Long-term Intervention with Pravastatin in Ischemic Heart Disease; SSSS, Scandinavian Simvastatin Survival Study; WOSCOPS, West of Scotland Coronary Prevention Study; HPS, Heart Protection Study.)

There may be evidence of cardiac failure (third heart sound, bilateral basal crackles, and possibly peripheral edema due to fluid retention).

Important points when diagnosing angina are:

- A sudden increase in exertional angina may be due to rupture of an atheromatous plaque in the coronary artery, which causes a step decrease in its luminal diameter; the condition may progress to full infarction.
- Esophageal pain is also relieved by nitrates.
- Chest pain on exertion can also be musculoskeletal in origin—obtain objective evidence of myocardial ischemia before giving an opinion.
- Any form of chest discomfort, even if atypical, could be angina, especially if it is related to effort.

People often wonder why a person who has never experienced any angina can suddenly have a massive heart attack resulting in death, while other patients can have stable angina for years without a MI. Remember: it is often a clot or thrombus that completely occludes the artery, causing a stoppage of blood flow and ischemia. In the case of a sudden MI without previous ischemia a plaque that was occluding only 50% of the lumen by itself can rupture and cause a thrombus to be formed, leading to 100% occlusion and the resultant MI. A person with stable angina may have a plaque that occludes 70–80% of the blood vessel, causing angina only when the heart needs more blood flow (which the mostly occluded blood vessel cannot provide). The plaque may be stable and not rupture—no rupture and no 100% occlusion.

Why are some plaques more stable than others? This is the billion dollar question. Early tests show that statins increase the stability of plaques (therefore statins may offer cardioprotection in patients with normal cholesterol), although much more research needs to be done in this area.

Investigation of angina pectoris

Resting electrocardiography

A normal resting EKG may occur even in individuals who have very severe angina.

Signs of angina on the resting EKG include:

- T wave flattening.
- T wave inversion.
- ST segment depression.
- Partial or complete left bundle-branch block.

Stress testing

There are many methods of stress testing. All aim to place the myocardium under stress and increase oxygen demand and therefore precipitate ischemia, which can be detected in a number of ways.

Remember that precipitation of ischemia is potentially hazardous; therefore, all these tests should be performed with facilities for resuscitation close at hand.

Exercise electrocardiography

The patient is made to walk on a treadmill that becomes incrementally faster and steeper at fixed time intervals. EKG monitoring is used throughout the test, and the presence of horizontal ST depression of greater the 1 mm suggests the presence of angina. (ST depression > 2 mm strongly suggests angina.) Exercise EKGs are only 70% specific and 70% sensitive and are less reliable in women than men.

Stress myocardial perfusion imaging

The exercise test is performed as above, but a radionucleotide is injected at peak exercise and the patient is encouraged to continue exercising for at least another 30 sec. This allows perfused myocardium to pick up the radionucleotide (any ischemic myocardium will not pick it up due to poor perfusion). Images of tracer uptake are performed at this stage and also after rest some time later (when the ischemia has resolved and the affected myocardium has had a chance to take up the tracer). Comparison of the two images provides information about the site of reversible ischemia.

Pharmacological nuclear stress testing

This is used for patients who are unable to exercise adequately due to peripheral vascular disease, arthritis, or chronic obstructive airways disease or asthma.

Agents used include dobutamine, dipyridimole, and adenosine, the rate of which is determined by the patient's own hemodynamic response to the drug.

Stress echocardiography

Imaging of the cardiac muscle at rest and immediately after exercise or dobutamine allows accurate definition of areas of dysfunction secondary to ischemia. In addition, any valve disorders and left ventricular hypertrophy can be diagnosed.

Coronary angiography

This is used in patients who have positive stress tests and in patients who have negative stress tests in whom the diagnosis of angina is still suspected since stress tests may give false-negative results. Coronary angiography is the most specific and sensitive test of coronary artery anatomical lesions.

An arterial puncture is made under local anesthetic in the femoral, brachial, or radial artery, and a guide wire is passed under X-ray control to the aortic root. A series of catheters is used to locate the right and left coronary ostia, and radiopaque dye is injected into each in turn. Images are taken from several angles to obtain a full view of all branches of the two coronary arteries.

Information about left ventricular function is obtained by injection of dye into the left ventricle rapidly to fill it. The rate at which the dye is expelled and the pattern of left ventricular contraction can be seen and gives an assessment of function (This is called a ventriculogram). While it is very useful in showing LV function, it does take a large dye load to produce. In patients with renal failure whose condition can be worsened by the dye, consider skipping this part of the catheterization.

Rapid pacing during cardiac catheterization may provoke ischemia as judged by:

- ST depression.
- Increase in left ventricular end-diastolic pressure.
- Lactate evolution into the coronary sinus.

Syndrome X

This is the term given to a group of patients (mostly middle-aged women) who have the following characteristics:

- Symptoms of angina pectoris.
- Positive exercise EKG.
- Normal coronary arteries at coronary angiography.

Possible causes for this are:

- Coronary artery spasm.
- Microvascular abnormalities.

The treatment for this syndrome consists of nitrates and calcium channel blockers, and the prognosis is good.

Management of angina pectoris

Management of angina involves two areas that are addressed simultaneously:

- Management of any modifiable risk factors.
- Management of the angina itself.

Management of the risk factors

Patients at all stages who smoke should be actively discouraged from continuing to smoke. All health professionals should be involved, and positive encouragement, advice on the complications of smoking, referral to a smoking-cessation clinic, and information about self-help groups should be made available to smokers.

Hypertension should be diagnosed and aggressively treated until the blood pressure is below 120/80 mm Hg, if possible. Many hypertensive patients are undertreated, and regular follow-up is required to ensure that this does not happen.

Diabetes mellitus should be tightly controlled, and often endocrinology follow-up is needed to ensure that control is well maintained.

Hypercholesterolemia should also be treated (Fig. 13.3). Some centers recommend that patients who have coronary artery disease should maintain total cholesterol under 200 mg/dl, with low-density lipoprotein (LDL) maintained below 70 mg/dl. Others may have slightly higher or lower recommended levels. Statin therapy should be considered in all patients with coronary artery disease regardless of baseline LDL and cholesterol levels. Patients should also be referred to the dietitian for American Heart Association lipid-lowering diet. The trials mentioned in Fig. 13.2 should be read because they have dramatically altered the way hypercholesterolemia is treated.

Treatment of the angina

Drug therapy

The main drugs used in the treatment of angina are aspirin, beta blockers, calcium channel blockers, and nitrates.

Aspirin

Aspirin acts to reduce platelet aggregation, which is a risk factor for the development and progression of atherosclerotic plaques.

Beta blockers

These agents are negatively inotropic and chronotropic and therefore reduce myocardial oxygen demand, swinging the balance of demand and supply. They are also effective antihypertensive agents and in some patients can perform a dual role, thus reducing the need for multiple drug therapy. Remember that beta blockers are contraindicated in:

- Unstable heart failure (they can cause severe problems in patients with new-onset pulmonary edema).
- Asthma.
- Peripheral vascular disease—a relative contraindication; the more $beta_1$-selective agents may be used (e.g., bisoprolol).

Other side effects include:

- Nightmares—use a nonfat soluble agent (e.g., atenolol).
- Loss of sympathetic response to hypoglycemia—use a more cardioselective agent.
- Postural hypotension—especially in elderly patients, who should start on a small dose initially.
- They may also worsen depression in some patients.
- Impotence and loss of libido.

Calcium channel blockers

The slowing of calcium influx to the myocardial cells results in a negative inotropic response. The blockade of calcium channels in peripheral arteries results in relaxation and therefore vasodilatation. This dual effect improves blood flow. The blockade of calcium channels in the atrioventricular node increases the refractory period and therefore slows the heart rate. Agents in this group have actions on one or more of

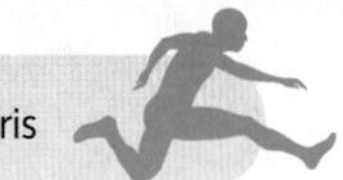

Drugs used to treat hypercholesterolemia						
Drug	**Notes**	**Examples**	**Action**	**Indication**	**Adverse effects**	**Information from clinical trials**
HMG CoA reductase inhibitors	Mainstay of treatment; generally well tolerated, effective; taken once daily	Simvastatin, pravastatin, atorvastatin, fluvastatin, rosuvastatin	Inhibition of HMG CoA reductase, the rate-limiting intrahepatic enzyme in cholesterol synthesis; intracellular cholesterol levels fall, upregulation of apolipoprotein B and E receptors on cell surface, resulting in increased clearance of these from the blood; LDL cholesterol levels fall	Most effective cholesterol-lowering agents available and so first-line therapy	Hepatotoxicity (LFTs should be checked before therapy and then every 6 months); myositis: patients may complain of muscle tenderness (creatine kinase should be checked and, if significantly elevated, the agent should be discontinued)	Many studies show that statins reduce cardiovascular mortality of patients who have and do not have a previous history of coronary artery disease (e.g., SSSS study, CARE study, WOSCOPS, and LIPID study)
Fibric acid derivatives	Also reduce fibrinogen	Clofibrate, gemfibrozil, fenofibrate	Increased lipoprotein lipase activity, leading to decreased VLDL; there is a significant reduction in blood triglyceride levels and a less significant decrease in blood cholesterol concentration; there is also reduced platelet aggregation	If statins not tolerated or contraindicated or severe hypertriglyceridemia is present	Nonspecific gastrointestinal symptoms; occasional myositis, especially if combined with statin	Helsinki Heart Study showed that, when compared with placebo, gemfibrozil reduced cardiovascular mortality in hypercholesterolemic men at 5-year follow-up
Bile acid sequestrants		Cholestyramine	Interrupt enterohepatic recycling of bile them in the gut, from where they are excreted in feces; bile acid synthesis increases, resulting in decreased intracellular cholesterol and therefore upregulation of apolipoprotein B and E receptors	Some familial hyperlipidemias	Gastrointestinal (e.g., reflux, nausea)	Reduces lipids, but no mortality rate data

Fig. 13.3 Drugs used to treat hypercholesterolemia. (CAD, coronary artery disease; HMG CoA, 3-hydroxy-3-methylglutaryl coenzyme A; LDL, low density lipoprotein; LFTs, liver function tests; VLDL, very low density lipoprotein; SSSS, Scandinavian Simvastatin Survival Study.)

Drugs used to treat hypercholesterolemia—cont'd						
Drug	**Notes**	**Examples**	**Action**	**Indication**	**Adverse effects**	**Information from clinical trials**
Nicotinic acid	Rarely tolerated		Decreases hepatic synthesis of VLDL	Some familial hyperlipidemias	Flushing, dizziness, headache, palpitations, pruritus, nausea, vomiting, impaired liver function, rashes	
Vitamin E	Normal vitamin		Antioxidant action counteracts LDL effects in arterial wall		None in μg or mg doses	Ongoing
Fish oil	Normal component of diet	Maxepa omega 3	Populations on traditional high fish oil diets have low incidence of coronary disease		Nausea, belching	Ongoing
Folic acid	Normal vitamin		Decreases homocysteine		None	Ongoing
Ezetimibe			Reduces intestinal cholesterol absorption		None	Ongoing

Fig. 13.3 *Continued*

these areas, and this affects the way they should be used:

- Nifedipine dilates both coronary and peripheral vessels and can be used as an antihypertensive and antianginal drug. Main side effects are flushing, reflex tachycardia, and ankle edema.
- Diltiazem dilates coronary arteries and has some negative inotropic and chronotropic effects. It is therefore a good antianginal drug. It has less effect on peripheral vessels. It causes less flushing and edema and no reflex tachycardia.
- Verapamil has almost no peripheral effects; its main effects are on the atrioventricular node and myocardium. Therefore, it can be used as an antianginal agent but is used mainly as an antiarrhythmic. It also acts as a negative ionotrope, decreasing the contractile strength of the myocardium.
- Amlodipine is a long-acting agent with actions similar to those of nifedipine. It is an effective antianginal and antihypertensive agent.

Nitrates

These act by conversion to nitric oxide, which is a potent vasodilator (mimicking the endothelial release of nitric oxide). The vasodilatation affects:

- Veins—shifting blood from the central compartment (heart, pulmonary vessels) to peripheral veins.
- Arteries—reducing arterial pressure.
- Coronary arteries—improving myocardial perfusion.

There are a variety of preparations:

- Sublingual—nitroglycerin (NTG) can be taken sublingually, from where they are absorbed and rapidly enter the blood. There is no risk of tolerance. NTG tablets should be changed every 6 months because they have a short shelf-life. Sublingual sprays do not have this problem. If they do not cause a burning sensation under the patient's tongue, they are too old to be beneficial.

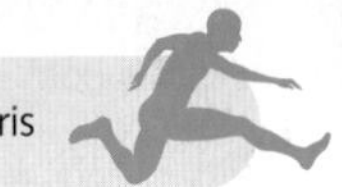

- Transdermal—these take the form of patches or cream that allow the drug to be absorbed through the skin. Care should be taken to vary the location of the application each day.
- Oral nitrates (isosorbide mononitrate, isosorbide dintrate—these may be taken in once, twice, or three times daily dosages.

All nitrates cause headache and flushing because of their vasodilatory action. Tolerance may develop to the oral and transdermal preparations; therefore, a nitrate-free period of 6 hours should be arranged by removing patches overnight or taking the twice daily preparations at 8 AM and 2 PM.

Angiotensin converting enzyme (ACE) inhibitors

ACE inhibitors work to decrease afterload and blood pressure. They are also very beneficial in diabetic patients who have microalbuminuria. Currently they are not first-line agents to treat angina because their benefit in this situation is still under investigation. However, they are still very beneficial due to their proven efficacy in patients with prior MIs. Possible side effects include hyperkalemia and a chronic, dry cough in some patients.

Management plan for angina pectoris

A possible plan of action is therefore:

- Prescribe all patients aspirin.
- Prescribe a beta blocker if not contraindicated.
- If beta blockade fails to control the symptoms or is contraindicated, there is a choice to either start a calcium antagonist or consider an ACE inhibitor if the patient has had been a prior MI. Be prepared to add a long-acting nitrate if the effect is still insufficient.

Revascularization

There are two main ways of improving myocardial blood supply, and coronary angiography is required to make the judgment:

- Percutaneous transluminal angioplasty (PTCA) forces the lumen open by means of an inflated intraluminal balloon; this can be reinforced by stenting.
- Coronary artery bypass graft surgery (CABG).

When diagnosing ischemia, remember that:

- Angina patients have additional ischemic episodes that do not cause pain—called "silent ischemia" and detectable on Holter monitoring.
- Silent ischemia is more common in diabetics who have autonomic neuropathy.
- Drug therapy needs to be tailored to the characteristics of the individual patient.

Percutaneous transluminal coronary angioplasty

PTCA achieves revascularization by the inflation of a small balloon placed across a stenotic lesion. The procedure is carried out in the catheterization laboratory under local anesthetic. In many centers cardiac catheterization with PTCA, with or without stenting, is the standard of care for acute MIs. A patient who presents with a STEMI will proceed almost directly to the catheterization lab, where the blockage will be opened and stent(s) placed.

A guide wire is passed into the aorta via the femoral or brachial artery and the balloon catheter is passed over it. Once the balloon catheter has been positioned across the stenotic plaque to be treated, the balloon is inflated.

Advantages of PTCA

The advantages of this technique over coronary artery bypass grafting (CABG) are as follows:

- No general anesthetic is needed.
- The patient does not need a cardiopulmonary bypass.
- Patients unfit for CABG can still be treated.
- Patients who have clotting disorders or who have recently had thrombolysis can be treated in an emergency setting.
- If PTCA is unsuccessful, CABG can still be performed (whereas a second CABG operation carries a much higher risk).

Disadvantages of PTCA

Patients who have left main stem disease are unsuitable for PTCA, as are patients who have multivessel disease and tortuous vessels. Patient selection is therefore important.

The restenosis rate is much higher than with CABG—approximately 30% within the first 6 months after PTCA. Coated stents and irradiated stents are currently under investigation. The hope is that their use, combined with platelet-inhibiting drugs (such as clopidogrel and GIIb/IIIa inhibitors, discussed later) will decrease the restenosis rate.

Complications of PTCA

These include:

- Myocardial infarction—secondary to thrombosis, spasm of the coronary artery, or dissection of the coronary artery by the balloon.
- Coronary artery perforation.
- Arrhythmias.
- Dye reactions.
- Hemorrhage or infection at the puncture site.

PTCA with coronary artery stenting

In the past 10 years the use of stents in conjunction with PTCA has dramatically increased. These have been shown to reduce the risk of restenosis after PTCA.

Stents are flexible, cylindrical structures made of metal, usually with a mesh or coil design. They are initially loaded in a compressed form over the deflated balloon and expand when the balloon is inflated at the site of stenosis.

Thrombosis at the site of stenting may occur and is partly prevented by the use of intravenous heparin and antiplatelet aggregation agents (Fig. 13.4).

Coronary artery bypass grafting

Coronary artery bypass grafting aims to achieve revascularization by bypassing a stenotic lesion using grafts.

The patient undergoes full general anesthesia, and the heart is exposed using a median sternotomy incision and sternal retractors.

Cardiopulmonary bypass is achieved by inserting a cannula into the right atrium and another into the proximal aorta. The two cannulas are connected to the bypass machine, which oxygenates the venous blood from the right atrium and feeds it back to the aorta.

The heart is stopped by using cooling and cardioplegic solutions.

Vein grafts harvested from the great saphenous vein or arterial grafts are used to bypass the occlusive coronary lesions.

A number of arteries may be used for grafting, including:

- Left and right internal mammary arteries.
- Radial arteries.
- Gastroepiploic artery.
- Inferior epigastric artery.

Antiplatelet agents used to prevent thrombosis following PTCA with or without stenting

Class of drug and examples	Action	Side effects
Aspirin	Irreversible inactivation of cyclooxygenase—within platelets. This enzyme is needed for the production of thromboxane (a stimulator of platelet aggregation)	Gastritis (possibly with ulcer formation and bleeding), renal impairment, bronchospasm, rashes
Platelet ADP receptor blockers (e.g., clopidogrel)	When activated, the adenyl cyclase-coupled ADP receptor causes binding of fibrinogen to the platelet and initiation of thrombus formation —this is irreversibly inhibited by these agents	Hemorrhage, diarrhea, nausea, neutropenia, hepatic dysfunction
Platelet membrane glycoprotein IIIb/IIIa receptor inhibitors (abciximab is a monoclonal antibody that binds to and blocks this receptor)	The Gp IIa/IIIb platelet receptor binds fibrinogen, von Willebrand's factor, and other adhesive molecules—blockade therefore inhibits platelet aggregation and thrombus formation	Hemorrhage

Fig. 13.4 Antiplatelet agents used to prevent thrombosis following PTCA with or without stenting. (ADP, adenosine diphosphate.)

The last two in this list are used much less often than the first two.

Arterial grafts have the advantage of much lower rates of reocclusion.

Complications of CABG

These are:

- Death—mortality rates are approximately 1% in good centers.
- Myocardial infarction, stroke, peripheral thromboembolism.
- Wound infection.
- Complications related to cardiopulmonary bypass—these are related to the hemodilution involved and the exposure of the blood to manmade materials in the oxygenating process. Examples include clotting and pulmonary abnormalities and impaired cognitive function.

Minimally invasive CABG

Minimally invasive CABG (MICABG) is a new technique that involves a smaller incision, usually a left anterior minithoracotomy. The left or right internal mammary artery is used to graft the occluded vessel (usually the left anterior descending coronary artery because it is situated within easy reach).

Cardiopulmonary bypass is not used. Instead, the heart is slowed with beta blockers and a specifically designed instrument is used to immobilize the small area under the anastomosis.

Benefits of MICABG Compared with traditional CABG, MICABG has the benefits of:

- A rapid recovery because of smaller scar.
- No need for cardiopulmonary bypass.

Disadvantages of MICABG Compared with traditional CABG, MICABG has the following disadvantages:

- It sometimes takes longer to perform.
- Multiple stenoses cannot be bypassed; the procedure is currently suitable for patients who require only one or two grafts.
- Lesions of the right coronary or circumflex artery are more difficult to graft.

Unstable angina

This condition is one of the acute coronary syndromes. The pathophysiology underlying unstable angina involves rupture of an atherosclerotic plaque within the coronary artery and the subsequent formation of a thrombus over this. The result is a rapid reduction in the size of the lumen of the vessel. A marked change in symptoms occurs. The patient who has angina on exertion only suddenly develops an increase in severity of the pain and eventually pain at rest.

Troponin levels (troponin T or troponin I) are routinely measured. A raised troponin level suggests myocardial necrosis, and the patient is said to have sustained a myocardial infarction rather than unstable angina.

Management

The management plan summarized by the mnemonic MAN HO BAG (**m**orphine, **a**spirin, **n**itrates, **h**eparin, **o**xygen, **b**eta blockers, **A**CE inhibitor, **g**lycoprotein IIa/IIIb inhibitor) should be followed:

- Admit the patient to the coronary care unit or monitored bed for observation and strict bed rest. Remember that if the thrombus extends and completely occludes the vessel lumen, a myocardial infarction will occur.
- Provide analgesia with intravenous morphine (2.5–5mg) if required to calm the patient and relieve pain. Give a beta blocker if not contraindicated. Decrease the heart rate to less than 85bpm to lessen oxygen demand.
- Give aspirin—it has been shown to reduce the incidence of myocardial infarction and death in patients who have unstable angina (325mg soluble aspirin).
- Give an intravenous infusion of nitrates (e.g., NTG 0.5–2mg/hour or until chest pain resolves)—to dilate the coronary arteries and reduce the load on the heart by peripheral vasodilatation and venodilatation. The blood pressure will drop so it should be carefully monitored.
- Give oxygen as needed.
- Give intravenous heparin as a 24-hour infusion (or subcutaneous low-molecular-weight heparin) to prevent further thrombus formation. Intravenous heparin has the disadvantage that the activated partial thromboplastin time needs to be monitored to ensure that it does not become too high and lead to hemorrhage. Low-molecular-weight heparins are given at doses according to patient weight, and no such measurements are required. Evidence suggests that the low-

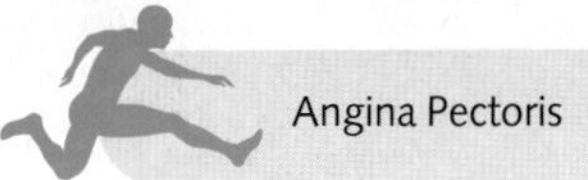

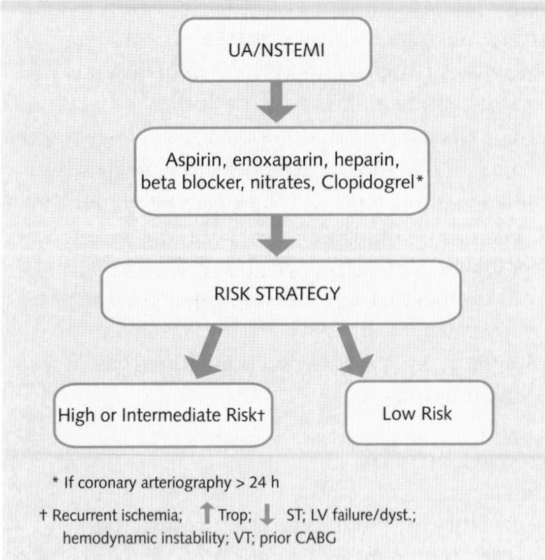

Fig. 13.5 Initial approach to patients with unstable angina/NSTEMI. (Trop. = troponin. LV = left ventricular, dysf. = dysfunction, VT = ventricular tachycardia, CABG = coronary artery bypass graft.)

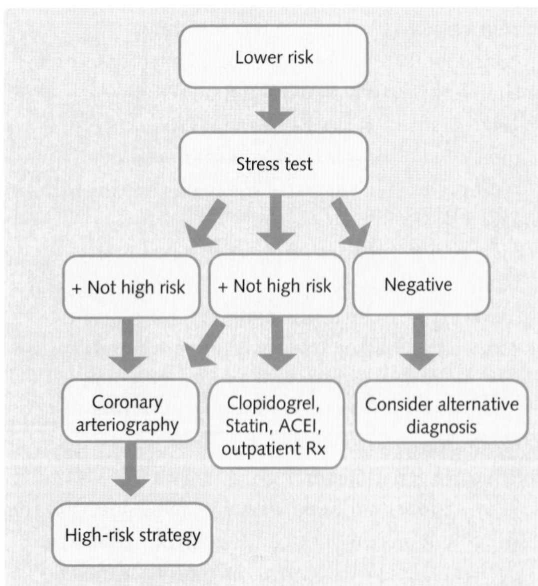

Fig. 13.6 Approach to lower risk patients with unstable angina/NSTEMI. (ACEI = angiotensin-converting enzyme inhibitor.)

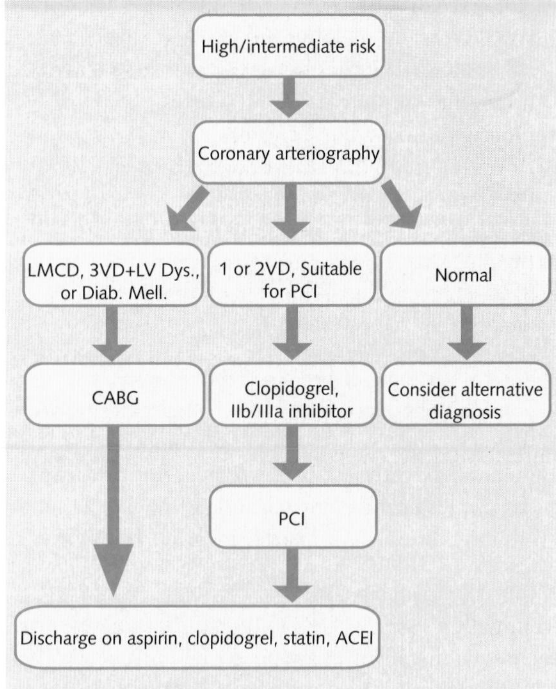

Fig. 13.7 Approach to higher/immediate risk patients with unstable angina/NSTEMI. (LCD = left main coronary disease, 3VD = three vessel disease, LV Dys. = left ventricular dysfunction, Diab. Mell. = diabetes mellitus, 2VD = two vessel disease, CABG = coronary artery bypass graft, PCI = percutaneous coronary intervention, ACEI = angiotensin-converting enzyme inhibitor.)

molecular-weight heparins are more effective than intravenous heparin.

- Consider antiplatelet medications and/or G IIb/IIIa inhibitors.
- Arrange early angiography if appropriate.

Algorithms summarizing the approach to patients with unstable angina and NSTEMI are presented in Figs 13.5, 13.6, and 13.7.

Heparins

The heparins consist of a highly heterogeneous group of compounds—all are proteoglycans, but they differ in their constituent sugar units and in molecular weight.

Heparin acts to alter antithrombin, which becomes much more effective in inhibiting thrombin and the coagulation factors Xa and IXa.

The problems with heparin administration for unstable angina are as follows:

- To maintain a constant effect, heparin must be given as an intravenous infusion. Therefore, the patient must be an inpatient and remian relatively immobile.
- During this time the activated partial thromboplastin time must be regularly monitored to ensure that the effect of heparin is not too little (rendering the drug ineffective) or too great (leading to a risk of hemorrhage).
- Side effects of heparin include increased risk of bleeding and thrombocytopenia; osteopenia is seen in patients who take long-term heparin.

Low-molecular-weight heparins form a more uniform group of heparins with 13–22 sugar residues. They have high bioavailibility after subcutaneous injection and a longer half-life. They also have a more predictable anticoagulant effect than conventional heparin.

The benefits of low-molecular-weight heparin are:

- They can be given as twice daily subcutaneous injections instead of as a continuous infusion.
- The dose is adjusted according to patient weight, and the anticoagulant effect is sufficiently predictable that regular monitoring is not required.
- There is a lower risk of osteoporosis and thrombocytopenia.

14. Acute Myocardial Infarction

Definition of acute myocardial infarction

Acute myocardial infarction (MI) is the term used for cell death secondary to ischemia. The most common cause of MI is atherosclerotic narrowing of the coronary arteries. The immediate precursor to MI is rupture of an atherosclerotic plaque and the formation of thrombus over the plaque, resulting in rapid occlusion of the vessel.

Depending upon the rate of vessel occlusion (if an atherosclerotic plaque grows slowly over months, collateral vessels develop and protect the myocardium) and the degree of occlusion of the vessel by thrombus, a number of clinical conditions can result from plaque rupture. These conditions are termed the acute coronary syndromes.

Acute MI is the most serious of this spectrum of acute illnesses (Fig. 14.1). World Health Organization (WHO) criteria for diagnosing acute MI includes the occurrence of any two of the following: (1) chest pain, (2) EKG changes, and (3) elevated cardiac enzymes.

For simplicity, and to make the management algorithm work (see below), these are divided into two categories:

- ST elevation (STEMI).
- Non-ST elevation (NSTEMI).

All these syndromes present as severe central chest pain of typical cardiac type (see Chapter 1), and patients usually present at the emergency department with one of the following:

- Unstable angina: Unstable angina is usually defined as either the development of a patients angina symptoms at rest or an increase in frequency of previously stable angina or new onset angina. Cardiac enzymes are not elevated in these patients. Note that the only difference between unstable angina (UA) and a NSTEMI is the release of cardiac enzymes into the blood. Troponins are elevated in NSTEMI and negative in UA.
- Non-ST elevation MI—Myocardial necrosis is caused by thrombotic coronary artery occlusion in which myocardial cell death is confined to the endocardial layers and is not full thickness. It occurs either because the occluded artery is a relatively small branch, or because there is good collateral flow around the occluded vessel.
- ST elevation MI—this follows necrosis through the whole thickness of the ventricular wall, leaving permanent Q waves on the EKG (remember: Q wave means dead myocardium) (Fig. 14.2).

Clinical features of acute myocardial infarction

History

The history is very important because it provides clues about the severity of the infarction and the time of onset (important when deciding on therapy). The following are classical features of the history of acute MI. Remember that angina does is not always chest pain. The elderly, diabetics, and women can present with anginal equivalents. These range from nausea and GI upset to jaw or shoulder pressure. These equivalents, or rather an increase in their frequency, should be treated just as an change in the more typical chest pain angina.

Presenting complaint

The main presenting complaint is chest pain. The following characteristics are common:

- Usually severe in nature.
- Normally lasts at least 30min.
- Patients may make a fist and place it over their sternum. This is called Levine's sign. Patients typically describe the pain as pressure, or an "elephant is sitting on my chest."
- Usually tight, crushing, and bandlike in nature.
- Retrosternal in location.
- May radiate to the left arm, throat, neck, or jaw.
- Associated features include sweating, breathlessness, and nausea.
- Elderly patients may have relatively little pain but may present with features of left ventricular failure (profound breathlessness) or syncope.

Acute coronary syndromes in descending order of severity

- ST elevation infarction
- Non-ST elevation infarction
- Unstable angina due to coronary arterial thrombosis
- Widespread subendocardial ischemia
- Sudden increase in severity of exertional angina
- Severe angina episode in a patient who has exertional angina

Fig. 14.1 Acute coronary syndromes in order of severity.

Past medical history

Important features include a history of angina or intermittent chest pain that often increases in severity or frequency in the few weeks preceding this event.

Risk factors for ischemic heart disease are male sex, increased age, smoking, hypertension, diabetes mellitus, hypercholesterolemia, and positive family history. (Although some of these do not belong in this section of the H and P, it is important not to forget them and therefore easier to ask about them all together at the same time).

The patient may have a history of previous MIs or of cardiac intervention such as stress testing, angiography, percutaneous transluminal angioplasty (PTCA), or coronary artery bypass grafts (CABG).

Also ask about any contraindication for thrombolysis at this stage.

Examination

On inspection the patient is often extremely anxious, distressed, and restless. He or she may be in severe pain. Breathlessness suggests the presence of pulmonary edema, as does the presence of pink frothy sputum. The patient may be pale, clammy, and sweaty, suggesting a degree of cardiogenic shock. Look for scars of previous surgery. Also look for JVD, signs of chest trauma (e.g., a steering wheel imprint on the chest), or asymmetric leg swelling suggestive of a possible DVT and PE. Do not lose sight of the forest looking for the great big tall tree of a MI. Other problems, like those listed above plus acute aortic dissection, can kill patients faster than the MI that they are not really having.

Cardiovascular system

The pulse may be tachycardic secondary to anxiety or left ventricular failure, or it may be bradycardic in the case of an inferior MI in which the right coronary artery is occluded and the atrioventricular node (which is supplied by the right coronary artery in 90% of people) is affected.

The blood pressure may be normal. In some patients it may be high, and this rise may be due to anxiety. If there is cardiogenic shock, the blood pressure may be low.

The jugular venous pressure may be elevated in cases of congestive heart failure or in pure right ventricular infarction.

Examination of the precordium may reveal the following:

- A displaced diffuse apex in cases of left ventricular failure.
- In anterior infarction a paradoxical systolic outward movement of the ventricular wall may be felt parasternally.
- Audible murmurs.
- The murmur of mitral regurgitation—may occur as a new murmur due to rupture of the papillary muscle.
- A pericardial rub—may be audible in some patients because it is not uncommon for an MI to be complicated by pericarditis.
- A fourth heart sound (Fig. 14.3)—common in MI due to reduction of left ventricular compliance.
- A third heart sound—occurs in the presence of left ventricular failure.
- Further evidence of cardiac failure (e.g., bilateral basal crackles, peripheral edema and poor peripheral perfusion).

Investigation of acute myocardial infarction

Blood tests

Indicators of myocardial damage

Creatine kinase

The MB isoenzyme of creatine kinase (CK) increases and falls within 72 hours. (The source of CK-MB isoenzyme is cardiac muscle, whereas CK-MM is found in skeletal muscle and CK-BB in brain and kidney. Many laboratories provide only total CK measurements for routine use, but this value is not specific.) The CK-MB isoenzyme does not begin to increase until at least 4 hours after infarction and is therefore not used to make the initial diagnosis in most cases.

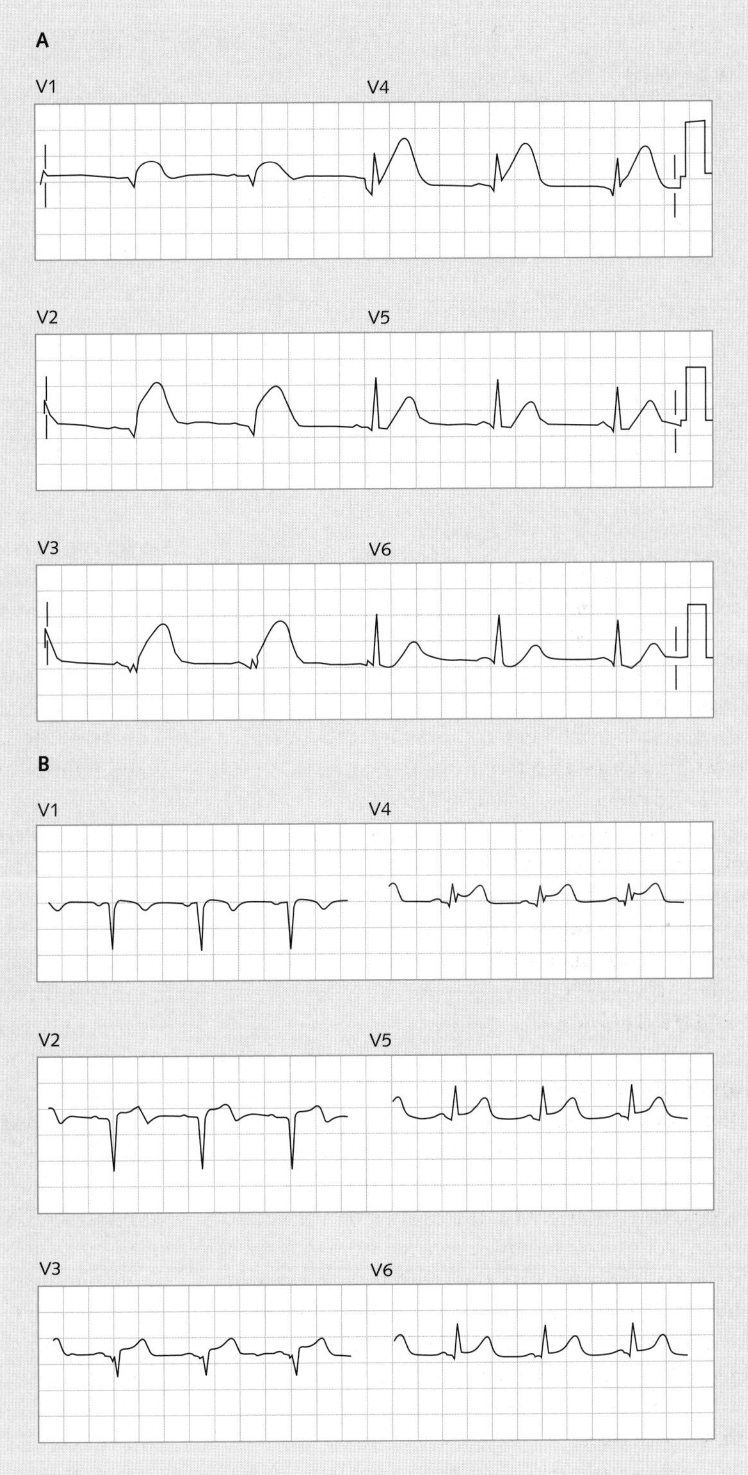

Fig. 14.2 (A) EKG showing acute anterior MI. (B) EKG 24 hours after anterior MI. Note the resolution of the ST elevation and the development of Q waves. The loss of the R wave in this EKG suggests that a significant left ventricle muscle mass has undergone necrosis.

Notes on third and fourth heart sounds			
Heart sound	**Mechanism**	**When heard**	**Causes**
Fourth	Represents atrial contribution to ventricular filling	Heard in any condition that causes a "stiff" left ventricular wall	Hypertension, aortic stenosis, acute myocardial infarction
Third	Rapid filling of the ventricle as soon as the mitral valve opens	Normal finding in young people and heard in conditions with fluid overload of the ventricle	Mitral regurgitation, ventricular septal defect, left ventricular failure, myocardial infarction

Fig. 14.3 Notes on third and fourth heart sounds.

Troponin

Troponin is more cardiospecific than the other indicators and increases rapidly, remaining elevated for 2 weeks. In patients who have unstable angina, marginally high levels of troponin indicate a high likelihood of subsequent infarction. Of note there are two types of troponin: T and I. Troponin T can be abnormally high in patients with chronic renal insufficiency despite no damage to myocardium.

Myoglobin

Myoglobin is a small heme molecule that is quickly leaked from damaged tissue due to its small size. It is currently being used in some EDs to help diagnose MIs because it can be detected much faster than the other cardiac injury markers (peak release is approximately 1 hour after injury). However, because of its half-life in the blood (under 10 minutes) and its lack of cardiac specificity, it has yet to widely replace CK-MB and troponin-I as the prime markers of cardiac injury.

Renal function and electrolytes

These are important in all patients who have MI. Renal function may be deranged or may worsen due to poor renal perfusion in cardiogenic shock. Hypokalemia may predispose to arrhythmias and must be corrected because acute MI is in itself a proarrhythmogenic condition. Always monitor urine output: if the patient is making urine, there must forward flow; if not, this may be a sign of cardiogenic shock.

Blood glucose

Diabetes mellitus must be aggressively controlled after MI, and all patients who have diabetes mellitus benefit from insulin therapy either using an intravenous sliding scale or, if their condition is stable, 4 times daily subcutaneous insulin.

Complete blood count

Anemia may precipitate an acute MI in a patient who has angina. There is often a leukocytosis after acute MI.

Serum cholesterol

This should be measured within 24–48 hours of an MI—otherwise it may be forgotten. Hypercholesterolemia is a risk factor for MI and should therefore be treated in all these patients. Cholesterol level falls to an artificially low level 24 hours after MI, so a true reading can be obtained only 2 months after MI.

Electrocardiography

The EKG is the main diagnostic test in acute MI (Fig. 14.4). It is therefore important to have a thorough knowledge of the EKG appearances of different types of MI. Delay in the diagnosis wastes precious time because cardiac catheterization should be performed as soon as possible for maximum benefit.

Classic EKG changes of a full-thickness MI are as follows:

- ST segment elevation—this is due to full-thickness myocardial injury and may appear within minutes of the onset of infarction; it is almost always present by 24 hours. The criteria for acute thrombolysis are a good history and ST segment elevation greater than 1 mm in two or more consecutive leads. However, emergency cardiac catheterization has been shown in multiple studies to be the treatment of choice for STEMI. Time is myocardium. Patients who are received in the ED with a STEMI should be routed to the catheterization lab as soon as possible. Reciprocal ST segment depression may be present at the same time and represents the mirror image of the ST elevation as seen from the opposite side of the heart.

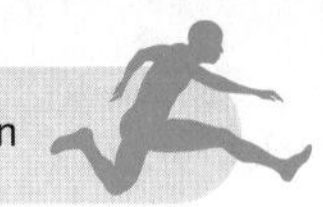

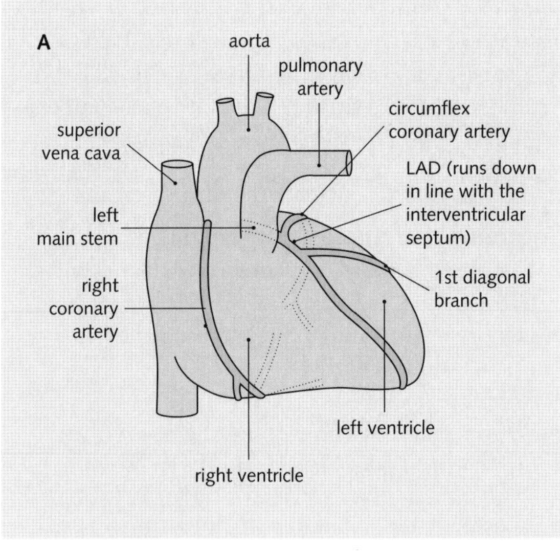

B Localizing EKG changes	
Location of MI	**EKG changes**
Anterior (LAD)	ST elevation in leads V1–4
Inferior (RCA or circumflex)	ST elevation in leads II, III, AVF coronary artery
Lateral (circumflex)	ST elevation in leads V4–6 coronary artery
Posterior (RCA or circumflex coronary artery)	Prominent R wave in V1 and V2 with ST depression (mirror image of anterior MI)
Anterolateral (proximal LAD) above diagonal branch	ST elevation V1–6
Right ventricular infarction (suspect in inferior or posterior MI)	Perform right-sided EKG using lead VI (as normal), leads V3–6 placed on the right side, limb leads as normal

Fig. 14.4 (A) Location of coronary arteries. Note the left anterior descending coronary artery branch (LAD) supplies the anterior aspect of the heart (the left ventricle and the septum), the right coronary artery (RCA) supplies the inferoposterior aspect, and the circumflex supplies the lateral part of the left ventricle. (B) Localizing EKG changes.

- Over 24 hours the ST elevation resolves and the T waves begin to invert.
- Q waves develop within 24–72 hours after MI.

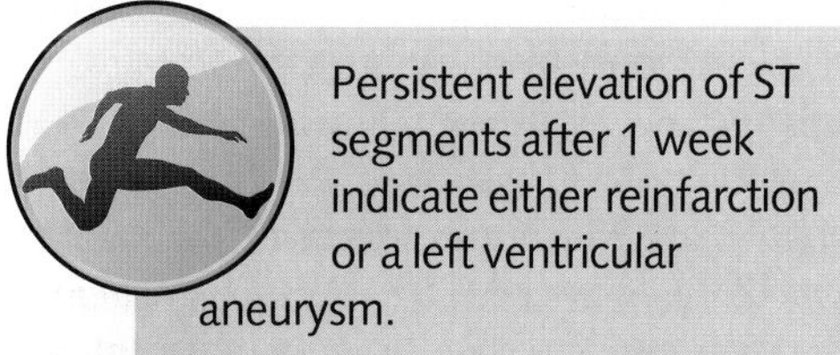

Persistent elevation of ST segments after 1 week indicate either reinfarction or a left ventricular aneurysm.

EKG changes in non-ST elevation myocardial infarction

These are variable, and the absence of Q waves does not necessarily indicate that full-thickness infarction has not occurred. (The conventional view was that this represented subendocardial damage only.)

The EKG changes tend to be in the form of persistent T-wave inversion accompanied by an increase in cardiac enzymes. New left bundle-branch block (LBBB) on EKG in the presence of chest pain suggests acute myocardial infarction and is also an indication for emergent cardiac catheterization.

Chest radiography

This should be performed on all patients who have acute MI. Points to note are:

- Widening of the mediastinum—suggests a likelihood of aortic dissection, which is an absolute contraindication for thrombolysis.
- Signs of pulmonary edema—signify the need for antifailure therapy (intravenous diuretics, oxygen, and possibly a nitrate infusion).
- An enlarged heart—suggests cardiac failure. Brain natriuretic peptide is also being used to determine if a patient is in heart failure. BNP is released from the ventricles when they are overexapanded in heart failure. A quick blood test can now determine if the ventricles are in failure.

Echocardiography

This is not a first-line investigation but is very useful in the first week to assess left ventricular function or investigate valve lesions (mitral regurgitation may occur after MI as a result of papillary muscle infarction).

Management of acute myocardial infarction

Acute MI is a medical emergency; therefore, you must know its acute management thoroughly (Fig. 14.5).

Acute management of acute MI

- Administer oxygen via a facial mask
- Give the patient soluble aspirin, 300mg, in water
- Establish IV access and connect patient to cardiac monitor
- If the patient is distressed or in pain, give IV morphine and arrange to take the patient to the cardiac catheterization laboratory
- Administer intravenous atenolol, 5mg over 10 minutes; if tolerated, repeat the dose after 10 minutes
- Continue to observe the patient in the coronary care unit

Fig. 14.5 Acute management of acute MI. (IV, intravenous; rt-PA, recombinant tissue plasminogen activator.)

Emergency cardiac catheterization

Over the past several years studies have shown that while lytic (= thrombolytic) therapy does decrease mortality, emergent catheterization with percutaenous coronary balloon angioplasty (PTCA) and possible stent placement is superior. More recent trials have shown that the time lost in transporting a patient with MI to a center that offers catheterization is not detrimental when mortality is compared with lytic therapy at the originating hospital. In the U.S. this modality is preferred to lytic therapy.

Thrombolytic therapy

A number of large prospective, double-blind, placebo-controlled trials have shown that thrombolysis reduces mortality rate after MI (e.g., the Italian GISSI trial and the International Study of Infarct Survival [ISIS] II study). Thrombolysis results in recanalization of the occluded vessel and restores coronary flow, which reduces infarct size and improves myocardial function if thrombolysis is administered within 24 hours of pain.

Thrombolytic agents

There are a number of thrombolytic agents (Fig. 14.6). The two most commonly used are streptokinase and recombinant tissue plasminogen activator (rt-PA). There are, however, an increasing number of new agents.

Two major trials, GISSI II and ISIS III, showed no increased benefit when different thrombolytic agents were compared. GISSI II compared streptokinase and t-PA; ISIS III compared streptokinase, rt-PA, and anisoylated plasminogen streptokinase activator complex (APSAC). These trials also showed that heparin provided no benefit. However, GUSTO I (Global Use of Strategies to Open Occluded Arteries) showed a small benefit with accelerated rt-PA followed by a heparin infusion over other regimens.

Contraindications to thrombolysis

- History of hemorrhagic cerebrovascular event—ever.
- History of any type of cerebrovascular event in past 6 months.
- Recent gastrointestinal bleed.
- Bleeding diathesis or warfarin therapy with an international normalized ratio (INR) over 1.5.
- Operation within past month—not an absolute contraindication, but you should consult a senior before proceeding.
- Pregnancy.
- Any other invasive procedure in the past month (e.g., organ biopsy, dental extraction)—consult a senior before proceeding.
- SBP > 180mmHg.

Indications for thrombolysis

Most centers consider a door to needle time of greater than 30min unacceptable. Ideally all patients should be thrombolysed within 70min of onset of pain to receive the greatest benefit.

All patients who satisfy the following criteria should be thrombolysed as soon as possible.

- History of chest pain lasting less than 24 hours.
- And one of the following—ST elevation greater than 1mm in standard leads or in two adjacent chest leads or new bundle-branch block on EKG.

Other agents used for acute myocardial infarction

Aspirin

The antiplatelet aggregation action of aspirin makes it effective in all acute coronary syndromes in which the primary event is clot formation. This drug has relatively few side effects and should be administered promptly to all patients as soon as the EKG is found to be positive.

Aspirin was found to reduce the mortality rate in the ISIS II study.

Antiplatelet medications

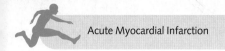

The mere fact that one of the most important medications given during an acute MI is aspirin

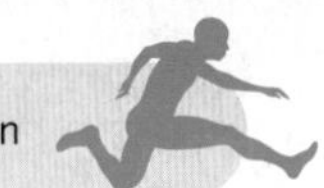

Overview of thrombolytic agents				
Agent	**Action**	**Half-life (min)**	**Administration**	**Other features**
Streptokinase	Binds to plasminogen to form a complex that activates to convert another molecule of plasminogen to plasmin; not clot-specific—will attack all plasminogen	18 (but 180 for streptokinase plasminogen complex)	Infusion of 1.5 million units over 1 hour	Allergic reactions, hypotension; previous streptokinase treatment renders subsequent doses less effective due to antibody production; hemorrhage
rt-PA	Binds to fibrin and complex converts plasminogen to plasmin; clot-specific—will act only in presence of fibrin	4–5 (circulating plasminogen and fibrinogen levels return to 80% of normal within 24 hours)	Infusion, often preceded by a bolus dose; accelerated t-PA—15mg bolus, then 50 over 30min followed by 35mg over 1hr (as in GUSTO trial)	Hemorrhage, very expensive
APSAC	A stable form of the streptokinase–plasminogen complex that is activated in injection	Long—100min; therefore can be given as a single dose; enables the drug to be used in the community and can therefore be administered earlier	30 units intravenously	Hypotension, hemorrhage, very expensive
The ideal thrombolytic agent	Very clot-specific, easily reversible in the event of hemorrhage; administration by intravenous bolus	Very short half-life for use in hospital as infusion (can be easily controlled) and long half-life preparation for community use where coronary care not easily accessible		Cheap, no antibody effects, derived from human protein so no anaphylaxis

Fig. 14.6 Overview of thrombolytic agents. (APSAC, anisoylated plasminogen streptokinase activator complex; rt-PA, recombinant tissue plasminogen activator.)

should underline the importance of antiplatelet medication in decreasing mortality. New medications that inhibit platelets in ways different from aspirin have recently been shown to be beneficial in keeping stents and arteries open. Clopidogrel, an adenylate cyclase inhibitor, is now standard care for patients receiving a stent during catheterization. The medication is prescribed for periods ranging from 3 months to lifelong in order to decrease the restenosis rate.

Glycoprotein (Gp) IIb/IIIa inhibitors affect platelet aggregation. Recent date have shown their usefulness in patients who will undergo catheterization and stenting within 24 hours of administration. As more research is done on these medications, they may be used in other situations.

Morphine

A powerful anxiolytic and analgesic, morphine is extremely effective in the patient who has cardiac pain. It has venodilating properties and is therefore also effective in patients with acute pulmonary edema.

Beta-blockers(beta-adrenoceptor antagonists)

These drugs were shown to reduce mortality rate acutely after MI in ISIS 1. The following are contraindications to the administration of beta blockers:

- Unstable or acute cardiac failure (beta blockers can worsen pulmonary edema).
- Bradycardia (heart rate < 60 beats/min).
- Hypotension (systolic blood pressure < 90 mmHg).
- Asthma.

Oxygen

Oxygen should be administered to all patients initially and then continued for all patients who have hypoxemia (i.e., arterial oxygen saturation 90%).

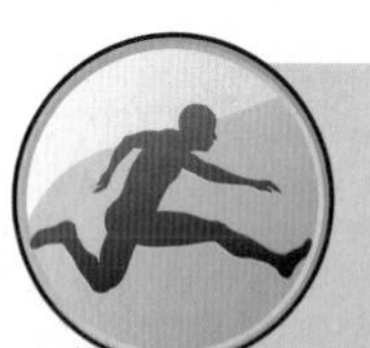

A quick note about inferior MIs: ST elevation in the inferior leads suggests the possibility of posterior/right-sided damage. Because of the possible damage to the right ventricle (RV) and /or the sinoatrial (SA) node, this may greatly change management. SA node damage can result in bradycardia and even bradicardic arrest. RV damage can lead to a precipitous drop in BP on administration of nitroglycerin. In the setting of RV damage the patient may become preload-dependent and require liters of fluid to retain a satisfactory BP.

Complications of an acute MI
Early (0–48 hours) Arrhythmias—VT, VF, SVT, heart block Cardiogenic shock due to left or right ventricular failure
Medium term (2–7 days) Arrhythmias—VT, VF, SVT, heart block Pulmonary embolus (4–7 days) Rupture of papillary muscle (3–5 days) Rupture of interventricular septum (3–5 days) Free wall rupture (3–5 days) (rupture of the above structures usually presents with acute cardiac failure and progresses rapidly to death; a few patients may survive after surgery)
Late (>7 days) Arrhythmias—VT, VF, SVT, heart block Cardiac failure Dressler's syndrome (3–8 weeks) Left ventricular aneurysm (after several weeks) Mural thrombosis and systemic embolization

Fig. 14.7 Complications of an acute MI. (SVT, supraventricular tachycardia; VF, ventricular fibrillation; VT, ventricular tachycardia.)

Drugs on discharge after MI
• Aspirin • Beta blocker • ACE inhibitor • Statin lipid-lowering drug—this should probably be given regardless of lipid levels because statins seem to modify the progress of atheroma independently • Clopidogrel • Eplerenone (when the EF is <45%) • Sublingual nitrates

Fig. 14.8 Drugs on discharge after MI. (ACE, angiotensin-converting enzyme).

Nonacute management

Complications may arise after acute myocardial infarction (Fig. 14.7). The following points of management must be observed. Particular points to look for on examination and questioning are:

- Chest pain—further pain indicates the possibility of another MI and should be investigated early with urgent coronary angiogram.
- Breathlessness or signs of cardiac failure—diuretics should be commenced and urgent echocardiography performed to exclude septal defect or mitral regurgitation secondary to papillary muscle rupture.
- New murmurs—a ruptured papillary muscle causes mitral regurgitation; a ruptured septum causes ventricular septal defect.
- Pericardial rub—pericarditis.
- Hypotension—drug-induced or secondary to cardiogenic shock.
- Bradycardia—heart block after an inferior MI (or very large anterior MI with septal necrosis).

The patient should have daily EKGs to look for arrhythmias, including heart block.

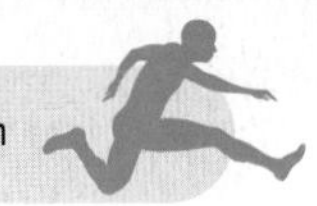

Panel A

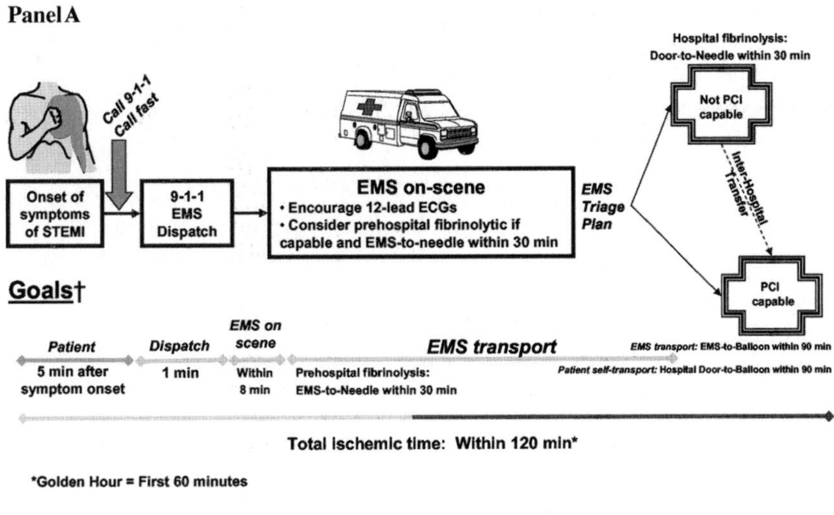

Panel B

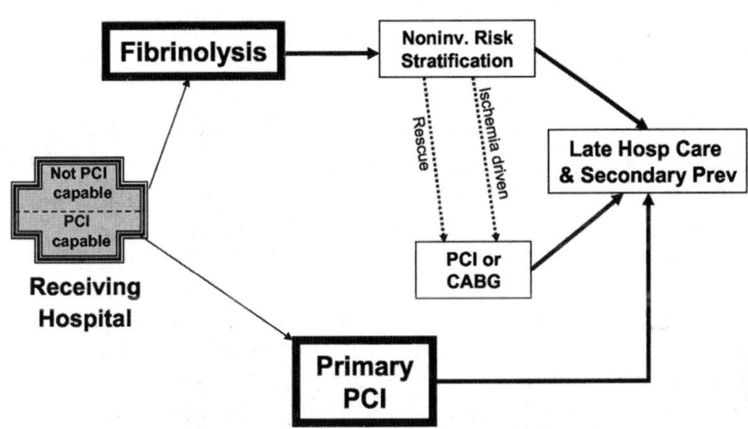

Fig. 14.9 Options for transportation of STEMI patients and initial reperfusion treatment. Panel A, *Patient transported by EMS after calling 9-1-1*: Reperfusion in patients with STEMI can be accomplished by the pharmacological (fibrinolysis) or catheter-based (primary PCI) approaches. Implementation of these strategies varies based on the mode of transportation of the patient and capabilities at the receiving hospital. Transport time to the hospital is variable from case to case, but the goal is to keep total ischemic time within 120 minutes. There are 3 possibilities: (1) If EMS has fibrinolytic capability and the patient qualifies for therapy, prehospital fibrinolysis should be started within 30 minutes of EMS arrival on scene. (2) If EMS is not capable of administering prehospital fibrinolysis and the patient is transported to a non-PCI-capable hospital, the hospital door-to-needle time should be within 30 minutes for patients in whom fibrinolysis is indicated. (3) If EMS is not capable of administering prehospital fibrinolysis and the patient is transported to a PCI-capable hospital, the hospital door-to-balloon time should be within 90 minutes. Panel B, *Interhospital transfer*: It is also appropriate to consider emergency interhospital transfer of the patient to a PCI-capable hospital for mechanical revascularization if (1) there is a contraindication to fibrinolysis; (2) PCI can be initiated promptly. (From Antman et al.: Management of Patients with STEMI. Executive Summary. J Am Coll Cardiol Aug. 4, 2004, Fig.1, with permission.)

A continuous cardiac monitor should be used for the first few days because fatal arrhythmias are common after MI (usually ventricular tachycardia or fibrillation).

Early mobilization (after 48 hours) is instituted to prevent venous stasis.

If the patient has had a large MI or there is clinical evidence of cardiac failure (and provided there is no renal failure or hypotension), an angiotensin-converting enzyme inhibitor should be introduced within 24-hours after MI. This improves outcome, as seen in the ISIS IV, GISSI III, and SAVE studies.

Hypercholesterolemia should be treated with a statin and the patient referred to a lipid management clinic for follow-up. Suitable dietary advice should be given. Recent evidence suggests that a statin should be given in any case because statins may have additional benefits after MI in addition to their lipid-lowering effect. The LIPID (Long-term Intervention with Pravastatin in Ischemic Heart Disease) study shows benefit with pravastatin in patients after MI who have a total cholesterol level before treatment as low as 4.0mmol/L.

Follow-up care should include:

- An exercise test at about 6 weeks after MI to assess the risk of further ischemia—if the test is positive, a coronary angiogram should be performed.
- Access to the rehabilitation program.

Cardiac rehabilitation

All good cardiac units have an integrated rehabilitation program available to all cardiac patients that consists of:

- Progressively increasing exercise level to a maintenance level of as much regular rapid walking as possible every day.
- Dietary advice, particularly emphasizing the value of fish and olive oil and fresh fruit and vegetables. Carbohydrate restriction for non-insulin-dependent diabetes mellitus and insulin resistance. Calorie restriction for patients who have diabetes mellitus or who are obese.
- Advice on medications (Fig. 14.8), their role in improving prognosis, and the importance of compliance.
- Advice from a clinical psychologist on how to cope with the illness.
- Group gymnasium sessions may help some patients by encouraging exercise and giving psychological support to each other.
- A subsequent support group may be continued as long as each individual patient finds it helpful; a doctor's input is important from time to time.

Summary of management of acute ST elevation myocardial infarction

An algorithm summarizing the management of acute ST elevation MI is given in Fig. 14.9.

Heart block after myocardial infarction

Ischemic injury may occur at any point in the conducting system, whether it be the sinoatrial node or the atrioventricular node or anywhere from the bundle of His downward. It is therefore not surprising that heart block after MI may be:

- First- or second-degree atrioventricular block.
- Complete heart block with atrioventricular dissociation.
- Interventricular block (complete or partial RBBB or LBBB).

Inferior MI is more commonly associated with atrioventricular block because the atrioventricular node is supplied by the right coronary artery in 90% of cases.

Anterior MI may cause heart block in the presence of marked septal necrosis (indicating a large anterior MI).

Management of post-myocardial infarction heart block

Patients who have Mobitz type II or complete heart block should have temporary pacing wires inserted as soon as possible.

The need for a permanent pacemaker depends upon the site of the MI.

Patients who have anterior MI and septal necrosis often need permanent pacing because the atrioventricular node rarely recovers.

Patients who have an inferior MI may not need permanent pacing because many recover normal function of the atrioventricular node. Current practice is to wait at least 2 weeks before deciding on a permanent system because recovery can take up to 3 weeks.

15. Supraventricular Tachyarrhythmias

Definition

Supraventricular tachyarrhythmias (SVTs) are fast rhythms characterized by narrow QRS complexes (unless aberrant conduction is present).

A tachycardia is defined as a rate of 100 beats/min or greater. In ascending order of atrial electrical dysfunction, these are:

- Sinus tachycardia.
- Atrial ectopics.
- Nodal ectopics.
- Atrial tachycardia.
- Junctional tachycardia and supraventricular re-entry tachycardia.
- Atrial flutter.
- Atrial fibrillation.

Sinus tachycardia

Points of importance are:

- The sinus node fires at over 100 beats/min.
- Every complex is preceded by a normal P wave.
- The PR interval is within normal limits and remains stable.

Causes

Causes of sinus tachycardia include:

- Fever.
- Thyrotoxicosis.
- Hypotension.
- Any form of stress (e.g., pain, anxiety, exertion).

These are all physiological responses. Rarely an inappropriate resting sinus tachycardia occurs. This is due to an abnormality of sinus node discharge or another atrial focus of activity located near the sinus node.

Premature atrial ectopics

These are seen on the EKG as a premature P wave (which may be normal or abnormal in appearance) followed by a prolonged PR interval (120ms). They are followed by a pause because the atrioventricular (AV) node is refractory.

Premature atrial ectopics can be precipitated by many conditions, including:

- Stress.
- Caffeine.
- Alcohol.
- Myocardial ischemia.
- Myocardial inflammation.

Treatment is not indicated unless the patient is very symptomatic in which case beta-blockers (beta-adrenoceptor antagonists) may be of some help.

Nodal and junctional ectopics

The AV node is a compact structure, and lying close to it is the AV junctional area. It is from this area and from the node itself that these ectopic beats originate. These structures have the ability to fire autonomously, but they have a slower rate of firing than the sinoatrial (SA) node; therefore, they are usually suppressed.

In some conditions impulses may arise ectopically from the AV node and junctional region. The impulse is conducted to the atrium, where a retrograde P wave is produced, and also to the ventricle, where a narrow complex QRS is produced (Fig. 15.1). (Depending upon the speed of conduction the P wave may occur just before, after, or simultaneously with the QRS.)

Again, treatment is not usually indicated.

Atrial tachycardia

Atrial tachycardia is a tachyarrhythmia generated in the atrial tissue. The atrial rate is 150–200 beats/min.

Because the origin of the tachycardia is not the SA node, the P wave morphology is different to normal. The P wave axis may also be abnormal. For example, when the atrial focus is in the left atrium, the P wave in lead V1 is positive.

Causes

The following may lead to atrial tachycardia:

- Structural heart abnormality (e.g., COPD, atrial septal defect).
- Coronary artery disease.
- Digitalis toxicity.

Investigation and diagnosis

On examination the pulse is rapid and of variable intensity:

- Jugular venous pressure may reveal many a waves to each v wave if there is a degree of AV block.
- EKG may show 1:1 conduction or variable degrees of AV block.
- It may be difficult to differentiate atrial tachycardia from atrial flutter.

Diagnosis may be aided by enhancing AV block and therefore making it easier to visualize the P-wave morphology and rate. There are two effective methods of doing this:

- Carotid sinus massage—increases vagal stimulation of the SA and AV node.
- Intravenous adenosine—results in transient complete AV block.

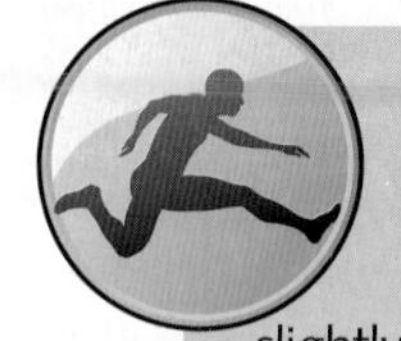

Remember that atrial flutter usually has an atrial rate of 300/min with a degree of AV block. Atrial tachycardia has a slightly slower atrial rate with abnormal P waves.

Management

The patient will present with palpitations. Any underlying cause should be treated (e.g., check digoxin levels and stop the drug).

Drugs used to treat atrial tachycardia include:

- Atrioventricular blocking drugs such as digoxin, beta blockers, calcium channel blockers—these slow the ventricular response rate but do not affect the atrial tachycardia itself).
- Class 1A (e.g., disopyramide), 1C (e.g., flecainide), or III (e.g., amiodarone) drugs (see p. 126) may be used in an effort to terminate the atrial tachycardia.

Electrical cardioversion is often successful.

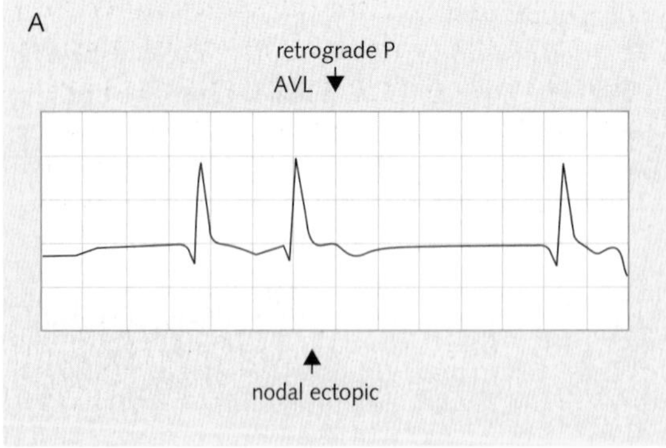

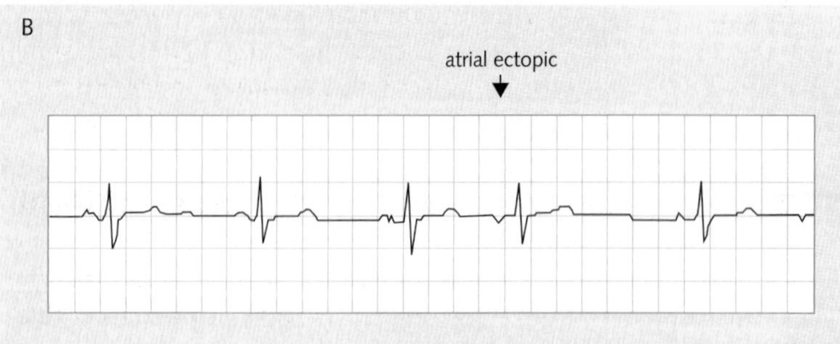

Fig. 15.1 (A) A nodal ectopic. The ectopic complex is similar to the normal QRS suggesting that it originates from the atrioventricular or junctional region. The P wave is retrograde and is seen just after the ectopic QRS superimposed on the T wave. The ectopic beat is followed by a compensatory pause. (B) EKG illustrating an ectopic atrial beat. Note that the premature atrial beat fires an abnormally shaped P wave and a normal QRS complex. A compensatory pause follows.

Atrioventricular junctional tachycardia

Tachycardias arising from the junctional area occur when there is a focus of activity with a discharge rate that is faster than that of the SA node. This is an abnormal situation and is usually due to ischemic heart disease or digitalis toxicity.

Clinical features

The following features are seen:

- Rate is usually up to 130 beats/min.
- Gradual onset.
- Terminates gradually.
- EKG shows a narrow complex tachycardia, occasionally with retrogradely conducted P waves. It is difficult to distinguish this from an AV nodal re-entry tachycardia and you will not be expected to do so. The main point is to realize that the junctional tissue may be a site of ectopic electrical activity.

Management

Treatment is aimed at the underlying cause:

- Antiarrhythmic agents such as digoxin, beta blockers, and calcium channel antagonists may be tried.
- Electrical cardioversion may be successful.

Atrioventricular nodal re-entry tachycardia

These tachycardias involve a re-entry circuit that lies in or close to the AV node and allows impulses to travel round and round triggering the ventricles and the atria (in a retrograde manner) as they go.

Clinical features

These tachycardias display the following features:

- Rate is 150–260 beats/min.
- Usually sudden onset and offset.
- QRS complexes are narrow unless there is aberrant conduction and the P waves may occur just before, just after, or within the QRS (it is not always easy to see these) (see Fig. 4.3C).

Causes of re-entrant tachycardia are caffeine, alcohol, and anxiety.

Diagnosis

Differentiation from atrial flutter and atrial fibrillation (AF) can be made by either:

- Performing carotid sinus massage or Valsalva maneuver.
- Giving intravenous adenosine.

These procedures block the AV node; therefore, the P waves of atrial flutter can be seen or the baseline fibrillation of AF can be seen. Blockade of the AV node in re-entrant tachycardia breaks the re-entry circuit and terminates the tachycardia in most cases.

Management

These tachycardias often terminate spontaneously with relaxation.

Vagal maneuvers such as carotid sinus massage and the Valsalva maneuver are often effective in terminating the tachycardia and patients can be taught to do these themselves.

In hospital the following treatments can be effective:

- Vagal maneuvers.
- Intravenous adenosine.
- Atrioventricular node-blocking agents (e.g., beta-blockers, digoxin, calcium channel blockers).
- Direct current (DC) cardioversion if less invasive methods have been unsuccessful.

In a patient who has recurrent troublesome AV nodal re-entry tachycardia, electrophysiological testing can locate the site of the abnormal circuit and this can then be ablated. This is a curative procedure. The main risk is AV node ablation resulting in complete heart block and requiring a permanent pacemaker.

Wolff–Parkinson–White syndrome

In this condition there is an abnormal connection between the atrium and the ventricle along which the impulse can travel. This is known as an accessory pathway. In Wolff–Parkinson–White syndrome the accessory pathway is known as the bundle of Kent.

Characteristics of the bundle of Kent

The bundle of Kent is capable of:

- Anterograde conduction—that is, it can conduct from the atrium to the ventricle; it is also capable of retrograde conduction.

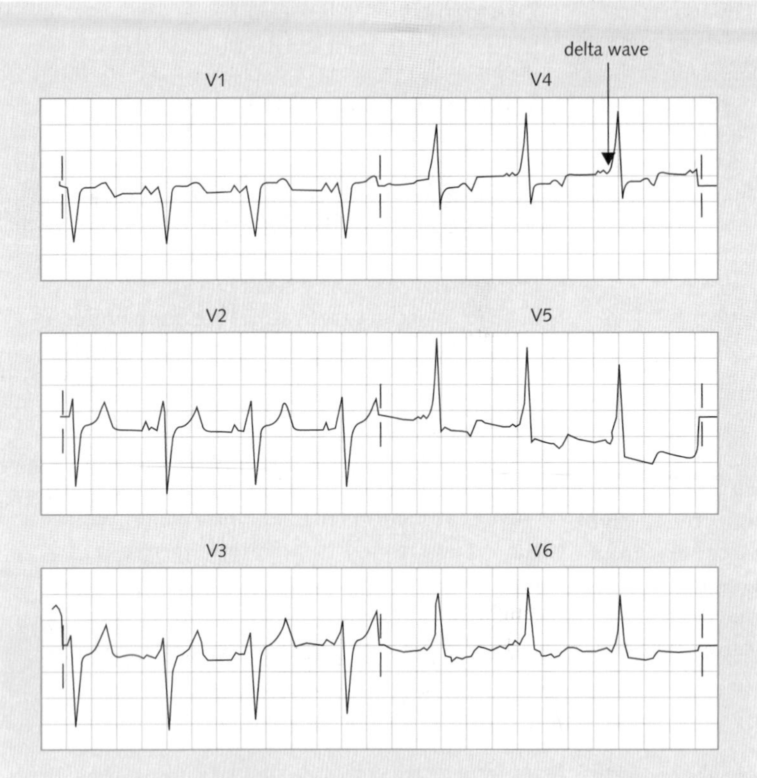

Fig. 15.2 Wolff–Parkinson–White syndrome. Note the short PR interval (0.08s) and the slurred upstroke of the QRS complex (the delta wave). This is caused by part of the impulse travelling down the accessory pathway and causing pre-excitation (early excitation) of the ventricle (represented by the delta wave). The rest of the impulse travels via the atrioventricular node and is represented by the main QRS complex.

- Conducting impulses faster than the normal His conductive tissue. Therefore, the ventricle is activated sooner than normal.

If, however, the impulse does not travel down the bundle of Kent, the P wave and QRS complex are normal. Therefore, it can be seen that the impulse can travel via two different routes from the atrium to the ventricle.

The impulse often travels both routes simultaneously; this results in a short PR interval and a slurred upstroke to the R wave (known as a delta wave; Fig. 15.2).

Tachycardias associated with Wolff–Parkinson–White syndrome

A number of tachycardias may occur:

- Orthodromic atrioventricular re-entry tachycardia (OAVRT)—the impulse is conducted from the atrium to the ventricle via the AV node, then back to the atrium via the accessory pathway. This results in a narrow complex tachycardia.
- Antidromic AVRT (AAVRT)—a similar tachycardia with conduction in the opposite direction (i.e., from the atrium to the ventricle via the accessory pathway) results in a wide complex tachycardia because the ventricle is depolarized from a point away from the bundle of His.
- Atrial fibrillation and atrial flutter may occur and may present a potential risk because the atrial impulses can be conducted rapidly via the accessory pathway giving ventricular rates of 300 beats/min or greater. This rapid ventricular rate predisposes to ventricular fibrillation.

Clinical features

Wolff–Parkinson–White syndrome is a congenital condition. Patients present with recurrent palpitations or syncope. Sudden death is a risk due to ventricular tachycardia. The accessory pathway may cease to conduct as patients grow older, but other patients continue to have problems.

Management

Treatment of Wolff–Parkinson–White syndrome is indicated only in patients who have recurrent tachyarrhythmias or who are symptomatic. Some patients have EKG evidence of the accessory pathway (short PR and delta wave) but no tachyarrhythmia; they do not require treatment.

First it is important to decide what type, OAVRT or AAVRT, is responsible. If it is difficult to determine, then err on the side of a wide complex tachycardia. There are a number of treatment options: the main ones to consider are drug therapy and ablation therapy.

Drug therapy

The aim of drug therapy is to slow conduction in the accessory pathway as well as to slow AV conduction. Drugs that do both are Vaughan Williams-Singh classification IA, IC, and III drugs (see p. 126).

AAVRT should be treated with procainamide; this is a common question on the wards and the boards. Even without terminating the abnormal rhythm, procainamide can usually slow the rhythm and improve hemodynamics. AV node-blocking agents, such as calcium channel blockers, beta blockers, digoxin, and adenosine, should not be used in these patients since they will block the AV node and encourage conduction down the accessory pathway. This is especially true of patients with Wolff–Parkinson–White syndrome and atrial fibrillation.

OAVRT should be treated, as noted above, with vagal maneuvers followed by adenosine or verapamil administration.

Drugs such as digoxin and verapamil are inappropriate in the treatment of WPW given the long half-life, difficulty in titration, and often acute nature of the arrythmias. Digoxin and-verapamil block the AV node but do not affect the accessory pathway, thus increasing the risk of rapid conduction of atrial fibrillation and flutter via the accessory pathway. For this reason, procainamide should be used in the acute termination of wide complex tachyarrhythmias associated with Wolff–Parkinson–White syndrome.

Remember that digoxin and verapamil should not be used as single agents in the treatment of tachycardias in Wolff–Parkinson–White syndrome.

Ablation therapy

Ablation may be surgical or electrical:

- Electrical ablation (or radiofrequency catheter ablation) is performed after the accessory pathway has been located by electrophysiological testing. This procedure is usually performed under light sedation using local anesthetic before inserting the electrodes. Ablative therapy using a radiofrequency catheter has a success rate around 90% depending on where the accessory pathway is situated.
- Surgical ablation is rarely performed but may be useful if electrical ablation is not successful.

Atrial flutter

Atrial flutter has the following characteristics:

- Atrial contraction rate is regular and is 250–350 beats/min (usually 300 beats/min).
- Ventricular response may be 1:1 (300 beats/min), 2:1 (150 beats/min), 3:1 (100 beats/min), etc.
- Severity of the symptoms depends upon the ventricular response rate (i.e., a rapid ventricular response is likely to cause palpitations, angina, and cardiac failure).

Causes include:

- Structural heart disease (e.g., valve disease, cardiomyopathy).
- Pulmonary disease (e.g., pulmonary embolus, pneumothorax, infection).
- Toxins (e.g., alcohol, caffeine).

Investigations and diagnosis

The EKG findings are (Fig. 15.3):

- Regular sawtooth atrial flutter waves (P waves).
- Narrow QRS complexes (unless there is coexistent bundle-branch block).

Diagnosis is confirmed by performing AV nodal blocking maneuvers (e.g., adenosine or carotid sinus massage). This slows the ventricular response so that the sawtooth P waves are revealed on the EKG.

Management

Cardioversion back to sinus rhythm is the best treatment, but if this is not possible then slowing of the ventricular rate will provide symptomatic relief and protect against cardiac failure. Direct current cardioversion using a synchronized shock will rapidly and safely restore sinus rhythm in some cases. Class IA, IC or III drugs (see p. 126) may be useful:

- To chemically cardiovert to sinus rhythm. When DC cardioversion is unsuccessful.
- To maintain sinus rhythm after successful electrical cardioversion.

When cardioversion is not possible or not sustained, AV-blocking agents are used to slow the ventricular response rate (class II, class IV, or digoxin).

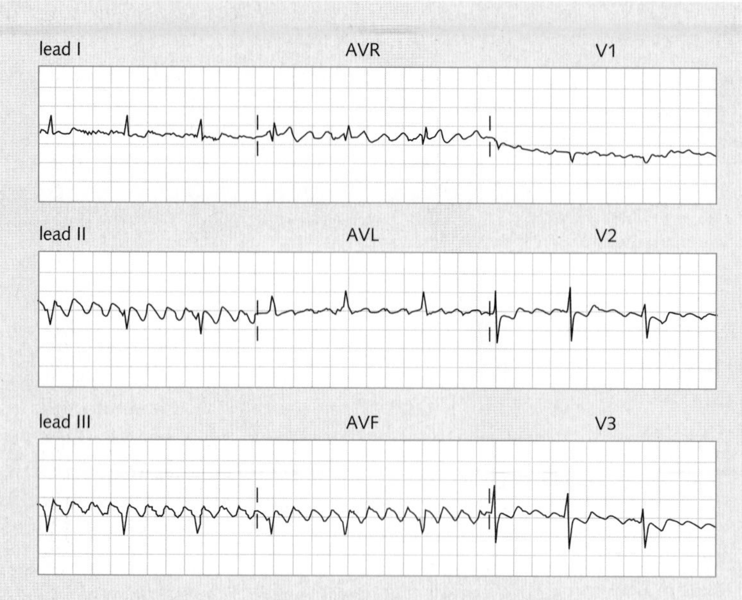

Fig. 15.3 Atrial flutter. Note the sawtooth F waves at a rate of just over 300 beats/min and the ventricular response of 4:1. Leads II and V1 often show P waves best (but not in this case).

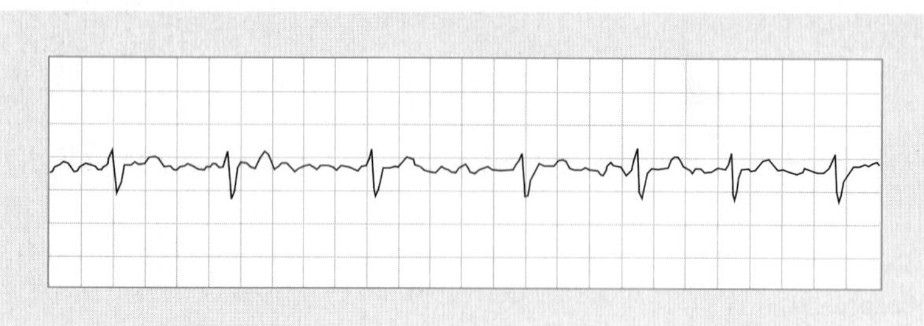

Fig. 15.4 Atrial fibrillation. Note the irregular baseline and the lack of P waves. The rhythm is irregularly irregular.

Because of the increased risk of thrombus formation in atrial flutter, anticoagulation is recommended before DC cardioversion, as with atrial fibrillation.

Atrial fibrillation

Atrial fibrillation has the following features:

- It is a common arrhythmia found in over 10% of the population above the age of 80.
- Disorganized random electrical activity in the atria results in a lack of effective atrial contraction.
- Stasis of blood in the atria predisposes to thrombus formation and embolic episodes.

Causes

Common causes are as follows:

- Ischemic heart disease.
- Valvular heart disease, especially mitral valve disease.
- Hypertensive heart disease.
- Pulmonary disease (e.g., embolus, infection, pneumothorax).
- Any form of sepsis.
- Thyrotoxicosis.
- Alcohol excess—holiday heart syndrome. Holiday heart syndrome is the occurrence of supraventricular arrhythmias (usually atrial fibrillation or atrial flutter) following an alcoholic binge and is usually transient.

Investigations and diagnosis

The EKG shows no P waves and an irregular baseline with a variable ventricular response rate (hence the irregularly irregular pulse; Fig. 15.4). Ventricular response ranges from 90 to 170 beats/min but may

ACC/AHA guidelines for minimum evaluation of atrial fibrillation

1. History and physical examination, to define:
   - The presence and nature of symptoms associated with AF
   - The clinical type of AF (first episode, paroxysmal, persistent, or permanent)
   - The onset of the first symptomatic attack or date of discovery of AF
   - The frequency, duration, precipitating factors, and modes of termination of AF
   - The response to any pharmacological agents that have been administered
   - The presence of any underlying heart disease or other reversible conditions (e.g., hyperthyroidism or alcohol consumption)
2. Electrocardiogram, to identify:
   - Rhythm (verify AF)
   - LV hypertrophy
   - P-wave duration and morphology or fibrillatory waves
   - Pre-excitation
   - Bundle-branch block
   - Prior MI
   - Other atrial arrhythmias
   - To measure and follow the RR, QRS, and QT intervals in conjunction with antiarrhythmic drug therapy
3. Chest radiograph, to evaluate:
   - The lung parenchyma, when clinical findings suggest an abnormality
   - The pulmonary vasculature, when clinical findings suggest an abnormality
4. Echocardiogram, to identify:
   - Valvular heart disease
   - Left and right atrial size
   - LV size and function
   - Peak RV pressure (pulmonary hypertension)
   - LV hypertrophy
   - LA thrombus (low sensitivity)
   - Pericardial disease
5. Blood tests of thyroid function: for a first episode of AF, when the ventricular rate is difficult to control, or when AF recurs unexpectedly after cardioversion
6. Additional testing. One or several tests may be necessary:
   - Exercise testing
     If the adequacy of rate control is in question (permanent AF)
     To reproduce exercise-induced AF
     To exclude ischemia before treatment of selected patients with a type IC antiarrhythmic drug
   - Holter monitoring or event recording
     If diagnosis of the type of arrhythmia is in question
     As a means of evaluating rate control
   - Transesophageal echocardiography
     To identify LA thrombus (in the LA appendage)
     To guide cardioversion
   - Electrophysiological study
     To clarify the mechanism of wide-QRS-complex tachycardia
     To identify a predisposing arrhythmia such as atrial flutter or paroxysmal supraventricular tachycardia
     To seek sites for curative ablation or AV conduction block/modification

Fig. 15.5 ACC/AHA guidelines for minimum evaluation of atrial fibrillation (AF).

be faster or slower. The actual AF rate may be from 300 to 600 beats/min. Because of the absence of atrial contraction, there are no a waves in the jugular venous pressure waveform and no fourth heart sound. Figure 15.5 summarizes the AHA/ACC guidelines for the minimal evaluation of patients with atrial fibrillation.

Management

The likelihood of successful cardioversion depends upon:

- Persistence of the underlying cause (e.g., a patient who has untreated mitral stenosis is unlikely to cardiovert successfully, whereas a patient who has angina treated with medication or angioplasty is).

American College of Chest Physicians recommendations or anticoagulation in chronic nonvalvular atrial fibrillation*

Risk group/status	Annual risk (%)	Recommendation
Low risk	1	Aspirin, 325 mg/day
One moderate risk factor	1–4	Aspirin or warfarin (target INR = 2.5; range = 2.0–3.0)
High or >1 moderate risk factor	8–12	Warfarin (target INR = 2.5; range = 2.0–3.0)

Patients are classified into the following risk groups (in accordance with data from Albers GW, Dalen JE, Laupois A, et al.: *Chest* 2001;119:1948 and Lip GYP: *Lancet* 1999;353:4):

Low risk: age under 65 years with no clinical or echocardiographic evidence of cardiovascular disease (no history of embolism, hypertension, diabetes, or other clinical risk factors).

Moderate risk: age 65–76 years, diabetes, or coronary heart disease with preserved left ventricular function.

High risk: patients with risk factors including previous transient ischemic attack; systematic embolus or stroke; history of hypertension; clinical evidence of valve disease (rheumatic mitral valve disease or prosthetic valve); heart failure or impaired left ventricular function on echodardiography; thyroid disease; or age ≥75.

* Long-term anticoagulation with warfarin is recommended only in patients with no contraindications.
The combined use of aspirin and warfarin is not recommended.

Fig. 15.6 American College of Chest Physicians recommendations for anticoagulation in chronic nonvalvular atrial fibrillation.

- Duration of the atrial fibrillation (i.e., the longer the duration the smaller the chance of cardioversion).

Treatment options are similar to those of atrial flutter:

- DC cardioversion (often requiring higher energy than for atrial flutter) may cardiovert the patient into sinus rhythm.
- Pharmacological agents from groups IA, IC, and III (see p. 126) can be used to cardiovert or to maintain sinus rhythm after electrical cardioversion.
- Patients who have resistant atrial fibrillation may be treated with an AV node-blocking agent to slow the electrical response (group II or IV drugs or digoxin).

Anticoagulation and atrial fibrillation

Atrial fibrillation carries an increased risk of thromboembolism because of cerebrovascular and peripheral embolization in particular. Benefits of anticoagulation must be balanced against risk of hemorrhage before the decision to anticoagulate is made (Fig. 15.6). The following points must be recognized:

- Patients who have structural heart disease (e.g., valve lesion, dilated left ventricle) and atrial fibrillation have a higher risk of thromboembolic complications than those who have lone atrial fibrillation (i.e., with no obvious underlying cause).
- Patients who have other risk factors for thromboembolism (e.g., hypertension, diabetes mellitus, previous cerebral embolus) have a higher risk of thromboembolism.
- Older patients who have atrial fibrillation are at a greater risk.
- Warfarin reduces the risk of cerebral embolus by approximately 60–80%.
- Aspirin reduces the risk of cerebral embolus by approximately 40%.

Anticoagulation should be carefully monitored, especially in the elderly. As mentioned above, this group of patients has a higher risk of hemorrhage with anticoagulation. The international normalized ratio (INR) should be maintained between 2 and 3. The importance of maintaining an INR between 2 and 3 is shown in the finding that two-thirds of patients with ischemic stroke while on warfarin had an INR < 2.

Anticoagulation and cardioversion of atrial fibrillation

There is an increased risk of thromboembolism after cardioversion of atrial fibrillation to sinus rhythm. This is thought to be due to the formation of atrial thrombus before cardioversion and the persistence of inefficient contraction in certain parts of the atrium

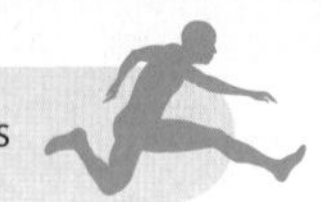

(e.g., left atrial appendage) for a few weeks after apparently successful cardioversion. Therefore, there is a risk of intracardiac clot forming for a few weeks, even after successful cardioversion. Points to note are as follows:

- If the atrial fibrillation is of recent onset (within 48–72 hours), it is reasonable to anticoagulate the patient with intravenous heparin and cardiovert straight away.
- If the patient has a longer history, full anticoagulation should be given (warfarin with an INR of 2–3) for at least 4 weeks before cardioversion and continued for 1 month after cardioversion.
- In patients in whom emergency cardioversion is required (i.e., patients who have severe heart failure secondary to atrial fibrillation), cardioversion should be performed with heparin cover immediately.
- Transesophageal echocardiography is a reliable way of excluding intracardiac clot and can be used to see whether it is safe to proceed to cardioversion immediately in an unanticoagulated patient.

Investigation of patients who have supraventricular arrhythmias

The following investigations are appropriate for all patients who have an SVT:

Blood tests

These include:

- Electrolytes—hypokalemia may predispose to tachyarrhythmias and also to digoxin toxicity.
- Thyroid function tests.
- Complete blood count—anemia may precipitate ischemia.
- Liver function tests, particularly γ-glutamyltransferase, which is abnormal in patients who have excess alcohol intake.

Electrocardiography

Features that may be evident include:

- The arrhythmia.
- Ischemic changes—these are usually accentuated during a tachycardia due to increased cardiac oxygen demand.
- Hypertensive changes.
- Pre-excitation.

24- or 48-hour electrocardiography

This may be useful in identifying paroxysmal tachyarrhythmias.

Chest radiography

Notable features may include:

- Cardiomegaly or pulmonary edema.
- Valve calcification.

Echocardiography

This may be useful because:

- Valve lesions and dilated cardiac chambers may be identified.
- Transesophageal echocardiography will exclude intracardiac clot.

Electrophysiological studies

These are useful for arrhythmias when it is difficult to identify the mechanism and any possible focus or accessory pathway suitable for ablation.

Atrioventricular nodal blocking maneuvers

These are used diagnostically and therapeutically:

- Diagnostically—they slow the ventricular response and enable P wave morphology to be seen.
- Therapeutically—they are used to terminate arrhythmias with re-entry circuits involving the AV node.

The following maneuvers are appropriate:

- Carotid sinus massage.
- Valsalva maneuver—straining against a closed glottis.
- Adenosine administration (rapid intravenous injection).

Carotid sinus massage

This increases vagal tone and so prolongs AV node conduction time. The patient should be lying comfortably with the neck extended. Carotid bruits must be excluded (carotid artery occlusion may cause a stroke if the opposite side is heavily diseased).

The patient should preferably be connected to a 12-lead EKG, running all 12 leads simultaneously. If

Electrophysiological actions of anti-arrhythmic drugs						
VWS class of drug	**Examples**	**Site of action**	**Sinus node rate**	**Atrial conduction rate**	**AV node refractory period**	**Ventricular conduction rate**
IA	Quinidine, procainamide, disopyramide	Block fast sodium channels	No effect	Decreased	Increased	Decreased
IB	Lidocaine, mexiletine, tocainide	Block fast sodium channels	No effect	No effect	Not much effect (may slightly increase or decrease)	Decreased
IC	Flecainide, propafenone	Block fast sodium channels	Reduced	Decreased	Increased	Decreased
II	Atenolol, metoprolol, sotalol, propanolol	Block beta-adrenergic receptors	Reduced	No effect	Increased	No effect
III	Amiodarone, sotalol, bretylium	Block potassium channels; mechanism not entirely understood	Reduced	Decreased	Increased	Decreased
IV	Verapamil, diltiazem	Block slow calcium channels	Small reduction	Slightly reduced	Increased	No effect
Digoxin		Blocks Na/K ATPase	No effect	Increased	Increased	Slows AV conduction

Fig. 15.7 Electrophysiological actions of antiarrhythmic drugs. VW, Vaughan Williams-Singh; AV, atrioventricular; Na, sodium; K, potassium; ATPase, adenosine triphosphatase.

only a few leads are running, the P waves may not be seen.

Initial gentle and then firm pressure is applied to the carotid pulse just below the angle of the jaw. Remember—never do this on both sides simultaneously.

Pressure is applied for a maximum of 5–10sec.

Adenosine administration

Again the patient should be supine and connected to a 12-lead EKG continuous trace. Warn the patient that he or she may experience chest pain, flushing, and dyspnea for a few seconds after administration.

Establish intravenous access in a good-sized vein (antecubital fossa is ideal). Start with 3mg rapid intravenous injection, follow with a rapid normal saline flush of 20ml. If there is no response, this may be repeated with incrementally higher doses up to 12mg.

Actions of adenosine

Adenosine activates potassium channels and hyperpolarizes the cell membrane. It acts to slow AV conduction time.

The half-life of adenosine is very short (6sec), and it can be safely used to differentiate ventricular tachycardia from SVT with aberrant conduction. After adenosine the P waves will be revealed in SVT, or the SVT may be terminated.

If verapamil is used for this purpose, there is a risk of fatal myocardial depression in patients who have ventricular tachycardia.

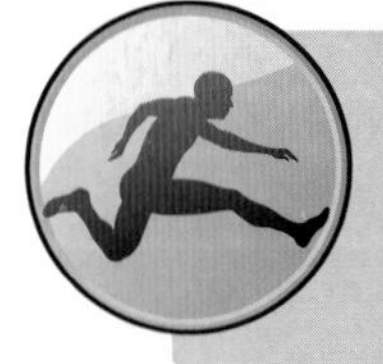

Adenosine may precipitate bronchospasm and should be avoided in asthmatic patients.

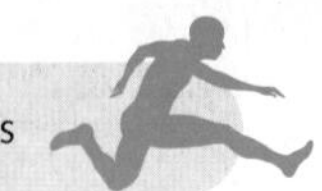

Pharmacokinetics and adverse effects of antiarrhythmic drugs					
Drug	**Route of administration**	**Half-life**	**Mode of excretion**	**Interactions**	**Adverse effects**
Procainamide (IA)*	Oral, IV, or IM	3–5 hour	Renal	Amiodarone reduces clearance	Skin rashes, Raynaud's syndrome hallucinations; toxicity—cardiac failure, long QT, ventricular tachyarrhythmias
Lidocaine (IB)	IV (extensive first-pass metabolism in liver)	1–2 hour	Hepatic	Cimetidine reduces clearance	Myocardial depression, cardiac failure, long QT; toxicity—dizziness, confusion, paraesthesia
Flecainide (IC)	Oral, IV	20 hour	Renal (partly hepatic)	Cimetidine reduces clearance	Myocardial depression, ventricular arrhythmias (a major problem, especially in patients who have ischemic heart disease)
Atenolol (II)	Oral, IV		Renal	May precipitate asthma or peripheral ischemia	Myocardial depression, bronchospasm, asthma, or peripheral vasoconstriction
Sotalol (II) and (III)	Oral, IV	10–15 hour	Renal	May precipitate asthma or peripheral ischemia	Myocardial depression, long QT, ventricular tachyarrhythmias
Amiodarone (III)	Oral, IV	3–6 weeks	Hepatic	Reduces digoxin excretion, reduces warfarin excretion (need to watch INR closely)	Pulmonary fibrosis, liver damage, peripheral neuropathy, hyper- or hypothyroidism, corneal microdeposits, photosensitivity, myocardial depression (but safe in cardiac failure), long QT
Verapamil (IV)	Oral, IV	3–7 hours	Renal	Reduces digoxin excretion	Myocardial depression, constipation
Digoxin	Oral, IV	36–48 hours	Renal	Amiodarone, verapamil, and propafenone decrease renal clearance; erythromycin increases absorption; captopril decreases renal clearance	Toxicity—heart block, atrial tachycardia, ventricular arrhythmia, xanthopsia

Fig. 15.8 Pharmacokinetics and adverse effects of antiarrhythmic drugs. Note that a common complication of all antiarrhythmic agents is bradycardia, which may be severe. Care must always be used when increasing dosage or combining more than one agent. (IM, intramuscular; INR, international normalized ratio; IV, intravenous.)
* Vaughan Williams-Singh class in parenthesis.

Drugs used to treat tachyarrhythmias

The older Vaughan Williams-Singh classification is still sometimes used:

- Class I—inhibitors of sodium current (i.e., like a local anesthetic).
- Class II—beta-adrenergic receptor antagonists.
- Class III—inhibitors of repolarization, which prolong the action potential and refractory period.
- Class IV—inhibitors of calcium current.
- Digitalis glycosides.

A summary of the electrophysiological actions of antiarrhythmic drugs is given in Fig. 15.7. It can be seen from this that class 1A, 1C, and III drugs affect conduction in the atrial and ventricular tissue. They are therefore useful for cardioverting many rhythms to sinus by breaking re-entry circuits or reducing the excitability of ectopic foci. Class III drugs have the added advantage of slowing AV conduction and therefore slowing ventricular response as well.

Class II and IV drugs and digoxin act as AV node blockers. This is useful in slowing the ventricular response and will cardiovert rhythms that are caused by re-entry circuits involving the AV node (e.g., AV nodal re-entry tachycardias and AV re-entry tachycardias).

A summary of the pharmacokinetics and side effects of antiarrhythmic agents is shown in Fig. 15.8.

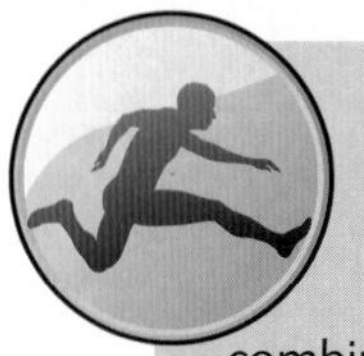

All antiarrhythmic agents can cause bradyarrhythmias and extreme caution should be exercised when using them in combination.

16. Ventricular Tachyarrhythmias

Definition

A ventricular tachyarrhythmia is an abnormal rapid rhythm that originates in the ventricular myocardium or the His–Purkinje system.

Ventricular tachyarrhythmias are wide complex—the QRS complex is greater than 0.12sec in duration or three small squares on a standard EKG trace.

There are four basic types of ventricular tachyarrhythmia:

- Premature ventricular contractions.
- Ventricular tachycardia.
- Torsades de pointes (which can stem from hypocalcemia, hypokalemia, or hypomagnesemia).
- Ventricular fibrillation.

Premature ventricular contractions (PVCs)

PVCs have certain EKG characteristics (Fig. 16.1) such as:

- They occur before the next normal beat would be due.
- They are not preceded by a P wave.
- The QRS complex is abnormal in shape and has a duration of greater than 120ms.
- They are followed by a compensatory pause so that the RR interval between the normal beats immediately preceding and immediately following the ectopic beat is exactly twice the normal RR interval.

Clinical features

It is thought that PVCs occur in over half the normal population. This prevalence increases with age. These extra beats do not necessarily imply underlying heart disease.

Most people are entirely asymptomatic; others may complain of missed or extra beats. Alternatively, others may experience thumping or heavy beats because the beat immediately following the ectopic does so after a compensatory pause during which there is a prolonged filling time, resulting in an increased stroke volume plus post-extrasystolic potentiation of contractility.

A number of precipitating causes of ventricular premature beats are recognized, including:

- Low serum potassium.
- Excess caffeine consumption.
- Febrile illness.
- Underlying cardiac abnormality (e.g., recent myocardial infarction, cardiomyopathy, mitral or aortic valve disease).

Management

The clinical significance of PVCs is unclear, and the general rule is that in a patient who has no underlying cardiac abnormality no treatment is needed unless symptoms are severe (in this situation a small dose of beta blocker should suppress ectopic activity).

In the post-myocardial infarction setting, there is currently much controversy about the significance of, and need to treat, PVCs. There is no evidence currently that treatment of PVCs after myocardial infarction reduces mortality rate. Current opinion, therefore, seems to be that if hypokalemia is treated, no antiarrhythmic agents are indicated to treat PVCs in the post-myocardial infarction patient.

Ventricular tachycardia (VT)

VT is defined as three or more consecutive ventricular beats occurring at a rate greater than 100 beats/min (Fig. 16.2). Again, the complexes are abnormal and their duration is longer than 120ms. VTs that last greater than 30 seconds are termed "sustained VT," and those lasting less than 30 seconds are termed nonsustained VT (NSVT).

Clinical features

Patients occasionally tolerate this rhythm well and experience only palpitations or rarely nothing at all. More commonly the reduction in cardiac output caused by this arrhythmia causes dizziness or syncope. Common precipitants include hypokalemia and acute myocardial infarction.

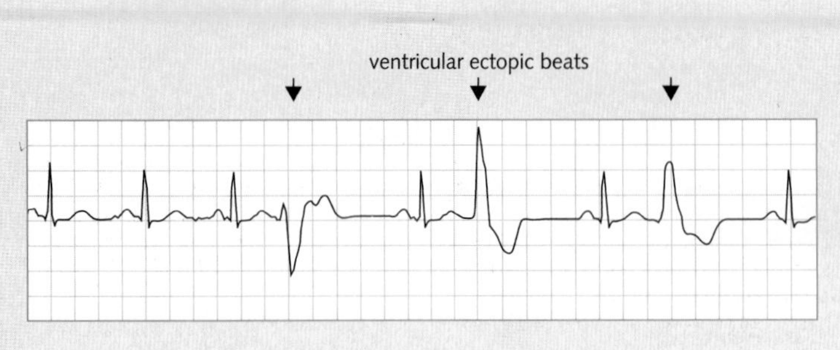

Fig. 16.1 Premature ventricular contactions, which are indicated by arrows.

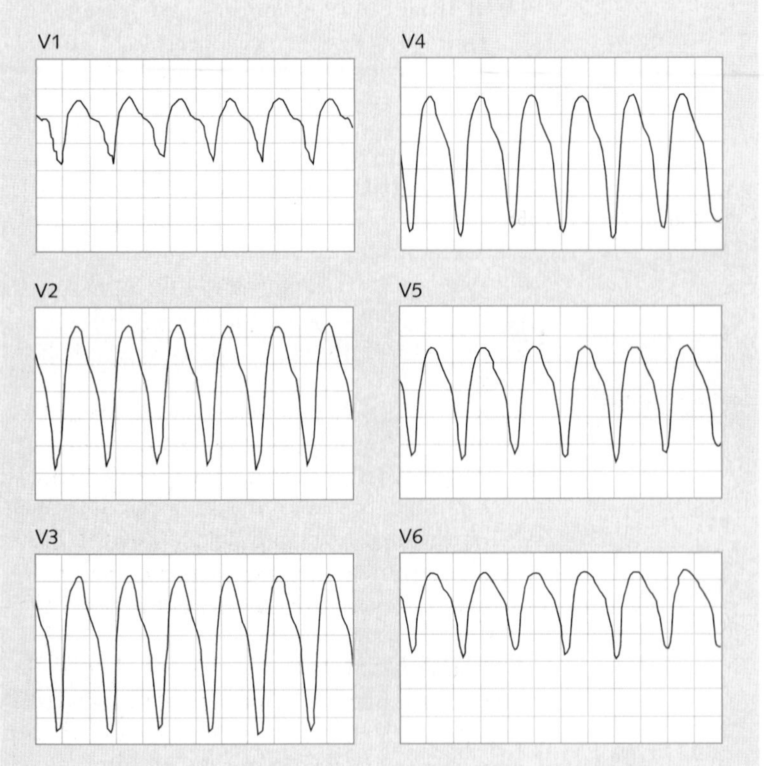

Fig. 16.2 EKG illustrating ventricular tachycardia. Note the concordance shown in the chest leads. No fusion or capture beats seen.

Diagnosis

The main differential diagnosis for VT is supraventricular tachycardia with aberrant conduction (or bundle branch block) (Fig. 16.3). This causes much confusion and concern amongst residents and medical students alike. It helps if you remember the following points:

- Both arrhythmias are potentially fatal so treat each with respect.
- The use of carotid sinus massage or adenosine may briefly block the atrioventricular node and therefore slow the ventricular response in supraventricular tachycardia (it will have no effect on VT).
- Never use verapamil to slow the ventricular response in this situation: the negative inotropic effect of this drug could have disastrous effects if the rhythm is in fact VT causing rapid development of heart failure.

Management

Ventricular tachycardia is very dangerous and, if allowed to continue, will result in cardiac arrest. Treatment must therefore be prompt. The nature

Differences between VT and SVT with BBB		
Arrhythmia	**VT**	**SVT with BBB**
QRS duration	>140ms	Variable
AV association	AV dissociation (no relationship between P waves and QRS)	P waves, if seen, are associated with the QRS
Variety of complexes	Capture beats (where a P wave is followed by a normal QRS); fusion beats (where a normal sinus beat occurs simultaneously with a ventricular beat, the resulting complex having an intermediate appearance that is a combination of the two component beats)	No capture or fusion beats
EKG pattern	May be RBBB or LBBB	Usually RBBB
Concordance	Present (the QRS complexes retain the same axis throughout the chest leads)	Absent (some QRS complexes will be positive, others will be negative)
QRS waveform	May vary from beat to beat	Constant

Fig. 16.3 Differences between ventricular tachycardia (VT) and supraventricular tachycardia (SVT) with bundle-branch block (BBB). (AV, atrioventricular; LBBB, left BBB; RBBB, right BBB.)

of the treatment depends upon the clinical scenario.

- Patient conscious with intermittent episodes of VT—treatment should be with drugs.
- Patient conscious with ongoing VT—triggered (synchronized) direct current (DC) cardioversion under general anesthetic.
- Patient compromised and unconscious with ongoing VT—triggered (synchronized) DC cardioversion according to ACLS guidelines (see Chapter 17).

It is vital to correct hypokalemia promptly for all patients who have ventricular arrhythmias. Potassium may be given orally or in a very dilute form via a peripheral vein; in the emergency setting, larger doses of potassium can be given via a central line with careful monitoring of cardiac rhythm and serum potassium levels. *Warning:* intravenous potassium can cause ventricular fibrillation.

Ventricular fibrillation (VF)

VF is irregular rapid ventricular depolarization (Fig. 16.4). There is no organized contraction of the ventricle, therefore the patient has no pulse. This arrhythmia rapidly causes loss of consciousness and cardiorespiratory arrest. EKG finding typically show disorganized wide complexes or varying amplitude and rate that decrease in duration until asystole occurs.

Clinical features

The most common cause of VF is acute myocardial infarction. VF is also seen at the end-stage of many disease processes and signifies the presence of severe myocardial damage (this is sometimes called secondary VF and usually results in death despite resuscitation attempts). It may be precipitated by:

- A PVC.
- Ventricular tachycardia.
- Torsades de pointes.

Management

VF must be treated promptly with simple (nonsynchronized) DC cardioversion (the resuscitation protocol is discussed in Chapter 17).

Antiarrhythmic agents are used prophylactically in certain patients who are at risk of recurrent episodes of VF.

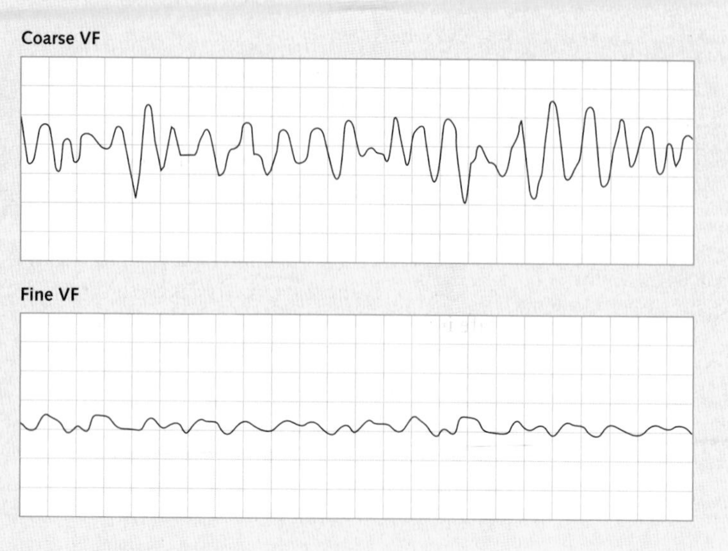

Fig. 16.4 Ventricular fibrillation (VF) may have a coarse or a fine pattern.

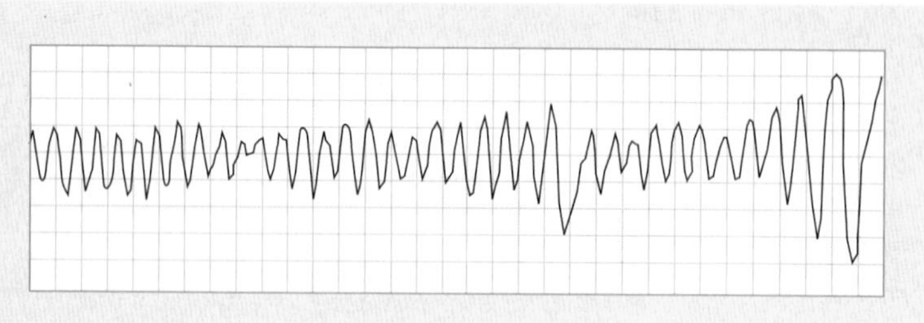

Fig. 16.5 Torsades de pointes. Note the irregular rhythm and twisting axis.

Torsades de pointes

This rhythm is usually self-terminating, but can occasionally lead to VF and death. It is an irregular, rapid rhythm with a characteristic twisting axis on the EKG (Fig. 16.5). Between episodes the EKG shows a long QT interval.

The QT interval corresponds to the time from depolarization to repolarization (beginning of the Q wave to end of T wave, i.e., action potential duration) and varies according to the heart rate. Therefore, a long QT interval is approximated by a corrected QT interval (QTc) of greater than 0.44s. QTc = QT/square root of RR interval.

Clinical features

The patient usually feels faint or loses consciousness due to a drop in cardiac output. Attacks are much more likely to occur during periods of adrenergic stimulation (e.g., fear). There are many possible causes, all of which cause a prolonged QT interval (Fig. 16.6).

Management

Treatment of torsades de pointes differs from that of the other ventricular arrhythmias and is as follows:

- Identify and treat any precipitating factors (stop offending drugs, correct electrolyte imbalance).
- Atrial or ventricular pacing to maintain a heart rate of no less than 90 beats/min prevents lengthening of the QT interval. Intravenous isoprenaline may also be used to reduce the QT interval.
- In congenital long QT syndromes high-dose beta blockers may be used, and there is increasing use of permanent pacemakers and cardiovertor defibrillators.

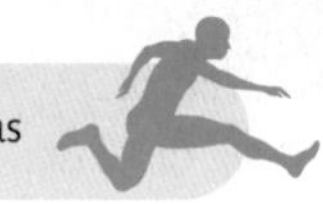

Causes of long QT interval	
Cause	**Examples**
Congenital	Jervell and Lange-Nielsen syndrome (autosomal recessive and senorineural deafness) Romano-Ward syndrome (autosomal dominant, no deafness)
Drugs	Class 1A (e.g., quinidine, procainamide) Class 3 (e.g., amiodarone, sotalol) Tricyclic antidepressants (e.g., amitriptyline) Phenothiazines (e.g., chlorpromazine) Terfenadine
Electrolyte abnormalities	Hypokalemia Hypomagnesemia Hypocalcemia
Others	Acute myocardial infarction Central nervous system disease Mitral valve prolapse Organophosphate insecticides

Fig. 16.6 Causes of long QT interval.

- Aside from magnesium sulfate and sodium bicarbonate, do not use antiarrhythmic drugs.

Drugs used to treat ventricular tachycardia and ventricular fibrillation

In the acute situation, if the patient is unconscious or has no cardiac output, DC cardioversion is used initially at 200J. If the arrhythmia persists, further resuscitation is carried out according to the ACLS protocol (Chapter 17).

The drugs used to treat ventricular tachyarrhythmias other than torsades de pointes fall into two main classes:

- Class I.
- Class III.

In the acutely ill patient who has VT or VF, intravenous antiarrhythmic agents are given after sinus rhythm has been established by DC cardioversion (Fig. 16.7). They are given in the form of an infusion, usually in an attempt to stabilize the myocardium. Amiodarone and lidocaine are commonly used, but the latter is dangerously negatively inotropic.

The exact drug chosen depends upon the individual. The following are some considerations worth noting:

- Because amiodarone has many long-term side effects, caution must be used when prescribing it and the patient needs careful follow-up.
- Amiodarone is a good choice for the patient who has cardiac failure because it has been shown to be safe in heart failure.
- If given intravenously, amiodarone must be given centrally because it is extremely damaging to peripheral veins.
- Amiodarone has a very long half-life (25 days), and oral loading takes at least 1 month. Intravenous loading is faster.
- In a patient who has no contraindication for beta-blockers, sotalol is a good long-term agent because it has none of the long-term side effects of amiodarone.
- Flecainide is an effective agent, but it is avoided in patients who have suspected ischemic heart disease, which is thought to increase its proarrhythmic effects.

The Vaughan Williams-Singh classification of antiarrhythmic drugs allows agents to be grouped according to their mode of action on the myocardium and also makes selection of appropriate agents for the treatment of any given arrhythmia more straightforward; however, see also the Sicilian Gambit classification.

Nonpharmacological treatments of ventricular tachyarrhythmias

Nonpharmacological treatments are used in patients who have recurrent VT or VF because:

- If successful, complete cure is achieved without the need for drugs.
- Localization of the arrhythmogenic focus is becoming possible in more cases due to increased understanding of the mechanisms of these arrhythmias.

The two methods commonly used are:

- Radiofreqency ablation.
- Implantable cardioverter defibrillator (ICD).

Main features of common antiarrhythmic drugs					
	Class I	**Class II**	**Class III**	**Class IV**	**Digoxin**
Examples	IA—quinidine, procainamide, disopyramide; IB—lidocaine, mexiletine, tocainide; IC—flecainide, propafenone	Beta blockers (e.g., atenolol, bisoprolol, metoprolol); sotalol also has some class III activity	Amiodarone, sotalol, bretylium	Calcium channel blockers (e.g., diltiazem, verapamil)	Not classified by the Vaughan Williams-Singh system
Mode of action	Variable action on the His–Purkinje system	Increase AV node refractory period	Increase both AV node and His–Purkinje refractory period	Increase V node refractory period	Slows AV conduction; increases AV node refractory period, positively inotropic
Adverse effects	Quinidine—nausea, diarrhea; procainamide—development of antinuclear antibodies and SLE; flecainide—higher incidence of proarrhythmic effects than other class I drugs; all may lengthen QT and cause torsades; all are negatively inotropic	Negatively inotropic, may induce bronchospasm, exacerbation of peripheral vascular disease	Amiodarone—pulmonary fibrosis, hypo/hyperthyroidism, hepatic toxicity, cutaneous photosensitivity; corneal microdeposits (reversible), peripheral neuropathy; sotalol—as for other beta blockers; both may lengthen QT and cause torsades	Verapamil and diltiazem—complete AV block, negatively inotropic	Nausea, vomiting if blood levels too high, visual disturbances (xanthopsia), complete heart block

Fig. 16.7 Main features of common antiarrhythmic drugs classed using Vaughan Williams-Singh classification. (AV, atrioventricular; SLE, systemic lupus erythematosus.)

Radiofreqency ablation

This involves localization of the proarrhythmic focus using intracardiac electrodes introduced via a central vein, followed by the use of radiofrequency energy to cauterize the myocardium in that area. The successful result is the ablation of the focus, therefore rendering the patient cured and no longer needing antiarrhythmic agents. This technique is commonly used in patients who have Wolff–Parkinson–White syndrome (a supraventricular arrhythmia) who are young and have a discreet accessory pathway that can be localized easily. Ventricular arrhythmias can also sometimes be ablated.

Implantable cardioverter defibrillators

Implantable cardioverter defibrillators (ICDs) are now increasingly used in the treatment of sustained or life-threatening ventricular arrhythmias because they have been shown in some studies to prolong survival. ICDs are slightly larger than a permanent pacemaker and are implanted in the same way (i.e., the box is situated under the pectoralis major muscle on the patient's nondominant side and the leads are positioned in the atrium and ventricle). The device can sense VT and VF and can attempt to cardiovert the arrhythmia by pacing the ventricle or by delivering a DC shock.

The implantation and subsequent programming and monitoring of these devices should be performed in specialist centers. In addition, patients often need counseling and advice because the sensation when the ICD discharges a shock can be extremely unpleasant and comes without warning. This results in marked psychological problems in some patients.

17. Cardiac Arrest and Resuscitation

Cardiopulmonary arrest results in a rapid decline in oxygen delivery to the brain. Permanent disability or death results if the period of cerebral hypoxia lasts longer than 3 minutes.

Cardiopulmonary resuscitation (CPR) is the term used to describe the maintenance of adequate breathing and circulation in a patient who cannot do so for him- or herself. The aim of CPR is to restore respiration and adequate cardiac output as soon as possible to prevent death or permanent disability. CPR involves two types of protocol:

- Basic cardiovascular life support (BCLS)—no special equipment required.
- Advanced cardiovascular life support (ACLS)—requires specialist skill and equipment.

In any type of resuscitation protocol the following three areas must be assessed and supported in order of priority:

- Airway.
- Breathing.
- Circulation.

Basic cardiovascular life support

BCLS refers to the maintenance and support of airway, breathing, and circulation without the aid of any specialized equipment (Fig. 17.1). The aim of BCLS is to maintain adequate ventilation and cardiac output until the underlying cause can be reversed.

There are a number of points to note relating to Fig. 17.1:

- If trauma to the cervical spine is a possibility, the airway should be maintained without tilting the head.
- If there are two operators, one should go for help as soon as possible. If there is only one, it is generally agreed now that the victim can be left and the operator should go for help once it has been established that the victim is not breathing. If, however, the victim is a child, or if collapse was due to trauma or drowning, then 1 min of CPR should be given before the operator goes for help. In these situations the collapse is likely to be due to respiratory arrest, and the rescue breaths, if given early, will improve prognosis.
- Each rescue breath, is given by mouth-to-mouth inflation with the nose occluded and should deliver approximately 500ml of expired air into the lungs of the victim. The operator should watch the chest wall of the victim to ensure that it rises and falls with each breath. Each breath will take approximately 1–1.5sec. It is important to allow the chest wall to fall back completely before taking the next breath.
- Assessment of the carotid pulse should take no more than 10sec.
- If there is no pulse, chest compressions are performed by placing the heel of the hand over the lower half of the sternum two fingerbreadths above the xiphoid process. Enough pressure should be applied to depress the sternum 4–5cm and no more. The operator should be vertically above the victim's chest, and the arms should be kept straight. The rate of compressions should be 100/min. After each compression the pressure should be released and the chest wall allowed to rise back up.

Principle of chest compressions

The current theory suggests that chest compression increases intrathoracic pressure, which propels blood out of the thorax. The veins collapse, whereas the arteries remain patent. Therefore, flow is in a forward direction. The function and features of the recovery position are shown in Fig. 17.2.

Management of upper airway obstruction by foreign material

The management of choking in a conscious victim, although not strictly BCLS, is extremely important because it is a common occurrence both in the community and in the hospital, where aspiration of stomach contents or blood may occur (Fig. 17.3).

Points to note in the management of choking:

- If the patient becomes cyanosed, immediate positive action is needed with administration of oxygen and back blows followed by the Heimlich maneuver.

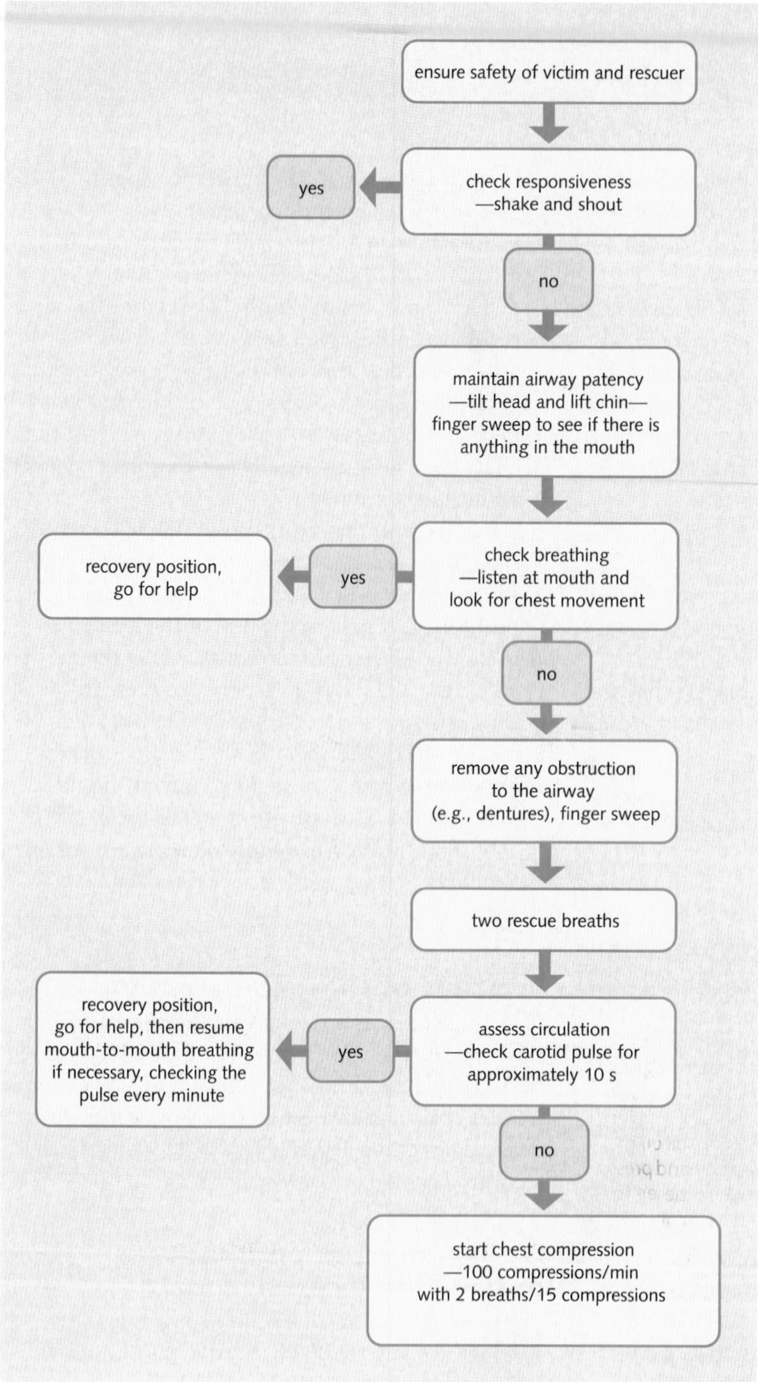

Fig. 17.1 Algorithm for adult basic life support.

- Back blows are performed during expiration either with the patient standing or sitting and with the head bent down below the level of the chest.
- Heimlich maneuver—this may be performed with the patient standing, sitting, or lying down. Sharp upward pressure is applied in the midline just beneath the diaphragm with the operator behind the patient. This procedure may result in damage to abdominal viscera and should not be attempted in small children or pregnant women.

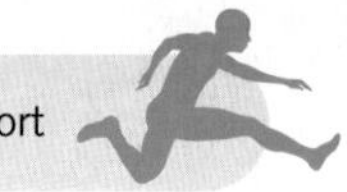

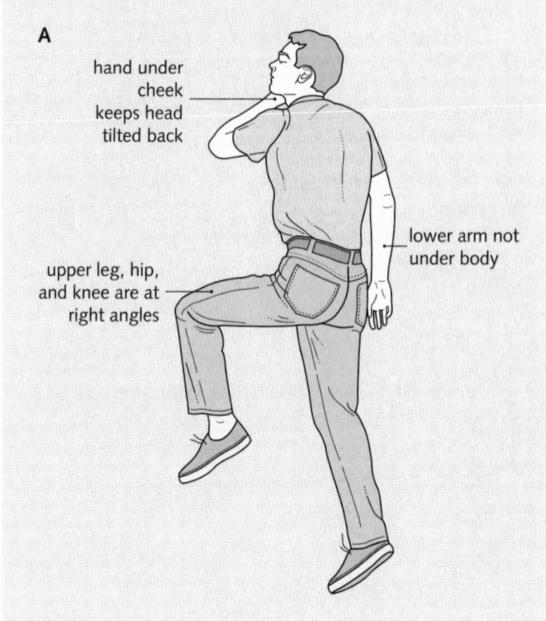

B	Function and features of the recovery position
Function	Keeps airway straight Allows tongue to fall forward and not obstruct airway Minimizes risk of aspiration of gastric contents
Main features	Remove victim's glasses Ensure airway is open by lifting chin Kneel beside victim Tuck one hand under the victim's buttock (arm should be straight with palm facing up) Bring other forearm across patient's chest and hold back of hand against the victim's nearest cheek With your other hand bring far leg into a bent position with foot still on the ground and keeping the hand pressed against the cheek pull on the leg to roll the victim towards you onto his or her side The upper leg should be adjusted so both the hip and the knee are at right angles
Special notes	The patient should not be lying on his or her lower arm The hand under the cheek keeps the head tilted back so the airway remains open

Fig. 17.2 (A) The recovery position viewed from above. (B) Function and features of the recovery position.

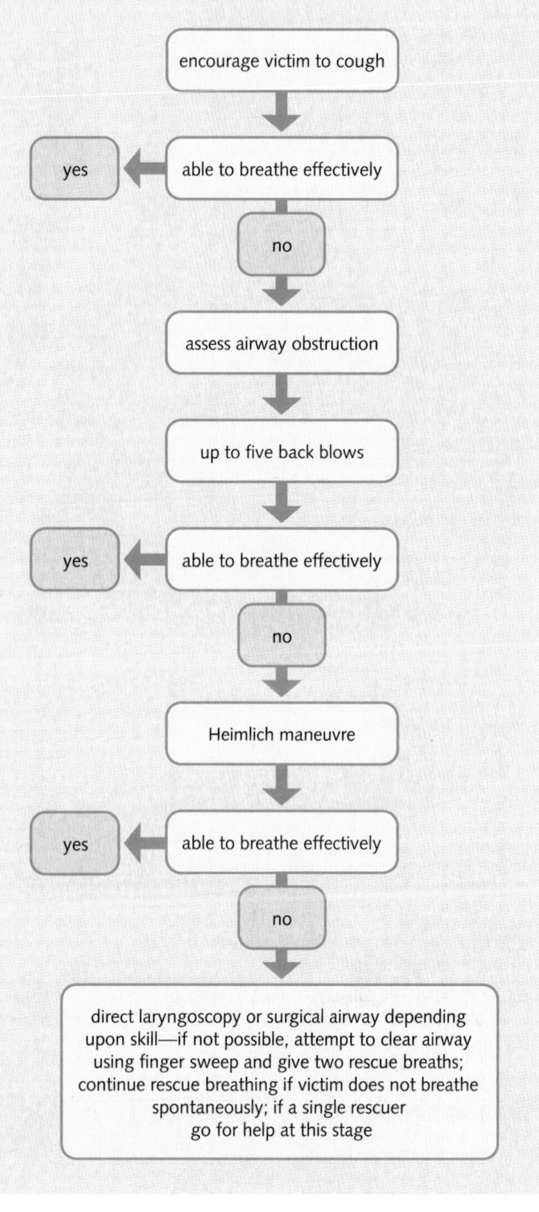

Fig. 17.3 Algorithm for the management of choking.

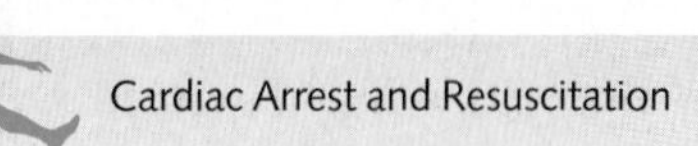

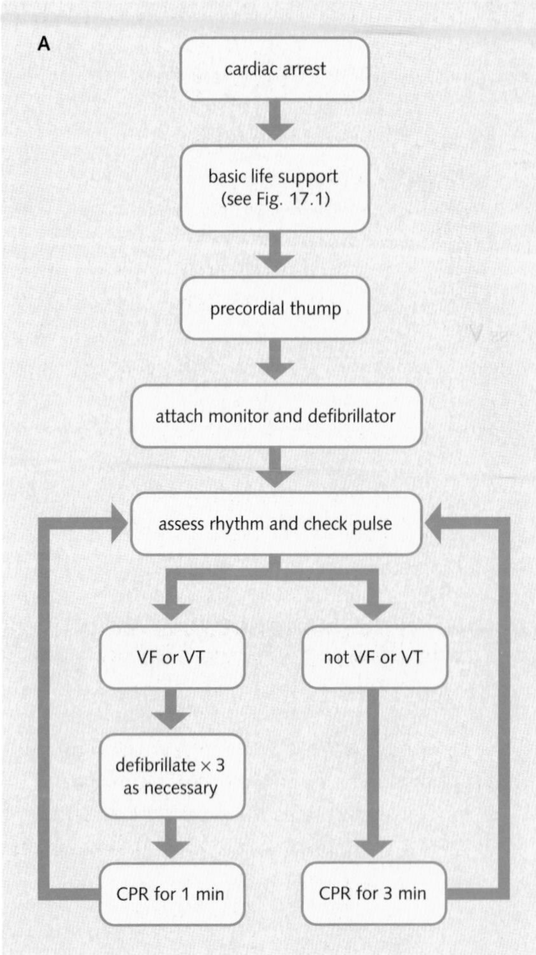

B Management aspects to consider during CPR

Correct reversible causes
Check electrode and paddle positions and contact
Check airway and oxygen
Ensure there is intravenous access
Apply DC shock if patient in VF
If the patient remains in shock, give adrenaline every 3 min
Consider giving antiarrhythmics, atropine
Consider pacing
Consider buffers

C Potentially reversible causes of cardiac arrest

Hypoxia
Hypovolemia
Hyper/hypokalemia
Hypothermia
Tension pneumothorax
Tamponade
Toxic or therapeutic disturbance
Thromboembolic or mechanical obstruction

Fig. 17.4 (A) Algorithm for advanced cardiovascular life support. (VF, ventricular fibrillation; VT, ventricular tachycardia.) (B) Management aspects to consider during CPR. (C) Potentially reversible causes of cardiac arrest.

Advanced cardiovascular life support

The ACLS method of resuscitation requires specialist training and equipment and has recently been reviewed and modified (Fig. 17.4). For the most current updates consult www.cpr-ecc.americanheart.org.

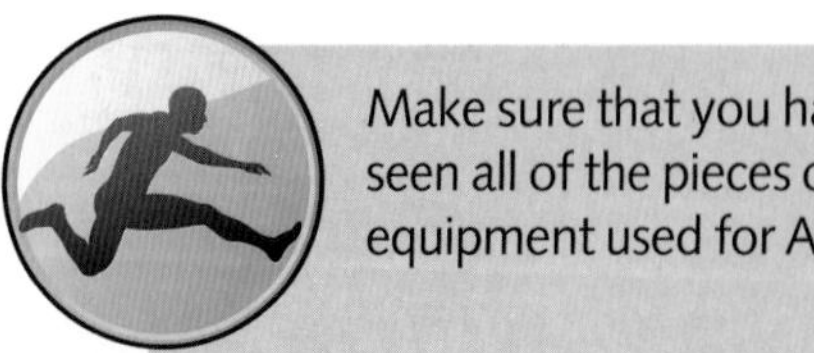

Make sure that you have seen all of the pieces of equipment used for ACLS.

Airway ventilation and protection

During these cycles of CPR:

- Adequate ventilation must be established.
- The airway must be protected by an operator (preferably an anesthesiologist) who remains at the patient's head.

The optimal method of protecting the airway is by insertion of a cuffed endotracheal tube. This device minimizes the risk of aspiration of the gastric contents and allows effective ventilation to be carried out. Endotracheal intubation can be a hazardous procedure and a laryngeal mask airway is an alternative.

Intravenous access must also be established either via a large peripheral vein or preferably via a central vein.

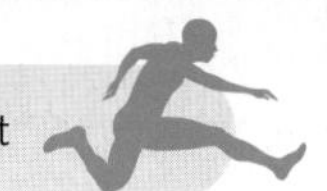

Placement of defibrillator paddles

Placement of the defibrillator paddles is important because only a small proportion of the energy reaches the myocardium during transthoracic defibrillation and every effort should be made to maximize this:

- The right paddle should be placed below the clavicle in the midclavicular line.
- The left paddle should be placed on the lower rib cage on the anterior axillary line.

> Regardless of the setting it is crucial that BCLS is commenced immediately and, once a cardiac monitor is available, that defibrillation of VT/VF is administered immediately. It is these two factors that affect the eventual outcome of resuscitation.

The VT/VF arm of the ACLS algorithm

The three initial shocks are usually 200, 200–300, and 360J. All subsequent shocks are usually 360J. After each shock the monitor should be watched:

- If the rhythm remains VF/VT, the CPR and defibrillation sequence should be followed for four cycles.
- If the arrhythmia persists at this stage, antiarrhythmics can be used. Intravenous lidocaine or amiodarone can be used, as can other agents. (No one agent has been found to be better in this situation.)
- If the monitor shows a flat line after defibrillation, this does not necessarily mean that asystole has occurred. It is not uncommon for a period of myocardial stunning to occur after defibrillation, and the screen should be watched for one full sweep.
- If the flat line (asystole) persists, CPR should be carried out for 1 min before epinephrine (1 mg IV push, repeated every 3–5 min) is given to allow the period of stunning to pass. If this is not successful, atropine (1 mg IV push, repeated every 3–5 min to a total of 0.04 mg/kg) can then be given.

The non-VT/VF arm of the ACLS algorithm

This arm includes asystole, pulseless electrical activity (PEA), and profound bradyarrhythmias. Prognosis for patients in this arm is much poorer than in the VF/VT arm. Defibrillation is not required unless VT/VF supervenes and 3-min cycles of CPR are given. During the 3 minutes possible underlying causes must be excluded or treated:

- Asystole is treated initially with intravenous atropine at a maximum total dose of 3 mg and intravenous adrenaline, 1 mg. During subsequent cycles of CPR adrenaline may be repeated, but not the atropine.
- Bradyarrhythmias are treated initially with atropine in the same way. Patients who have bradyarrhythmia may benefit from insertion of a temporary pacing wire.

PEA occurs when there is a regular rhythm on the monitor (that is not VT), with no cardiac output arising from it. Underlying causes must be sought because they may be easily treated. The following are possible underlying causes of PEA:

- Hypovolemia—rapid administration of intravenous fluids required.
- Electrolyte imbalance (e.g., hypokalemia, hypocalcemia).
- Tension pneumothorax—suspect in trauma cases or after insertion of central line; also seen spontaneously in fit young men. Look for absence of chest movements and breath sounds on one side. Treat with cannula into the pleural space at the second intercostal space in midclavicular line followed by insertion of chest drain.
- Cardiac tamponade—suspect in trauma cases and post-thoracotomy patients. Rapid insertion of pericardial drain is needed.
- Pulmonary embolism—if strongly suspected, thrombolysis should be administered.

18. Bradyarrhythmias

Definition of bradyarrhythmias

The bradyarrhythmias (Fig. 18.1) are slow rhythms.

Sinus bradycardia

Sinus bradycardia occurs when the resting heart rate is less than 60 beats/min when the patient is awake. In most cases it is asymptomatic and of no consequence (Fig. 18.2). Sinus bradycardia is common in children and endurance athletes.

Any increase in vagal tone can cause a decrease in the heart rate. This can be caused by many factors, including increased intracranial pressure, athletic activity, sleep apnea, and drugs that act on the AV node. Symptoms may occur in pathological situations and rarely in sinus bradycardia with no obvious cause. They may take the form of:

- Syncope (Stokes–Adams attacks).
- Hypotension.
- Dyspnea due to cardiac failure.

In these circumstances treatment of the bradycardia with intravenous atropine or insertion of a temporary pacing wire may be indicated to speed the heart rate until the underlying condition is treated. The pacing wire may be ventricular or atrial because the atrioventricular node is conducting impulses normally.

Sinus node disease

The sinoatrial (SA) node is the natural cardiac pacemaker. It is a crescent-shaped structure and is approximately 1mm by 3mm in size. The location of the SA node is at the junction of the right atrium and the superior vena cava just below the epicardial surface.

Impulses are generated at the sinus node. The rate is determined by both vagal and sympathetic tone. The impulses are then conducted via the atrial myocardium to the atrioventricular (AV) node.

Disease of the SA node may be due to:

- Infiltrative diseases and infections, sarcoid, amyloidosis, TB, lyme disease, infective endocarditis.
- Ischemia and infarction.
- Degeneration and fibrosis.
- Excessive vagal stimulation.
- Pericardial disease-pericarditis—given the close proximity of the pericardium to the SA node.
- Myocarditis.

This may result in pauses between consecutive P waves (>2sec). There are different degrees of SA node conduction abnormality:

- Sinoatrial exit block—there is an absence of the expected P wave, but the following one occurs at the expected time (i.e., the pauses are exact multiples of the basic PP interval).
- Sinus pause or sinus arrest (Fig. 18.3)—this occurs when the interval between the P waves is longer than 2sec and is not a multiple of the basic PP interval.

Tachybrady syndrome (sick sinus syndrome)

This is a combination of sinus node disease and abnormal tachyarrhythmias. Ischemia is a common cause for this syndrome, which occurs in the elderly.

- Tachybrady syndrome is often manifested by frequent unexplained atrial pauses that alternate with supraventricular tachycardias.
- At times the patient may be asymptomatic.

Management

Patients who have symptomatic sinus pauses or evidence of recurrent sinus pauses require permanent pacing with either an atrial pacemaker (if there is no evidence of AV node disease) or a dual chamber pacemaker. Ventricular pacemakers are usually reserved only for very frail and elderly patients or those who have atrial fibrillation because they do not improve prognosis and are associated with fatigue and lethargy (i.e., the pacemaker syndrome, which may result from the loss of the atrial component of cardiac output).

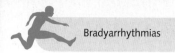

Bradyarrhythmias	
Bradyarrhythmia	**Features**
Sinus bradycardia Sinoatrial node disease and sick sinus syndrome	Heart rate 60 beats/min during the day prolonged PP interval, may be associated with tachyarrhythmias and, intermittently, tachybrady syndrome
First-degree heart block	PR interval >0.20sec
Second-degree heart block—Mobitz type I	Wenckebach phenomenon—progressive a prolongation of PR interval with eventual dropped beat
Second-degree heart block—Mobitz type II	Dropped beats, no prolongation of PR interval
Second degree heart block—2:1 heart block/3:1 heart block	Every second or third beat conducted; the rest are not
Complete heart block, third-degree heart block	Complete AV dissociation
Asystole	No beats conducted, no ventricular activity

Fig. 18.1 Bradyarrhythmias listed in ascending order of electrical dysfunction. (AV, atrioventricular.)

Causes of sinus bradycardia
Physiological Athletes Young adults During sleep (rate can drop to 35–40 beats/min)
Pathological Hypothermia Raised intracranial pressure Hypothyroidism Cholestatic jaundice Ischemic heart disease affecting the SA node (in 60% of patients the SA node is supplied by right coronary artery) Drugs (e.g., beta-blockers, antiarrhythmic agents, calcium channel blockers, adenosine, digoxin) In the elderly—due to fibrosis of SA node

Fig. 18.2 Causes of sinus bradycardia. (SA, sinoatrial.)

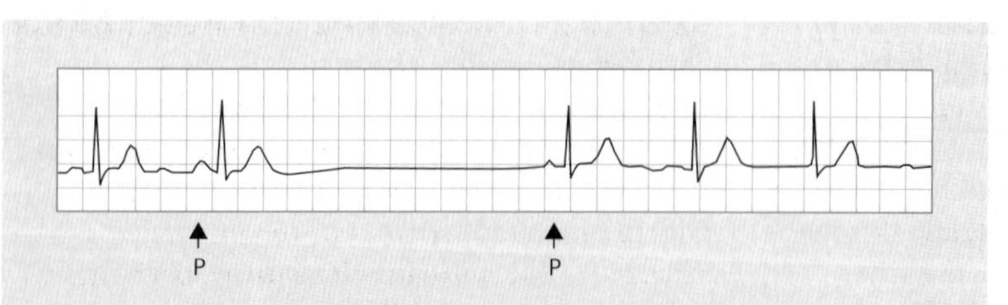

Fig. 18.3 Sinus pause or arrest. Note the interval of more than 2s between P waves.

Antiarrhythmic drugs may also be needed if the patient has sick sinus syndrome. It is important to insert a pacemaker before commencing these because they will make the SA node conduction defect worse.

Atrioventricular block

The AV node is a complex structure that lies in the right atrial wall on the septal surface between the ostium of the coronary sinus and the septal leaflet of the tricuspid valve; in 90% of patients the AV node is supplied by the right coronary artery. The rest are supplied via the circumflex coronary artery.

The AV node acts as a physiological gearbox conducting impulses from the atria to the ventricular conductive tissue.

First-degree atrioventricular block

In this conduction disturbance (Fig. 18.4) conduction time form the atria to the ventricles is delayed. This is shown by a prolonged PR interval that is longer than 0.22sec. Usually this is due to slowed conduction through the AV node, although the His system and even intra-atrial causes are also known. Heart block can be caused by any interference of the conduction system similar to any of the causes listed above for the SA node disease.

Prolonging conduction through the AV node by using vagal maneuvers or drugs can reassure that the AV node is responsible for the delay in conduction. If the long PR interval is associated with a bundle-branch block and a wide complex QRS, then the delay is usually not the AV node and the patient may need a pacemaker.

This condition does not require treatment in a healthy patient but should be watched because it may herald greater degrees of block (in approximately 40% of cases).

> In a patient who has infective endocarditis serial EKGs are performed to observe the PR interval. Prolongation of the PR interval can occur secondary to formation of a paravalvular abscess, and this usually heralds rapid development of complete heart block and valve dehiscence. In these patients progressive prolongation of the PR interval requires an urgent echocardiogram and temporary pacing wire.

Second-degree atrioventricular block

In this type of block some impulses are not conducted from the atria to the ventricles.

Mobitz type 1 heart block—Wenckebach phenomenon

Wenckebach phenomenon is characterized by progressive prolongation of the PR interval, eventually resulting in a dropped P wave. The cycle is then repeated. This is a common phenomenon and can occur in any cardiac tissue including the SA node.

Wenckebach phenomenon can occur in atheletes and children and is due to high vagal tone. It is usually benign and is not usually an indication for pacing.

When it occurs following an inferior myocardial infarction (RCA supplied in 90% of patients), pacing is not usually required unless it is symptomatic. In anterior myocardial infarction any newly developed heart block suggests massive septal necrosis and temporary pacing is required.

Mobitz type 2 heart block

The PR interval remains constant and P waves are dropped intermittently. This is almost always due to conduction abnormalities below the AV node, most likely in the His-Purkinje system.

This type of heart block carries a risk of progressing to complete heart block and requires insertion of a pacemaker.

2:1 or 3:1 heart block

This represents a more advanced degree of block and requires pacing because there is a high risk of complete heart block.

Third-degree or complete heart block

Complete heart block (Fig. 18.5) results in dissociation of the atria from the ventricles.

The EKG shows the P waves and the QRS waves are independent from each other. The P and QRS complexes are regular but bear no temporal relationship to one another. The pacing of the heart rate in complete heart block is within the intrinsic

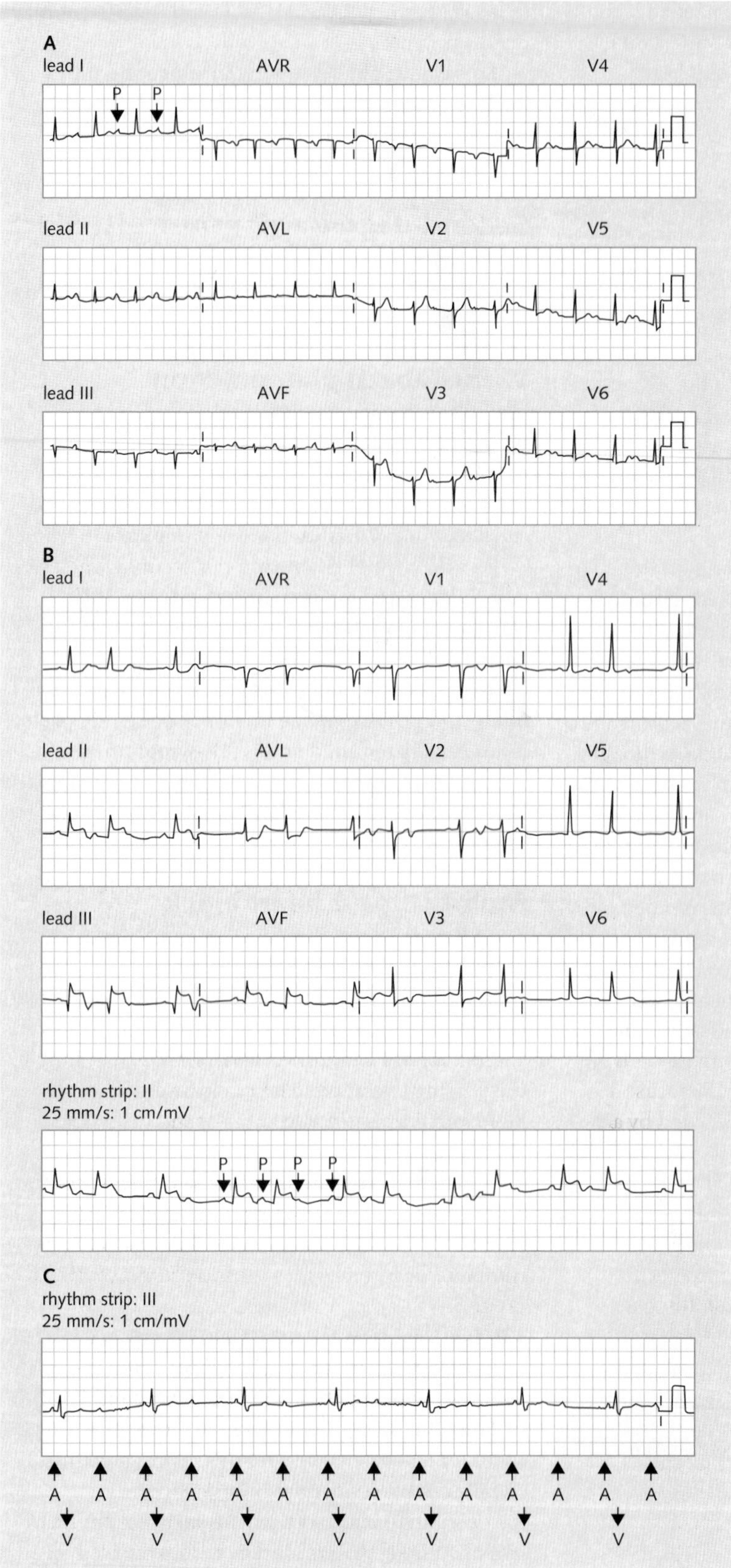

Fig. 18.4 EKGS of bradyarrhythmias. (A) First-degree heart block. Note the long PR interval. (B) Mobitz type 1 (Wenckebach) partial heart block caused by inferior myocardial infarction (raised ST segments in leads II, III, and AVF). (C) 2:1 heart block; arrows point to dropped P waves. There are two P waves (A) from the atrium for every QRS (V) from the ventricles.

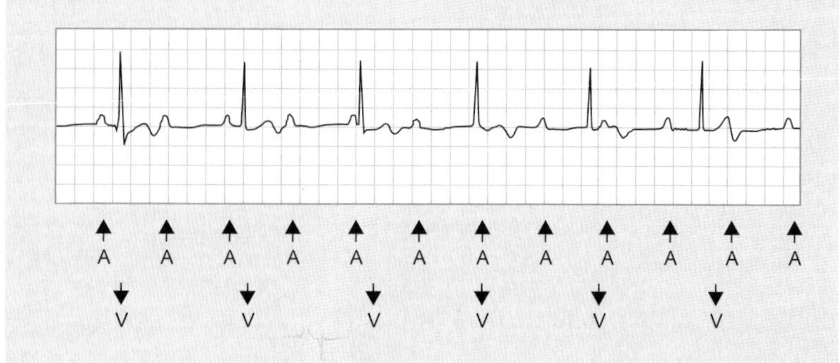

Fig. 18.5 Complete heart block. Atrial P waves (A) and ventricular QRS (V) complexes are completely dissociated.

pacemaker activity of the ventricle. The rate in acquired complete heart block is usually less than 40 beats per minute but can be faster in congenital complete AV block.

On examination there may be classical features:

- The first heart sound has a variable intensity.
- There are intermittent cannon waves in the jugular venous pulse. These correspond to a large a wave caused by the right atrial contraction against a closed tricuspid valve.

Management depends upon the underlying cause:

- After an inferior myocardial infarction a temporary pacemaker should be inserted. A significant proportion of these cases revert back to normal conduction within a few weeks and a permanent pacemaker is often not needed. If the heart block is due to drugs (e.g., beta-blockers) it may resolve once these are withdrawn.
- After an anterior myocardial infarction, or in any other situation, a permanent pacemaker will be required and should be inserted immediately (unless the patient is unstable in which case a temporary wire is inserted first followed by a permanent system some days later).

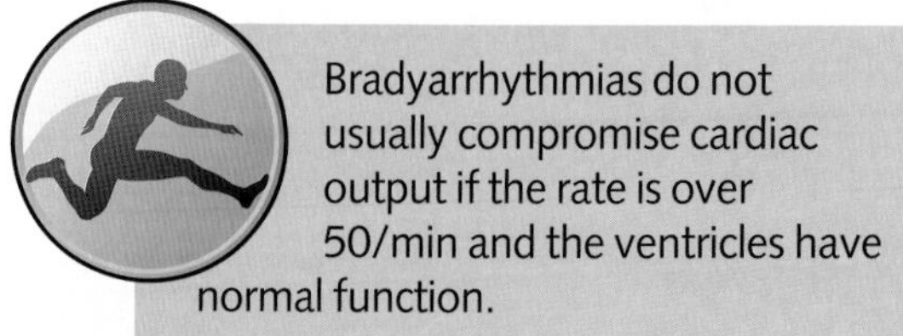

Bradyarrhythmias do not usually compromise cardiac output if the rate is over 50/min and the ventricles have normal function.

Bundle-branch block

Bundle-branch block is an interventricular conduction disturbance. The bundle of His arises

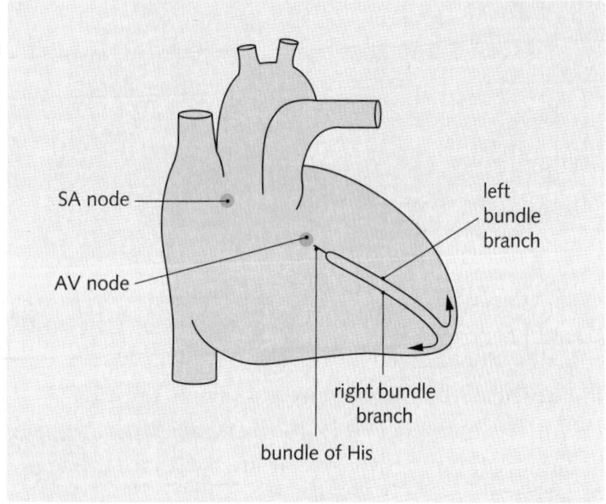

Fig. 18.6 Location of conductive tissue in the heart. (AV node, atrioventricular node; SA node, sinoatrial node.)

from the AV node and at the level of the top of the muscular interventricular septum it divides into left and right bundle branches (Fig. 18.6), which supply the left and right ventricles respectively. The left bundle divides again into anterior and posterior divisions.

Damage to one or more of these bundles due to ischemia or infarction (or any other condition disturbing electrical conduction; see SA node disease earlier in this chapter) results in a characteristic EKG picture as the pattern of depolarization of the ventricles is altered.

In either complete left (LBBB) or complete right bundle-branch block (RBBB) the QRS complex is widened to greater than 0.12sec.

Left bundle-branch block

In the normal situation the septum is depolarized from left to right. If the left bundle is blocked, the

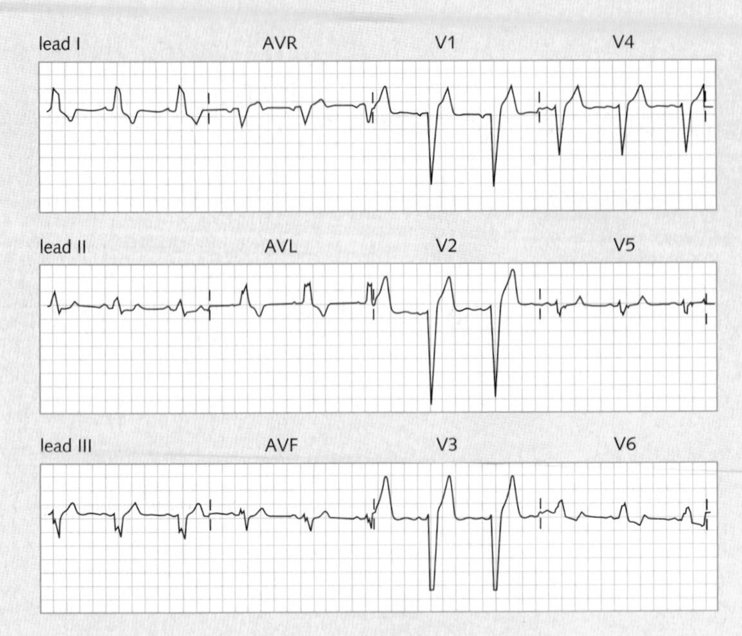

Fig. 18.7 Complete left bundle-branch block. This is characterized by widening of the QRS complex. The second half in time of the QRS is positive in I (to the left) and negative in V1 (posterior) (i.e. the delayed depolarization is to the left ventricle). Note the widened complexes and the M-shaped complexes in V6.

septum is depolarized from right to left and the right ventricle depolarized before the left. This results in the classical M-shaped complex in lead V6 (Fig. 18.7). The incidence of LBBB increases with age, and in older patients LBBB is associated with a cardiac event in 10 years.

Remember that V6 is on the left side of the chest and that a positive deflection occurs when current flows toward the lead. The initial upstroke is due to septal depolarization from right to left and therefore toward lead V6. Depolarization of the right ventricle occurs next, which is in a center-to-right direction and therefore causes a negative deflection. Finally, the left ventricle is depolarized, which is from right to left, causing the final upstroke. The incidence of LBBB is related to myocardial ischemia, and new LBBB should be treated as an MI, especially in the presence of cardiac markers or a positive clinical history.

It is possible to see isolated block of the left anterior or left posterior fascicles of the left bundle branch on the EKG. Left anterior hemiblock causes a left axis deviation on the EKG and left posterior hemiblock causes right axis deviation.

Right bundle-branch block

Right bundle-branch block occurs most commonly due to stretching/hypertrophy of the right ventricle secondary to cor pulmonale. Also, RBBB can occur acutely secondary to PE, MI, infection, or infiltrative disease.

This results in the classical RSR pattern in lead V1 and V2 (Fig. 18.8), which lies to the right of the left ventricle. The septum is depolarized from left to right as normal (resulting in an upstroke in V1), but as there is no conduction down the right bundle the left ventricle depolarizes first, which causes a current to the left resulting in a negative stroke in V1. Finally, the delayed right ventricular depolarization of the right ventricle occurs causing another upstroke in V1.

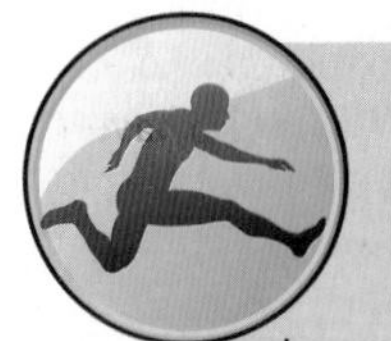

Bundle-branch block may progress to complete heart block; intermittent heart block should be suspected in patients who present with syncope and bundle-branch block.

Investigation of bradyarrhythmias

Electrocardiography

The EKG may show evidence of heart block. However, if the heart block is intermittent, the EKG may be normal.

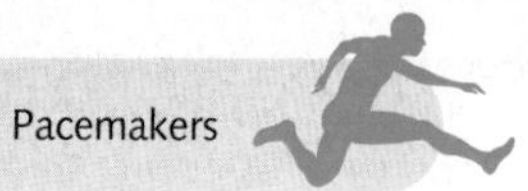

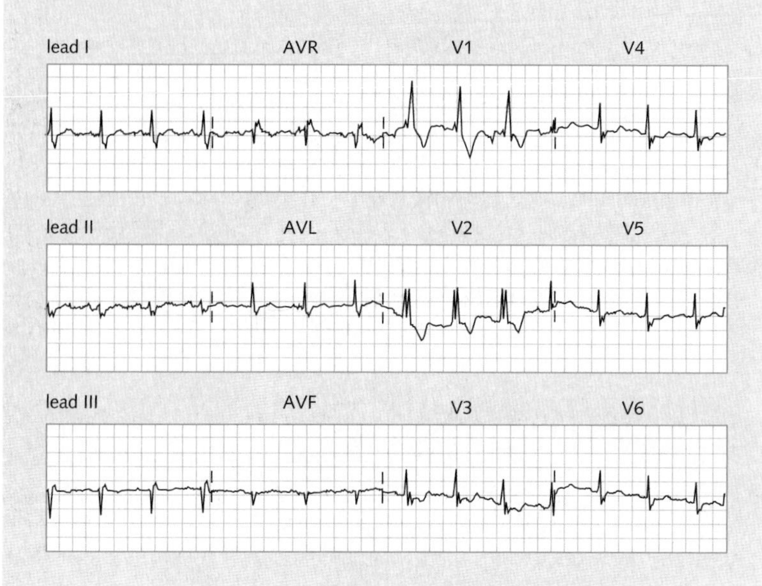

Fig. 18.8 Right bundle-branch block. Note the wide QRS. The late part of the QRS in time is negative in I (i.e. to the right) and positive in V1 (i.e. anterior). The delayed depolarization is to the right ventricle. Note the widened QRS complexes and the RSR pattern in V1 and V2.

In a patient who has unexplained syncope it is important to exclude intermittent conduction disturbances using continuous ambulatory EKG monitoring. These devices can be used to record the EKG over at least 24 hours continuously.

Blood tests

The following blood tests should be ordered:

- Serum electrolytes—for hypokalemia.
- Complete blood count/blood cultures—these can be used to diagnose infective endocarditis with pervalvular abscess and infiltration.
- Liver function and thyroid function tests—may reveal causes of sinus bradycardia.

Chest radiography

This may reveal cardiomegaly in patients who have ischemic cardiomyopathy or myocarditis. Pulmonary edema may be a result of the bradycardia.

Echocardiography

This may reveal regional wall hypokinesia due to areas of ischemia or infarction. This is especially relevant if it involves the septum.

Electrophysiological studies

These studies involve inserting multiple electrodes into the heart via the great veins and positioning them at various intracardiac sites. Electrical activity can then be recorded from the atria, ventricles, bundle of His, etc., to provide information about the type of conduction defect or rhythm disturbance. These studies are used mostly:

- To elucidate the mechanism of tachyarrhythmias.
- Therapeutically to terminate a tachyarrhythmia by overdrive pacing or shock.
- Therapeutically to ablate an area of myocardium thought to be propagating a recurrent tachyarrhythmia.
- Diagnostically to evaluate the risk of sudden cardiac death in patients who have possible ventricular tachyarrhythmias.
- Diagnostically to determine conduction defects in patients who have recurrent syncope.

Pacemakers

Indications for a permanent pacemaker

A pacemaker is used to deliver electric stimuli via leads in contact with the heart. The leads not only deliver energy but are also able to sense spontaneous electrical activity from the heart. The aim of inserting a pacemaker is to mimic as closely as possible the normal electrical activity of the heart in a patient who has a potentially life-threatening conduction disturbance. The indications for a permanent pacemaker are listed in Fig. 18.9.

Indications for temporary pacing

The following indications for temporary pacing are appropriate:

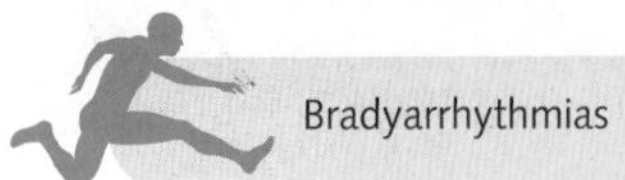

- All of the above (see Fig. 18.9) if no facility for permanent pacing is immediately available.
- Drug-induced symptomatic bradyarrhythmias—a temporary wire is used until the effect of the drug has worn off; for example, after a trial or overdose of a beta blocker (beta-adrenoceptor antagonist)).
- Heart block after inferior myocardial infarction.

Pacemaker insertion

Both temporary and permanent pacemakers are inserted via a venous route by introducing first a sheath and then a pacing wire into one of the great veins.

Permanent pacemakers are most often inserted into the cephalic, subclavian, or internal jugular veins. In an emergency situation a temporary wire may be inserted into the internal jugular, subclavian, or femoral vein.

In the case of the temporary pacemaker the pacemaker box sits externally. In the case of the permanent pacemaker it is buried under the fat and subcutaneous tissue overlying one of the pectoralis major muscles (usually on the patient's nondominant side).

Indications for a permanent pacemaker

Complete AV block—should be permanently paced whether symptomatic or not
Mobitz type 2 block and 2:1 and 3:1 block
Symptomatic bifascicular BBB (i.e., RBBB and left anterior or posterior hemiblock)
Trifascicular block, whether symptomatic or not (i.e., first-degree heart block, RBBB, and left anterior or posterior hemiblock, or first-degree block and LBBB)
Sinus node pauses with or without tachycardia
Symptomatic sinus bradycardia with no treatable cause
After inferior MI with persistent complete heart block or persistent Mobitz type 2 block after trial with temporary pacing wire for at least 2 weeks
After anterior MI with persistent complete heart block or persistent Mobitz type 2 block: trial with temporary pacing is unnecessary because conduction very rarely recovers
Symptomatic bradyarrhythmia following drug treatment of a serious tachyarrhythmia: continue the antiarrhythmic drug and combine with a permanent pacemaker

Fig. 18.9 Indications for a permanent pacemaker. (LBBB, left bundle branch block; MI, myocardial infarction; RBBB, right bundle branch block.)

Complications of pacemaker insertion

The following are recognized complications of pacemaker insertion:

- Complications of wire insertion such as pneumothorax, hemorrhage, brachial plexus injury (during subclavian vein puncture), arrhythmias as the wire is manipulated inside the heart, and infection (may progress to infective endocarditis).
- Complications of permanent pacemaker box positioning (e.g., hematoma formation, infection, and erosion of the box through the skin).
- Difficulties with the wire such as wire displacement and loss of ability to pace or sense (need to reposition wire), fracture of the wire insulation (usually due to tight sutures or friction against the clavicle—need to replace wire), and perforation of myocardium (uncommon unless after myocardial infarction when the myocardium is friable—need to reposition wire).

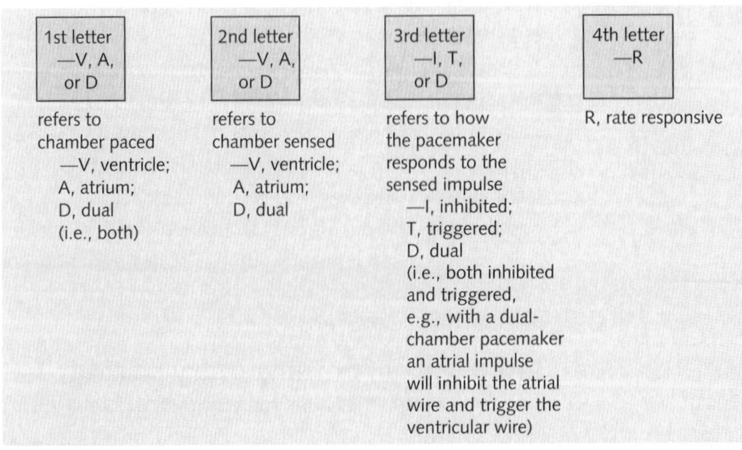

Fig. 18.10 Classification of pacemakers.

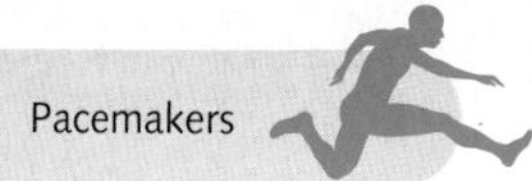

Types of pacemaker

Pacemakers are classified according to a four-letter code (Fig. 18.10).

Ventricular pacemakers stimulate ventricular contraction only and patients who have these have no atrial contribution to the cardiac output. The atrial contribution can, however, be very important (up to 25% of total cardiac output). It is generally accepted now that a dual chamber pacemaker should be fitted in patients in whom the atrium can be paced and sensed. The most common types of pacemakers are DDD or VVI.

Patients who have chronic atrial fibrillation cannot have an atrial wire because the constant random electrical activity cannot be appropriately sensed.

Pacemaker syndrome

Permanent single chamber right ventricular pacing in a patient who has intact atrial function can lead to atrial activation by retrograde conduction from the ventricle—so-called pacemaker syndrome. There is a cannon wave with every beat, pulmonary arterial pressure rises, and cardiac output is impaired. This is managed by replacing the pacemaker with a dual chamber device.

19. Heart Failure

Definition of heart failure

Heart failure is the inability of the heart to adequately perfuse metabolizing tissues. The most common cause is myocardial failure, which can be caused by a wide variety of disease states.

Myocardial failure may affect the left and right ventricles individually or both together. Left ventricular failure (LVF), if left untreated, will lead to right ventricular failure (RVF) due to high right ventricular pressure load. Occasionally heart failure occurs with no abnormality of myocardial function. This is due to a sudden excessivly high demand on the heart—so-called high-output heart failure (Fig. 19.1) or acute pressure load.

Some patients have an entity of heart failure termed "diastolic dysfunction," since the abnormality is caused by failure of the ventricle to relax during diastole. The vast majority of cases result from myocardial hypertrophy in response to hypertension. In addition, the following diseases can also cause diastolic dysfunction: long-standing hypertension, obstructive and nonobstructive hypertrophic cardiomyopathy, restrictive cardiomyopathy, and infiltrative cardiomyopathies.

Pathophysiology of heart failure

Normal myocardial response to work

During exercise and other stresses there is an increased adrenergic stimulation of the myocardium and cardiac pacemaker tissue. This results in tachycardia and increased myocardial contractility.

An increase in venous return causes an increased end-diastolic volume (preload) of the left ventricle resulting in stretching of the myocytes. This stretch causes an increase in myocardial performance—as predicted by the Frank–Starling law (Fig. 19.2).

> The terms "preload" and "afterload" are commonly used. Load is a force—in this case, the force in the wall of the cardiac chambers. Preload = diastolic force. Afterload = systolic force. Preload and afterload always change together because of the LaPlace relationship (e.g., increasing venous return increases volume and therefore systolic wall force). Vasodilatation shifts blood from the heart and decreases diastolic and systolic wall force.

At the same time vasodilatation in the exercising muscles reduces peripheral vascular resistance resulting in a marked increase in cardiac output with relatively little increase in systemic blood pressure.

The failing heart's response to work

The adrenergic system is already at an increased level of activity in heart failure in an attempt to boost cardiac output by increasing heart rate and ejection fraction. During stress this stimulation increases, but cardiac reserve does not permit a significant increase in contractility. The result is tachycardia with its increased energy consumption and a small increase in cardiac output (Fig. 19.3).

Similarly, the response to increased myocardial stretch is impaired in the failing heart. During stress the impairment results in inadequate contractile response and a large increase in pulmonary capillary pressure (back pressure). This predisposes to the development of pulmonary edema.

The elevated catecholamine activity may result in peripheral vasoconstriction. Cardiac output is redistributed toward vital organs (e.g., the brain and heart) with vasoconstriction in the skin and skeletal muscle. Therefore, the blood flow to less crucial organs is reduced, and this underperfusion leads to formation of lactic acid and weakness and fatigue—

Causes of high output heart failure
Thyrotoxicosis
Sepsis
Chronic anemia
Paget's disease of bone
Beriberi
Arteriovenous malformations
Congenital malformations
Pregnancy
Pheochromocytoma

Fig. 19.1 Causes of high-output heart failure.

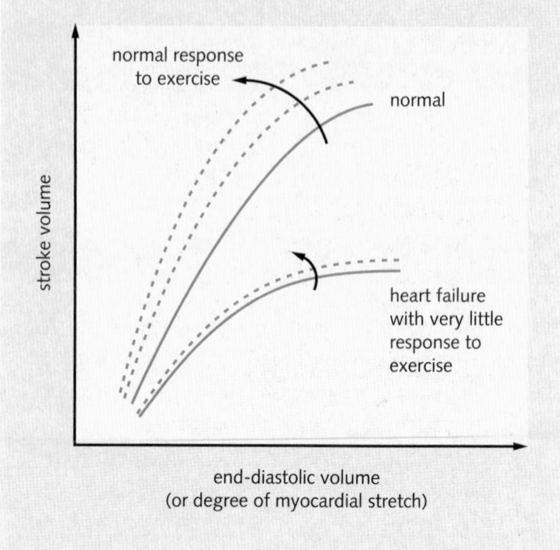

Fig. 19.2 Relationship between end-diastolic volume and stroke volume in normal and failing myocardium (Frank–Starling relationship).

classic symptoms in all patients who have heart failure.

The result is:

- An inadequate myocardial response to stress.
- Increased and wasteful myocardial energy consumption.
- Possible pulmonary edema.

Salt and water retention in heart failure

Salt and water retention causes the characteristic raised jugular venous pressure (JVP) and edema of congestive heart failure (CHF).

The renin–angiotensin system is activated in heart failure for two reasons:

- Stimulation of the $beta_1$-adrenergic receptors on the juxtaglomerular apparatus.
- Reduced renal perfusion leads to activation of the baroreceptors in the renal arterioles so stimulating renin production.

Renin acts to convert angiotensinogen to angiotensin I. The subsequent action of angiotensin-converting enzyme (predominantly in the lung) converts angiotensin I to angiotensin II.

Angiotensin II has a variety of actions:

- It is a potent vasoconstrictor.
- It may increase noradrenaline release (which in turn causes vasoconstriction and myocardial stimulation).
- It is the major stimulus for aldosterone release from the adrenal cortex. Aldosterone causes sodium retention in the distal convoluted tubule. Water is retained with the sodium resulting in increased intravascular volume, which leads to increased cardiac load, so exacerbating heart failure.

Other neurohumoral factors

Heart failure is still a relatively poorly understood field, and as our understanding improves, it becomes apparent that many different hormones and chemical messengers have a role to play. You will hear these hormones and messengers referred to as "neurohumoral factors." This term is fine to use so long as you appreciate that the identity of all these factors is not known and it is not known exactly how many there are. Natriuretic peptides, cytokines, and endothelin are thought to have a role in heart failure.

Natriuretic peptides

There are three such peptides known currently:

- Atrial natriuretic peptide (ANP).
- Brain natriuretic peptide (BNP).
- C-natriuretic peptide (C-NP).

Both ANP and BNP causes sodium excretion (natriuresis) resulting in water excretion and also peripheral vasodilatation, therefore reducing cardiac load. The exact role of C-NP is unclear.

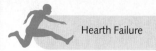

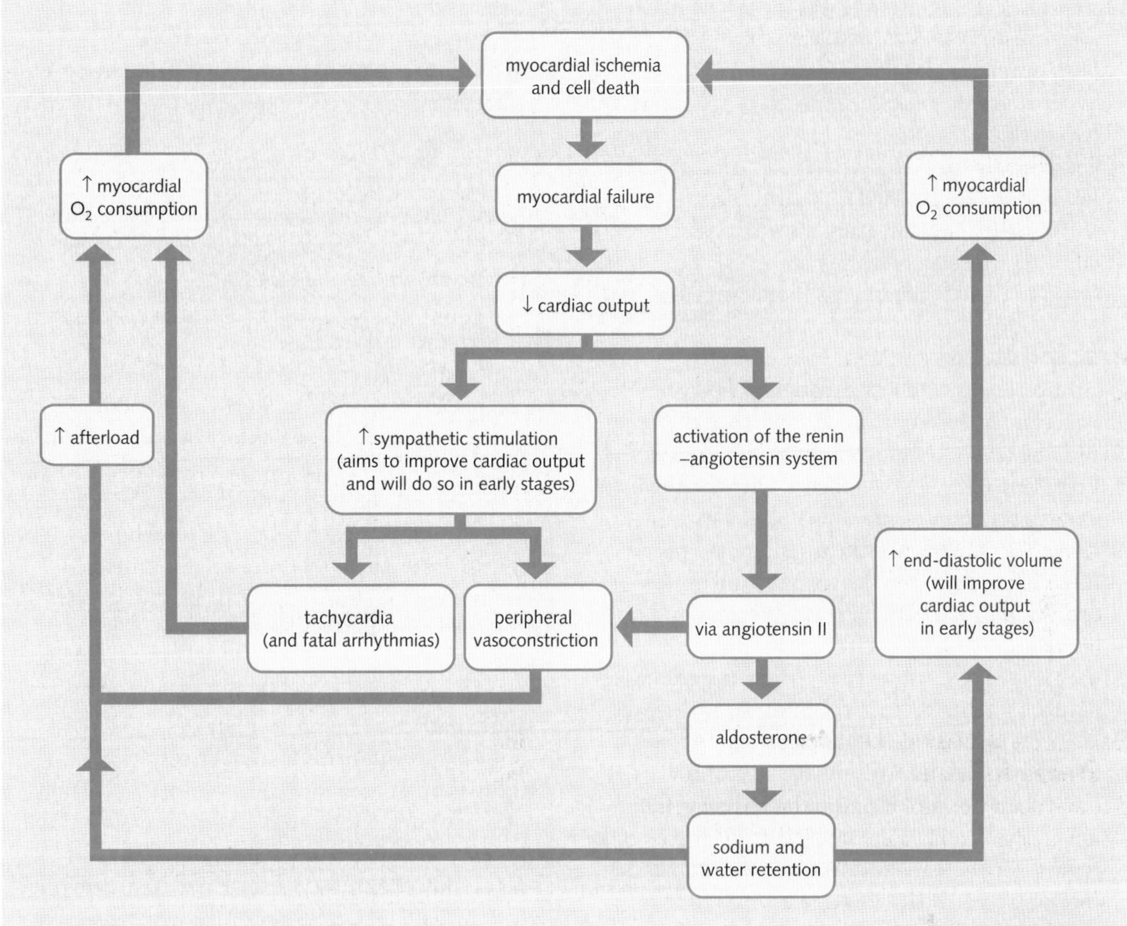

Fig. 19.3 Pathophysiology of heart failure.

Levels of all three peptides are increased in patients who are in heart failure. It is generally accepted that these peptides play a protective role in heart failure by attempting to break the vicious cycle illustrated in Fig. 19.3.

Cytokines

Cytokines (such as tumor necrosis factor alpha) are thought to be involved in causing cardiac dysfunction. Levels are increased in patients who have heart failure.

Endothelin

This peptide is a powerful vasoconstrictor. It is produced by endothelial cells and there are a number of different subtypes. Endothelin levels are raised in patients who have heart failure. The resulting increase in load may cause increased myocardial strain in heart failure.

Causes of heart failure

Nearly 5 million patients have heart failure in the U.S., and the number is rapidly growing, presumably secondary to new reperfusion techniques. Any cardiac disease can lead to heart failure, but a few common causes are:

- Ischemic heart disease—remember that a right ventricular infarction will give isolated RVF, which requires different acute management from LVF.
- Hypertensive heart disease.
- Valve disease—aortic valve disease will lead to CHF, as will MR. Remember that mitral

stenosis causes RVF but leaves the left ventricle unharmed.
- High output heart failure—secondary to hyperthryroidism, anemia, pregnancy, berberi, and AV shunt.
- Cardiomyopathy—most cases are idiopathic, but some are related to viral myocarditis, toxins/drugs, inflammatory disorders, and infiltrative diseases such as hemochromatosis, sarcoidosis, and amyloidosis (not common).

Precipitants

In most cases an acute exacerbation of heart failure is related to a precipitating event other than the underlying cause. Common precipitants are:

- Reduction of or noncompliance with therapy.
- Recent infection—especially pulmonary infection (to which patients with heart failure are prone). Infection increases metabolic rate and causes tachycardia, and both increase demand on the heart.
- Tachy- or bradyarrhythmias—these are common in such patients because the underlying diseases are often associated with arrhythmias. Atrial fibrillation with RVR results in a loss of the atrial component to cardiac output by reducing the efficiency of ventricular filling. Bradycardia requires an increase in stroke volume to maintain cardiac output with a lower heart rate and this may not be possible in the failing heart.

Clinical features of heart failure

The symptoms and signs of heart failure vary depending upon a number of factors:

- Severity of heart failure.
- Ventricles involved.
- Age of the patient.

Regardless of the cause of heart failure, it is possible to predict the effects of heart failure if the mechanics of pump failure are considered. The effects can be divided into forward and backward effects.

Forward effects

Forward effects refer to the failure of the pump to provide an adequate output. This applies to the left ventricle, resulting in:

- Poor renal perfusion, predisposing to prerenal failure.
- Poor perfusion of extremities, resulting in cold extremities.
- Increased lactic acid production in underperfused skeletal muscle, leading to weakness and fatigue.
- Hypotension.

Forward failure of the right ventricle results in reduced pulmonary flow, leading to dyspnea and underfilling of the left ventricle with consequent hypotension, and so on (as above).

Backward effects

The physiological response to a failing heart is to boost output, according to Starling's law, due to increasing end-diastolic volume. The sodium and water retention secondary to aldosterone will serve this function. As heart failure worsens, the pump fails to empty with each beat. This, combined with progressive salt and water retention, results in accumulation of blood in the atria and the venous system and therefore tissue congestion (CHF). There is also progressive dilatation of the ventricle. Again this applies to both left and right ventricles.

Left ventricular failure initially causes increased pulmonary venous pressure, which results in extravasation of fluid into the alveolar spaces and pulmonary edema formation. As the pressure in the pulmonary venous system rises the backpressure affects pulmonary arterial blood and eventually the right ventricle. Undertreated LVF, therefore, eventually leads to RVF.

Right ventricular failure causes increased backpressure in the venous system with resulting fluid extravasation at a number of sites:

- The peripheries—subcutaneous edema is felt in the legs and other dependent parts.
- The liver—tender hepatomegaly is a result of hepatic congestion and may lead to cirrhotic changes as well as an increase in LFTs and INR.
- The abdominal cavity resulting in ascites.

Although dividing heart failure into right and left ventricular failure seems complicated, it is worth taking the time to learn this distinction because it makes it much easier to logically work out the cause of a given set of signs and symptoms.

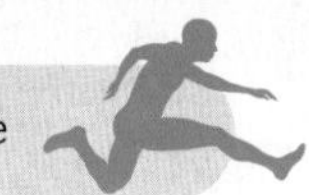

Symptoms

Dyspnea (shortness of breath), fatigue and weakness, nocturia, cough, epigastric discomfort, and anorexia are common in heart failure.

Dyspnea results from pulmonary edema, lactic acidosis, depressed respiratory muscle function, and reduced lung function. It may present in a number of ways:

- Exertional dyspnea—as heart failure worsens, the level of exertion required to cause dyspnea decreases until the patient is breathless at minimal exertion (e.g., when dressing or even when speaking). This is the most common complaint of patients with CHF.
- Orthopnea—the increased venous return when the patient lies flat is often too much for the failing heart to pump, resulting in the development of pulmonary edema. Patients who have severe LVF often sleep using several pillows to prop them up.
- RUQ tenderness—this can be caused by acute congestion of the liver.
- Paroxysmal nocturnal dyspnea—after being asleep for some time the patient is awakened by severe breathlessness, which is relieved only after standing or sitting upright. The cause is thought to be pulmonary edema due to gradual resorption of interstitial fluid overnight and nocturnal depression of respiratory function.

Fatigue and weakness result from reduced perfusion of skeletal muscles, and nocturia is due to the increased renal perfusion in the recumbent position.

Cough may be:

- A nocturnal dry cough due to bronchial edema or cardiac asthma (bronchospasm secondary to edema).
- Productive of pink frothy sputum due to pulmonary edema.

Cough is often overlooked as a symptom of heart failure with the patient being investigated for a respiratory cause instead. Always include heart failure in the differential diagnosis of cough. Pink, "frothy" sputum is sometimes considered the hallmark of pulmonary edema.

Epigastric discomfort occurs in cases of hepatic congestion. Anorexia (which may be caused by edema of the gut), ankle swelling (due to peripheral edema), and shortness of breath (due to inadequate pulmonary perfusion) may occur in a patient who has predominantly right-sided heart failure.

Severity of symptoms

The severity of heart failure symptoms can be determined by using the New York Heart Association guidelines.

- Class I: No symptoms.
- Class II: Heart failure symptoms with ordinary activity.
- Class III: Heart failure symptoms with minimal activity.
- Class IV: Heart failure symptoms at rest.

In addition, the American College of Cardiology and American Heart Association (ACC/AHA) have suggested a new set of guidelines that are less subjective and also include two classes of patients who lack the traditional diagnosis of heart failure but are at increased risk. The hope is that this new classification will enable more specific research based on the stage of heart failure.

- Stage A identifies the patient who is at high risk for developing HF but has no structural disorder of the heart.
- Stage B refers to a patient with a structural disorder of the heart but who has never developed symptoms of HF.
- Stage C denotes the patient with past or current symptoms of HF associated with underlying structural heart disease.
- Stage D designates the patient with end-stage disease who requires specialized treatment strategies such as mechanical circulatory support, continuous ionotropic infusions, cardiac transplantation, or hospice care.

Examination of patients who have heart failure

On observation the patient may be short of breath and cyanosed. Alternatively, if the heart failure is relatively mild there may be no obvious abnormality at rest, but the dyspnea may become apparent on exertion (e.g., when undressing before the examination).

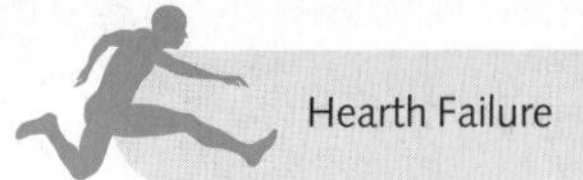

A	Consequences of left and right ventricular failure	
	LV failure	**RV failure**
Symptoms	Dyspnea secondary to pulmonary edema and lactic acidosis Fatigue due to poor cardiac output and lactic acidosis	Dyspnea secondary to poor pulmonary perfusion Fatigue due to poor LV filling (and therefore poor cardiac output and lactic acidosis)
Signs	Hypotension, cold peripheries, and renal impairment—all due to poor LV output LV 3rd heart sound—heard best at the apex Bilateral basal crackles Signs of CHF—severe chronic LV failure leads to fluid retention	Hypotension and cold peripheries due to poor LV filling (and therefore poor LV output) RV 3rd heart sound—very soft and best heard at the left lower sternal edge Elevated JVP Ascites, hepatic enlargement, and peripheral edema

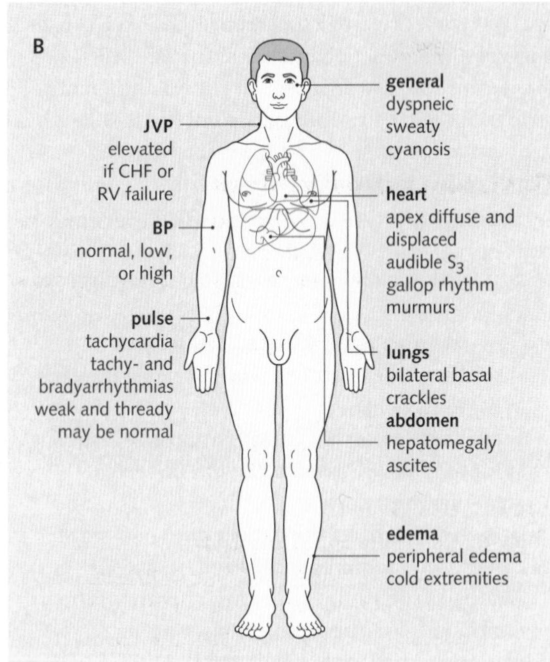

Fig. 19.4 (A) Consequences of left and right ventricular failure. One or the other will be dominant and the clinical picture varies accordingly. Often there are signs of both. (B) Clinical findings in a patient who has heart failure. (BP, blood pressure; CHF, congestive heart failure; JVP, jugular venous pressure; LV, left ventricle; RV, right ventricle.)

Cardiac cachexia is a term used to describe cachexia seen in patients who have chronic heart failure; this is due to:

- Gut edema and liver congestion, leading to anorexia.
- Increased metabolism due to increased work of breathing and increased cardiac oxygen consumption.

Cardiovascular system

On examination of the cardiovascular system (Fig. 19.4) note:

- Pulse—may be rapid, weak, and thready if there is considerable forward failure. Watch out for arrhythmias and pulsus alternans (alternate strong and weak beats), which is a sign of LVF. In addition, the extremities may be cool, pale, and cyanotic due to poor forward flow.

- Blood pressure—this may be normal, low in forward failure, or high in the hypertensive patient (remember that hypertension is a common cause of heart failure).
- Jugular venous pressure—this is elevated in CHF and pure right-sided failure (the normal jugular venous pressure is 2–3cm above the sternal angle). Often the JVP may be so high that the patient will need to be evaluated sitting upright.

If a raised JVP is nonpulsatile, consider superior vena caval obstruction. A pulsatile raised JVP with no edema means right heart failure. A pulsatile raised JVP with edema is usually due to congestive heart failure, but right heart failure is revealed if the JVP remains high after removal of the edema with diuretics.

- Carotid pulse—look for abnormal pulse character because it may reveal a possible etiology for the heart failure (e.g., aortic stenosis or regurgitation).
- Apex beat—may be displaced downward and laterally in a patient who has an enlarged left ventricle. A diffuse apex beat is a sign of severe left ventricular dysfunction. In addition, a right ventricular heave along the sternum can be often noted in right heart failure.
- Heart sounds—on auscultation there may be a third heart sound. Tachycardia combined with a third (or fourth heart sound) is referred to as a gallop rhythm.
- Murmurs—these may signify a possible cause of heart failure (e.g., aortic valve murmurs and mitral valve murmurs). Remember that mitral regurgitation may occur as a result of left ventricular dilatation and will therefore be caused by heart failure and not a cause of it in some cases.
- Peripheral edema—this may be elicited over the sacrum or over the ankle. Take care because edema may be tender. The extent to which the edema extends up the legs is an indication of the extent of the fluid overload.

Respiratory system

In addition to dyspnea and possible cyanosis the patient may have bilateral basal fine end-inspiratory crackles extending from the bases upwards. This is classical of pulmonary edema. Remember to look for signs of consolidation since infections are often the cause of heart failure decompensation.

In addition there may be pleural effusions and expiratory wheeze (secondary to cardiac asthma).

Dyspnea secondary to pulmonary edema is worse when the patient lies flat, and in severe cases the patient has to sit upright. In this situation it is reasonable not to ask the patient to sit at 45 degrees and to conduct the examination in the upright position.

Gastrointestinal system

In patients who have CHF or pure RVF there may be signs of hepatomegaly and ascites.

Take care when palpating the liver or attempting to elicit the hepatojugular reflex because CHF may result in tender hepatomegaly.

Investigation of heart failure

Blood tests

Electrolytes and renal function

Hypokalemia and hyponatremia are common findings in patients who are on diuretic therapy. There may also be renal impairment due to hypoperfusion or diuretic therapy. Hyponatremia may be found in patients who are not on diuretics due to sodium restriction and high circulating vasopressin levels (dilutional hyponatremia).

Hyperkalemia may be seen in patients who are being treated with potassium-sparing diuretics (e.g., amiloride, spironolactone) or angiotensin-converting enzyme (ACE) inhibitors (e.g., captopril, enalapril).

Cardiac markers

Patients who have heart failure that is due to ischemic cardiomyopathy may be having an MI that is causing the decompensation, or a new event may present in someone with previously diagnosed heart failure. This is important to keep in mind, especially if it has been some time since the patient's last stress test/catheterization.

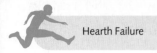

BNP
Useful in differentiating COPD from CHF.

Blood cultures
These can be used to direct antibiotic therapy if infection is exacerbating heart failure, or in diagnosing subacute endocarditis as the cause of acute valvular damage and heart failure.

Complete blood count
Chronic anemia may lead to heart failure. There may be a leukocytosis secondary to infection, which may exacerbate heart failure.

Liver function tests
Liver congestion may lead to impaired hepatic function, resulting in elevated hepatic enzymes and bilirubin.

Arterial blood gases
These show hypoxia, hypocapnea, and metabolic acidosis. The patient may require artificial ventilation if he or she is profoundly hypoxic.

Electrocardiography
This may be normal or may show ischemic or hypertensive changes. Look out for evidence of arrhythmias. If these are suspected, a 48-hour Holter should be performed.

Chest radiography
There may be cardiomegaly, indicating a dilated left ventricle. Sometimes a large left atrial knob can be visualized in left atrial enlargement. Pulmonary edema may be seen with prominent pulmonary veins, upper lobe blood diversion, and Kerley B lines (horizontal lines of fluid-filled fissures at the costophrenic angle).

Echocardiography
This is not usually an acute investigation, but it is extremely useful to evaluate the severity of LVF. It can also be used to rule out LV dysfunction and help diagnose diastolic dysfunction. The degree of left ventricular dilatation can be assessed as can the presence of pulmonary hypertension and right ventricular dilatation. Any valve lesions will be seen.

Dilatation and hypokinesis of the left ventricle predispose to the formation of intraventricular thrombus. Transthoracic echocardiography is not a reliable method for diagnosing this. If intraventricular thrombus is suspected, transesophageal echocardiography should be performed and the patient anticoagulated if intracardiac thrombus is found.

Management of heart failure

The most common clinical presentation seen in the outpatient clinic and on the wards is the patient who has chronic LVF or CHF (heart failure with fluid retention).

Before discussing these, two clinical situations should be covered because they are both emergencies.

These are

- Management of acute LVF.
- Management of acute RVF.

Management of acute left ventricular failure
This is a medical emergency that you will encounter in your first year as a house officer. You will be

> Acute left ventricular failure is a very common condition and is also a medical emergency. Rapid venodilatation is required to remove blood and fluid from the chest. It is therefore important that you know all the management steps, including drugs. Interestingly, IV diuretics also have vasodilatory properties. This may be why they are so effective in treating the initial presentation of heart failure.

Management of acute LVF	
Management in order	**Notes**
Sit the patient up	To reduce venous return to the heart
Administer 100% oxygen via a facial mask	Improvement of arterial oxygen tension will reduce myocardial oxygen debt and improve myocardial function
Establish peripheral IV access and administer:	
IV morphine 2.5–5mg	Morphine is a good anxiolytic and also a venodilator, thus reducing load
IV metoclopramide 10mg	Metoclopramide prevents vomiting secondary to morphine
IV furosemide 80–100mg	Furosemide is a venodilator; thus its initial effect is to reduce load It is also a powerful diuretic and will cause salt and water excretion thus reducing fluid retention By reducing load these drugs reduce the backpressure on the pulmonary circulation and hence relieve pulmonary edema by allowing resorption of fluid back from the extracellular to the intracellular space
Insert a urinary catheter	The patient will have a diuresis and is too ill to use a bed pan; also it is important to be able to monitor fluid output to detect renal impairment early
IV nitrates	Given as a continuous infusion; help by vasodilating both veins and arterioles and so reducing load; the dose is titrated to prevent hypotension (a common side effect of nitrates)
CPAP	Highly effective—it literally pushes fluid out of the alveoli back into the circulation; specialist equipment is required
Once the patient is stable, continue management as for chronic LVF	

Fig. 19.5 Management of acute left ventricular failure (LVF). (CPAP, continuous positive airway pressure; IV, intravenous.)

expected to administer all first-line treatment by yourself so it is important to know not only the drugs to use but also the doses and routes of administration.

The patient in acute LVF has pulmonary edema and is very breathless and distressed. He or she will be hypoxic and may cough up pink frothy sputum. Forward failure may be present, leading to hypotension.

Your aim is to relieve the pulmonary edema rapidly using IV diuretics.

If the patient has cardiogenic shock and is very hypotensive, inotropic agents/pressors may be needed and you should call your senior immediately because in this situation the blood pressure should be improved first.

Learn the management guide given in Fig. 19.5.

It is important in treating acute heart failure to find the cause. Often it is due to new ischemia. In this case, rapid transport to the catheterization lab often improves cardiac function by providing blood to dying or hibernating myocardium.

Management of acute right ventricular failure

Patients who have an inferior or posterior myocardial infarction may present with predominantly RVF. This is not common, but it is important to recognize the signs and to know how to treat it.

Remember Starling's law of the heart: the force of contraction is proportional to the stretch applied to the muscle. Basically it is often possible to improve function by increasing heart volume (unless the ventricle is severely dysfunctional, in which case this makes no difference).

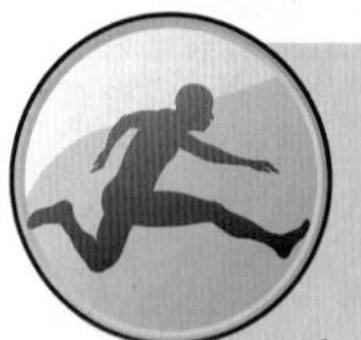

Treatment of acute RVF can be opposite to that of acute LVF. Fluid administration may be needed in RVF. In LVF the fluid needs to be removed.

Unlike left ventricular heart failure, isolated right ventricular failure is very rare and is more commonly found in association with left ventricular failure.

In the post-myocardial infarction patient dehydration, use of diuretics and nitrates is common. They conspire to reduce heart volume.

If right ventricular function is impaired, a reduced heart volume has the effect of reducing function, further resulting in poor left ventricular filling and hypotension. In fact, an impaired right ventricle requires greater than normal filling to maintain normal output. Therefore, a patient who has an inferior myocardial infarction and hypotension should be carefully assessed.

You must be aware that hypotension after inferior myocardial infarction may be secondary to the combination of right ventricular failure and relative underfilling of the right ventricle and that the treatment of this is careful fluid challenge with central venous pressure monitoring.

Provided that there is no evidence of pulmonary edema (suggesting the presence of significant left ventricular impairment) the correct management is a gentle fluid challenge (Fig. 19.6). If the patient is sick enough to be in the cardiac ICU, pulmonary artery catheters can be used to help assess the fluid status, though in recent years these have been found to be associated with increased mortality.

Management of chronic heart failure

In the treatment of chronic heart failure:

- The main agents used are angiotensin-converting enzyme (ACE) inhibitors, diuretics, nitrates, and digoxin.

Management of acute RVF

Management	Notes
Exclude pulmonary edema	Based on chest radiography, clinical examination, arterial oxygen levels; if present it indicates coexistent LVF, and a fluid challenge is unsafe in this situation without the use of inotropic agents
Assess right ventricular filling Infuse 100ml fluid (preferably colloid) over 10min and assess BP and CVP for improvement	Either look at the JVP or preferably insert central venous line and measure CVP
Continue gentle fluid challenges up to 300ml	CVP should rise; blood pressure should also rise; if not, then diagnosis of RVF is incorrect or RV function is severely impaired—need to perform echocardiography or insert Swan–Ganz catheter to confirm diagnosis by finding a low "wedge" pressure

Fig. 19.6 Management of acute right ventricular failure (RVF). The patient will be hypotensive and have had an inferior or posterior MI. (BP, blood pressure; CVP, central venous pressure; JVP, jugular venous pressure; wedge, pulmonary capillary pressure with a Swan–Ganz balloon inflated—it reflects left atrial and pulmonary venous pressure.)

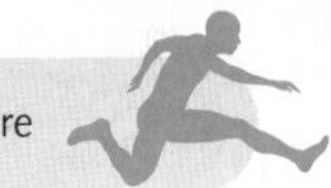

- Other agents used are hydralazine, beta-blockers (beta-adrenoceptor antagonists), and angiotensin II receptor blockers.

A dilated heart means chronic rather than acute heart failure.

Angiotensin-converting enzyme inhibitors

The role of the renin–angiotensin system in heart failure is discussed on p. 152. It is not difficult to see that inhibition of formation of angiotensin II may be beneficial by reducing systemic vasoconstriction and the sodium and water retention caused by aldosterone.

Angiotensin II increases efferent arteriolar tone and therefore increases glomerular filtration. Because ACE inhibitors remove this ability to regulate efferent arteriolar tone, the glomerular filtration rate declines and renal failure ensues in patients who have renal artery stenosis or any other condition in which renal blood flow is reduced (e.g., marked hypotension).

Examples of ACE inhibitors grouped according to which part of the molecule binds the zinc moiety of ACE are:

- Captopril—has a sulphydryl group.
- Enalapril, lisinopril, ramipril—carboxyl group.
- Fosinopril—phosphinic acid.

The ACE inhibitors have been shown to reduce the mortality rate for patients who have heart failure. They are the first-line drugs for all patients who have heart failure unless there is a specific contraindication (e.g., renal artery stenosis or profound hypotension). It is important that all patients leave the hospital on an ACE inhibitor, preferably one that has once daily dosing like lisinopril.

Clinical use of angiotensin-converting enzyme inhibitors

Angiotensin-converting enzyme inhibitors are usually started at low doses because they can cause first-dose hypotension. Patients most likely to suffer from this are:

- The elderly.
- Patients who are on high doses of diuretics.

The vast majority of patients who have heart failure do not require admission to hospital when starting ACE inhibitors. The first dose can be taken at night so that the patient is in bed for the duration of the first dose effect. This makes the risk of postural hypotension occurring extremely unlikely.

Once the dose has been established renal function and electrolytes should be checked 1 week later to ensure that no deterioration has taken place in renal function. Hyperkalemia is another complication, which is due to a reduction in aldosterone activity (aldosterone causes sodium absorption in exchange for potassium in the distal convoluted tubule). This is especially true of those taking potassium-sparing diuretics.

Other side effects of ACE inhibitors are:

- Cough—occurs in 5% patients. It is caused by inhibition of the metabolism of bradykinin (another function of ACE). Cough usually appears in the first few weeks of treatment. This is a side effect of all drugs in this class, and treatment needs to be switched to angiotension receptor blockade instead.
- Loss of taste (or a metallic taste) may occur.
- Rashes and angioedema.

Once the drug has been introduced, the dose should be increased to the recommended level if possible (e.g., captopril, 50mg 3 times/day; enalapril, 10mg twice daily).

Nitrates

The nitrates (e.g., isosorbide mononitrate and isosorbide dinitrate) are veno- and arteriolar dilators and therefore act by reducing preload and afterload load. Intravenous nitrates are useful in the treatment of the acutely sick patient with heart failure. Oral nitrates may provide some symptomatic relief in chronic heart failure. The combination of nitrates and hydralazine has been shown to reduce the mortality rate of heart failure, especially failure that is caused by valvular dysfunction.

Site of action and side effects of different diuretics		
Examples	**Site of action**	**Side effects**
Loop diuretics: furosemide, bumetanide	Thick ascending loop of Henle	Hypokalemia; exacerbation of gout
Thiazide diuretics: bendrofluazide, hydrochlorothiazide, metalozone	Distal convoluted tubule	Hyperglycemia, gout, elevated triglycerides and LDL, hypokalemia, hyponatremia
Potassium-sparing diuretics: amiloride, spironolactone	Collecting duct and distal convoluted tubule	Hyperkalemia—must not be used with ACE inhibitors

Fig. 19.7 Site of action and side effects of different diuretics. (ACE, angiotensin-converting enzyme inhibitor; low-density lipoprotein, LDL.)

Diuretics

Diuretics (Fig. 19.7) have not proven to reduce mortality in heart failure, but they have an important role in salt and water excretion. They provide symptomatic relief, and furosemide is extremely important in treating fluid overload in acute pulmonary edema.

Digoxin

Digoxin is a cardiac glycoside. This drug inhibits the sodium/potassium pump on the sarcolemmal and cell membranes. This adenosine triphosphate (ATP)-dependent pump has a role in transporting calcium out of the cell. Inhibition, therefore, prevents this, resulting in increased intracellular calcium concentration, which in cardiac muscle results in a positive inotropic effect.

In atrioventricular (AV) node tissue the effect of an increased calcium concentration is to prolong the refractory period and decrease AV node conduction velocity, thus slowing AV node conduction of the cardiac impulse—a negative chronotropic effect.

It is generally accepted that digoxin is an extremely useful drug in patients who have atrial fibrillation and heart failure, but no evidence suggests that the use of digoxin as an antifailure agent alone is effective in reducing mortality rates. Although digoxin has not been shown to decrease mortality in those with heart failure, it has been shown to improve symptoms and decrease the frequency of hospitalization.

Pharmacokinetics

Digoxin has a half-life of 24–36 hours, and it takes 3–4 weeks to reach a steady plasma level after oral loading. Intravenous loading speeds the process slightly because the time taken for absorption in the gut is bypassed. Forty percent of digoxin in the blood is protein-bound.

Excretion is predominantly renal (10% excreted in the stools), and digoxin should not be used in renal failure. In mild renal impairment the dose is reduced.

Side effects

Plasma levels of digoxin should be monitored and maintained at between 1 and 2ng/mL. Blood is taken 8 hours after an oral dose. Digoxin toxicity is more likely in patients who:

- Have renal failure.
- Are hypokalemic—digoxin competes with potassium for binding to the sodium/potassium ATPase.
- Are taking amiodarone or verapamil (which displace digoxin from protein-binding sites), erythromycin (which prevents inactivation of digoxin by gut bacteria), and captopril (which reduces renal clearance of digoxin). In addition, mild reactivity is known to occur between digoxin and propafenone, which can be a common combination in the treatment of AF.

Signs of digoxin toxicity are:

- Bradycardia, AV block, sinus arrest.
- Nausea and vomiting.
- Xanthopsia (yellow discoloration of visualized objects).

Angiotensin II receptor blockers

There are two types of angiotensin II receptors: AT1 and AT2. Losartan is a selective AT1 blocker and is

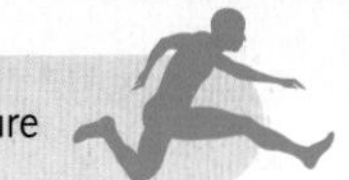

the first of these drugs to be established for use as an antihypertensive. Trials are currently underway to investigate its value in the treatment of heart failure.

The spectrum of activity is the same as that of ACE inhibitors, but the main advantage is that these drugs do not prevent the breakdown of bradykinin. Thus cough does not occur as a side effect.

Hydralazine

Hydralazine is a potent vasodilator, predominantly of arterioles; therefore, it reduces load, which acts to improve cardiac function. Side effects include flushing and a lupus-like syndrome.

Beta-blockers

Beta-blockers are effective treatment option in heart failure. As mentioned on pp. 151–2, the circulating level of catecholamines is high in heart failure. There is also a downregulation of beta receptors in response to this (perhaps the heart's way of protecting itself from the tachycardia and increased metabolic rate those results from sympathetic stimulation). Recent trials of metoprolol, bisoprolol, and carvedilol have shown benefit in their use in heart failure, perhaps for a number of reasons:

- Reduction in myocardial oxygen demand and ischemia.
- Decreased incidence of arrhythmias.
- Peripheral vasodilatation with non-selective beta-blockers that have some alpha blockade as well.
- Antioxidant effects (carvedilol and metoprolol).

Carvedilol, a nonselective beta-blocker with alpha-blocking activity, has been shown to reduce mortality rates in chronic heart failure by over 30%.

Beta blockers must be introduced with care to patients who have heart failure because they may cause the symptoms to deteriorate. There is still no evidence to suggest that they have efficacy in patients who have severe heart failure (i.e., dyspnea at rest) or acute heart failure. Patients who have heart failure should be stabilized with other drugs before prescribing beta-blockers.

Aldosterone-receptor blockers

In NYHA Class II/IV heart failure patients, spironolactone has been shown to increase mortality. More recently eplerenone has been shown to improve survival in post MI left ventricular dysfunction.

20. Cardiomyopathy

Definition of cardiomyopathy

Cardiomyopathy is heart muscle disease, often of unknown cause. There are three types of cardiomyopathy (Fig. 20.1):

- Dilated cardiomyopathy.
- Hypertrophic obstructive cardiomyopathy (HOCM).
- Restrictive cardiomyopathy.

Dilated cardiomyopathy

The heart is dilated and has impaired function. The coronary arteries are normal. Probable causes of dilated cardiomyopathy include:

- Alcohol.
- Viral infection (echovirus, coxsackievirus, and enteroviruses most likely).
- Untreated hypertension.
- Autoimmune disease.
- Thyrotoxicosis.
- Drugs/toxins (cocaine, adriamycin, cyclophosphamide, lead).
- Hemochromatosis.
- Familial syndrome.
- Peripartum status.
- Lyme disease.
- Chagas disease.
- Acquired immunodeficiency syndrome (HIV/AIDS).

Clinical features

Progressive biventricular heart failure leads to symptoms that were discussed in Chapter 19:

- Fatigue.
- Paroxysmal nocturnal dyspnea, orthopnea, dyspnea.
- Peripheral edema.
- Ascites.

Other complications secondary to the progressive dilatation of the ventricles include:

- Mural thrombi with systemic or pulmonary embolization.
- Dilatation of the tricuspid and mitral valve rings leading to functional valve regurgitation.
- Atrial fibrillation and other arrhythmias.
- Ventricular tachyarrhythmias and sudden death.

Investigation

Investigations to aid diagnosis are listed below.

Chest radiography

This may show:

- Cardiomegaly.
- Signs of pulmonary edema (upper lobe blood diversion, interstitial shadowing at the bases).
- Pleural effusions.

Electrocardiography

Electrocardiography may highlight:

- Tachycardia.
- Poor R wave progression across the chest leads.

Echocardiography

Points to consider with echocardiography include, can the dilated ventricles be easily visualized? And can the regurgitant valves be seen?

Occasionally intracardiac thrombus may be seen (transthoracic echocardiography is not a reliable method for diagnosing this, but it can be accurately diagnosed by transesophageal echocardiography).

Cardiac catheterization

This is important to exclude coronary artery disease (the most common cause of ventricular dysfunction).

Urine tests

Can be used to test for cocaine use.

Blood tests

Viral titers may be useful as well as thyroid function tests. Can also test for titers for Chagas and Lyme disease (*Trypanosoma cruzi*, *Borrelia burgdorferi*). Antinuclear antibody, C-reactive protein, and Anti-smith factors can be used to determine if the cardiomyopathy is autoimmune in origin.

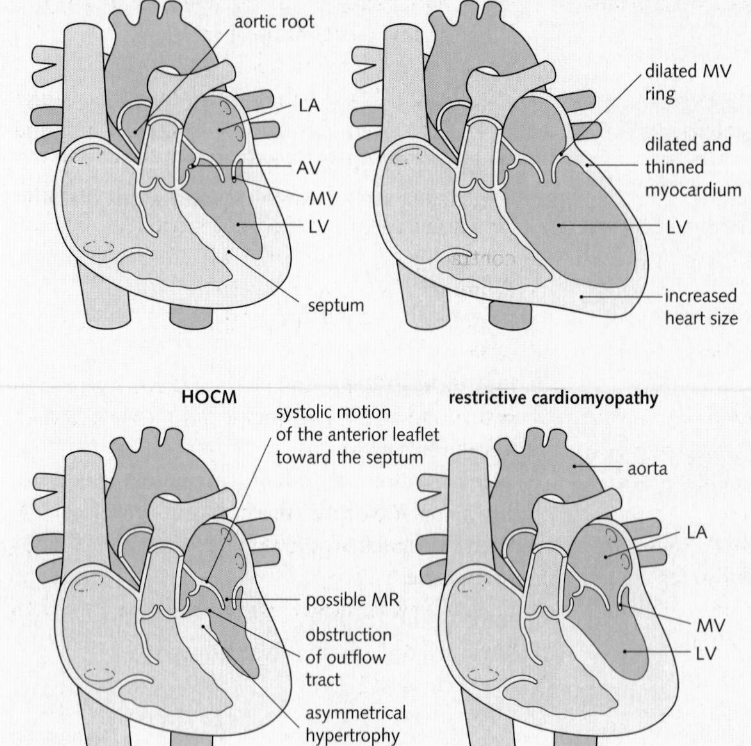

Fig. 20.1 Different types of cardiomyopathy. (AV, aortic valve; HOCM, hypertrophic obstructive cardiomyopathy; LA, left atrium; LV, left ventricle; MR, mitral regurgitation; MV, mitral valve.)

Management

The management plan follows four basic steps (the same applies for any other case of cardiac failure):

- Search for and treat any underlying cause (e.g., stop alcohol).
- Treat cardiac failure (diuretics, angiotensin-converting enzyme inhibitors, nitrates).
- Treat any arrhythmias. Patients with DCM are at an increased risk of sudden death. Use digoxin or amiodarone for atrial fibrillation, amiodarone for ventricular arrhythmias, including nonpharmacologic treatment with ablation for refractory cases of ventricular tachycardia (VT)/ventricular fibrillation (V), and pacer placement for heart block.
- Prevention of sudden death with placement of implantable cardioverter defibrillator (ICD) (CAT Trial) is not recommended, although a subset of patients who have recurrent VF, VF may be found to benefit from placement.
- Anticoagulate with warfarin to prevent mural thrombi.

If the cardiac failure does not respond to the above steps and the patient is a suitable candidate, cardiac transplantation may be a possible option.

Hypertrophic obstructive cardiomyopathy

This disorder is characterized by asymmetrical hypertrophy of the cardiac septum—the cardiac septum is hypertrophied compared to the free wall of the left ventricle. It is the most common cause of heart-related sudden death in those under 30 years old.

Hypertrophic obstructive cardiomyopathy is inherited as an autosomally dominant trait with equal sex incidence. The genetic abnormality is the subject of much current research, and it seems that different genes may be involved in different families.

The myocytes of the left ventricle are abnormally thick when examined microscopically. This makes left ventricular filling more difficult than normal and grossly disordered.

Clinical features

Symptoms usually begin in the third and fourth decades of life.

There are four main symptoms:

- Angina (even in the absence of coronary artery disease)—due to the increased oxygen demands of the hypertrophied muscle.
- Palpitations—there is an increased incidence of atrial fibrillation and ventricular arrhythmias in this condition.
- Syncope and sudden death, which may be due to left ventricular outflow tract obstruction by the hypertrophied septum or to a ventricular arrhythmia.
- Orthopnea/paroxysmal nocturnal dyspnea/dyspnea —due to the stiff left ventricle, which leads to a high end-diastolic pressure and can therefore lead to pulmonary edema.

The signs (Fig. 20.2) to watch for are:

- Jerky peripheral pulse—the second rise palpable in the pulse is due to the rise in left ventricular pressure as the left ventricle attempts to overcome the outflow tract obstruction.
- Double apical beat—the stiff left ventricle causes raised left ventricular end-diastolic pressure. The atrial contraction is therefore very forceful to fill the left ventricle. It is this atrial impulse that can be felt in addition to the left ventricular contraction that gives this classical sign.
- Prominent "a" wave in jugular.
- Systolic thrill—felt at the left lower sternal edge.
- Systolic murmur—crescendo and decrescendo in nature and best heard between the apex and the left lower sternal edge.

It may be difficult to differentiate between HOCM and aortic stenosis on examination. Use the following features to help:

- Pulse—slow rising in aortic stenosis, jerky or with a normal upstroke in HOCM.

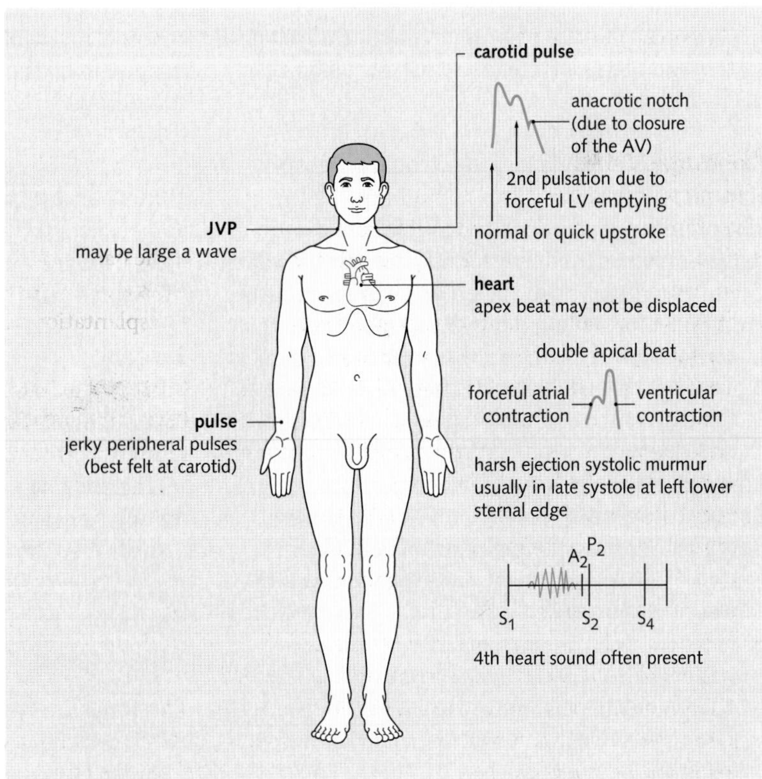

Fig. 20.2 Important clinical signs in hypertrophic obstructive cardiomyopathy. (AV, aortic valve; JVP, jugular venous pressure; LV, left ventricle.)

- Thrill and murmur—both found in the second right intercostal space in aortic stenosis and at the left lower sternal edge in HOCM.
- Variation of the murmur with Valsalva maneuver—this does not occur in aortic stenosis, but the murmur of HOCM is increased because the volume of the left ventricle is reduced by the maneuver and therefore the outflow obstruction worsens.

> Remember that the outflow obstruction of aortic stenosis is fixed and is present throughout systole, whereas the obstruction of HOCM is often absent at the start of systole and worsens as the ventricle empties.

Diagnosis and investigations

Electrocardiography

The EKG is usually abnormal in HOCM. The most common abnormalities are T wave and ST segment abnormalities; the signs of left ventricular hypertrophy may also be present. (Use of the clinical history and EKG can effectively narrow who will need echocardiography.)

Continuous ambulatory electrocardiography (Holter)

The presence of ventricular arrhythmias is common in patients who have HOCM and is a cause of sudden death. It is thought that the presence of ventricular arrhythmias on an ambulatory EKG monitor is a risk factor for sudden death and that an antiarrhythmic agent should be commenced. These tests are usually performed as part of a yearly screening program for these patients.

Echocardiography

This is the most useful investigation because it confirms the diagnosis and can be used to assess the degree of outflow tract obstruction. Characteristic echocardiography findings include:

- Increased mass of the left ventricle with asymmetric hypertrophy of the septum.
- Abnormal systolic anterior motion of the anterior leaflet of the mitral valve.
- Calcification of the mitral valve also frequently occurs.
- Left ventricular outflow tract obstruction.

Prognosis

Children who are diagnosed when they are less than 14 years of age have a poor prognosis and a high incidence of sudden death; 71% of those that die of sudden death are asymptomatic. Adults have a better prognosis, but they also have a higher mortality rate than the general population. Another outcome is progressive cardiac failure with cardiac dilatation.

Management

Drug management

As with aortic stenosis, vasodilators should be avoided because they worsen the gradient across the obstruction. Therefore, patients who have HOCM should not receive nitrates.

Beta-blockers are used because their negative inotropic effect acts to decrease the contractility of the hypertrophied septum and reduce the outflow tract obstruction.

Antiarrhythmic agents are important in patients who have ventricular and atrial arrhythmias. Patients who have atrial fibrillation should be cardioverted as soon as possible (patients who have a high left ventricular end-diastolic pressure rely on the atrial impulse to fill the left ventricle effectively). In addition, an ICD should be placed for any patient at risk for sudden death.

Dual chamber pacing

This reduces the outflow tract gradient by pacing the heart from the right ventricular apex and therefore altering the pattern of septal motion.

Surgery

Surgery is used only when all other treatments have failed. A myomectomy is performed on the abnormal septum.

There is a new catheter technique to infarct the septum by occluding the septal artery or by injecting a small amount of absolute alcohol.

Restrictive cardiomyopathy

This is the least common of the cardiomyopathies in developed countries, although it is much more common in third-world countries in Africa and

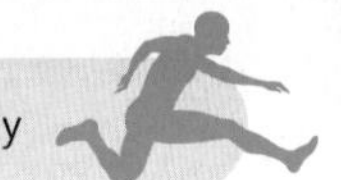

Southeast Asia due to increased fibrosis of the endocardium secondary to infection.

The ventricular walls are excessively stiff and impede ventricular filling; therefore, end-diastolic pressure is increased. The systolic function of the ventricle is often normal.

Presentation is identical to that of constrictive pericarditis, but the two must be differentiated because pericarditis is treatable with surgery.

Possible causes of restrictive cardiomyopathy include:

- Idiopathic/familial (limited to a small number of families).
- Storage diseases (e.g., glycogen storage diseases).
- Infiltrative diseases (e.g., amyloidosis, sarcoidosis)—most common cause in the U.S.
- Scleroderma.
- Endomyocardial diseases (e.g., endomyocardial fibrosis, hypereosinophilic syndrome, carcinoid).

Clinical features

The main features most commonly present as right-sided heart failure symptoms.

- Dyspnea, paroxysmal nocturnal dyspnea, and fatigue due to poor cardiac output.
- Peripheral edema and ascites.
- Elevated jugular venous pressure with a positive Kussmaul's sign (increase in jugular venous pressure during inspiration).

In addition, up to one-third of patients may present with a thromboembolic complication or conduction disturbance.

Management

Since the presentation is so similar to that of constrictive pericarditis (which can be treated with surgery), it is important to distinguish between the two. Often a history of pericarditis, TB, radiation, or surgery will favor constrictive pericarditis.

The condition usually progresses towards death relatively quickly; most patients do not survive 10 years after diagnosis. It is important that patients with cardiac amyloidosis be referred to specialized centers for management of their condition.

21. Pericarditis and Pericardial Effusion

Pericardium

The pericardium forms a strong protective sac around the heart. It is composed of an outer fibrous and an inner serosal layer with approximately 50ml of pericardial fluid between these in the healthy state.

Acute pericarditis

Figure 21.1 defines acute, subacute, and chronic pericarditis. Acute pericarditis is caused by inflammation of the pericardium or the fibrous sac that surrounds the heart (Fig. 21.1).

Clinical features

History

The chest pain of acute pericarditis is usually central or left-sided pleuritic pain that is sharp in nature and relieved by sitting forward. Aggravating factors include breathing, lying supine and coughing. A dull and constant pain that is similar to myocardial infarction may also occur and is important to remember.

Dyspnea may be caused by the pain of deep inspiration or the hemodynamic effects of an associated pericardial effusion.

Examination

The patient may have a fever and tachycardia.

A pericardial friction rub may be heard on auscultation of the heart. This is a high-pitched scratching sound (therefore heard best with the diaphragm). It characteristically varies with time and may appear and disappear from one examination to the next. It sounds closer to the ears than a murmur.

Investigation

Blood tests

These provide evidence of active inflammation—elevated white cell count, erythrocyte sedimentation rate (ESR), and C-reactive protein (CRP)—as well as clues about the underlying cause.

The following blood tests are appropriate:

- Purified protein derivative (PPD) test should be placed if TB is suspected.
- Complete blood count.
- ESR and CRP.
- Urea, creatinine, and electrolytes.
- Viral titers. HIV test should be included; other viral titers are often not helpful since the results will not affect treatment.
- Blood cultures.
- Autoantibody titers (e.g., antinuclear antibodies, rheumatoid factor).
- Cardiac enzymes—almost half of patients with proven pericarditis have mild elevations in troponin, suggesting myopericarditis.

Electrocardiography

Superficial myocardial injury caused by pericarditis results in characteristic EKG changes (Fig. 21.3).

- Concave ST segment elevation is usually present in all leads except AVR and V1.
- A few days later the ST segments return to normal and T-wave flattening occurs and may even become inverted.
- Finally, all of the changes resolve and the EKG trace returns to normal (this may take several weeks or, if the inflammation persists, many months).

Chest radiography

This is normal in most cases of uncomplicated acute pericarditis; however, a number of changes are possible:

- Malignancy can also cause pericarditis, especially if a widened mediastium or nodule is seen.
- A pericardial effusion may develop and if large will result in enlargement of the cardiac shadow, which assumes a globular shape.
- Pleural effusions may also be seen.

Echocardiography

This is the best investigation for confirming the presence of a pericardial effusion. In uncomplicated acute pericarditis, however, echocardiography may be normal.

A dissecting thoracic aortic aneurysm may occasionally present as acute pericarditis or a pericardial effusion. Therefore, be careful to look for a widened mediastinum of the chest radiograph; if this is suspicious, a computed tomography scan of the chest should be performed to avoid missing this diagnosis.

Acute, subacute, and chronic pericarditis
Acute pericarditis (<6 weeks)
Effusive
Fibrinous
Subacute pericarditis (>6 weeks to 6 months)
Chronic pericarditis (>6 months)
Effusive
Adhesive
Effusive–adhesive
Constrictive

Fig. 21.1 Acute, subacute, and chronic pericarditis.

Management

Any treatable underlying cause should of course be sought and treated appropriately. Most cases of pericarditis are viral or idiopathic. The main aims of management are therefore analgesia and bed rest. Non-steroidal anti-inflammatory agents are the most effective for this condition. Occasionally a short course of oral corticosteroids is required.

A pericardial effusion may be present. If large, or causing tamponade, the patient should be hospitalized for drainage. Analysis of the effusion may provide clues about the underlying cause of the pericarditis.

Dressler's syndrome

Dressler's syndrome is a syndrome of fever, leukocytosis, pericarditis, and pleurisy occurring more than 1 week after a cardiac operation or myocardial infarction. It can occur only if the pericardium has been exposed to the blood. Antibodies form against the pericardial antigens and then attack the pericardium in a type III autoimmune reaction. The incidence of this syndrome following MI is has declined since the advent of catherization and thrombolytic therapies and the decrease in the size of infarction.

Causes of acute pericarditis

Cause	Examples/comment
Viral infection	Coxsackievirus A and B, echovirus, Epstein–Barr virus, HIV
Bacterial infection	Pneumococci, staphylococci, Gram-negative organisms, *Neisseria meningitidis*, *N. gonorrhoeae*
Fungal infection	Histoplasmosis, candidal infection
Other infections	Tuberculosis
Acute MI	Occurs in up to 25% of patients 12 hours—6 days after infarction
Uremia	Usually a hemorrhagic pericarditis and may rapidly lead to cardiac tamponade; uremic pericarditis is an indication for hemodialysis
Autoimmune disease	Acute rheumatic fever, SLE, rheumatoid arthritis, scleroderma
Other causes	Neoplastic disease, other inflammatory diseases (e.g., sarcoidosis, Whipple's disease, Behçet's syndrome, Dressler's syndrome (i.e., post-cardiotomy syndrome))

Fig. 21.2 Causes of acute pericarditis. (HIV, human immunodeficiency virus; MI, myocardial infarction; SLE, systemic lupus erythematosus.)

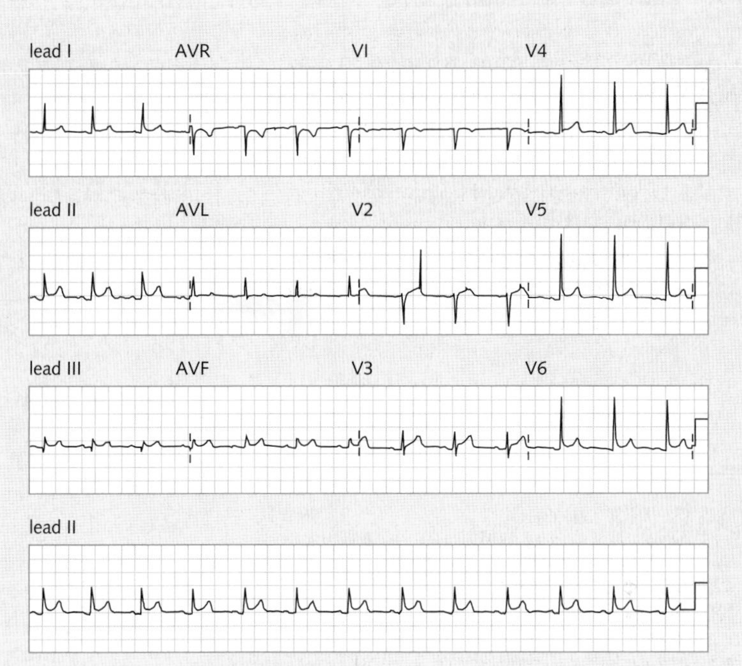

Fig. 21.3 EKG changes of pericarditis. Note the concave or saddle-shaped ST elevation seen in all leads except AVR.

Patients present with fever, malaise, and chest pain. They exhibit the classic signs of acute pericarditis. They may also have arthritis. Cardiac tamponade is not uncommon.

Chest radiography shows pleural effusions. Echocardiography may reveal a pericardial effusion.

Management consists of nonsteroidal anti-inflammatory agents and aspirin initially. Corticosteroids may be added if symptoms persist.

Causes of chronic restrictive pericarditis
Viral infection
Tuberculosis
Sarcoidosis
Post-surgery
Mediastinal radiotherapy
Mediastinal malignancy
Autoimmune disease

Fig. 21.4 Causes of chronic restrictive pericarditis. Note that any cause of acute pericarditis can persist and lead to chronic constrictive pericarditis. The diseases listed here, however, seem to be the most common causes.

Chronic constrictive pericarditis

Chronic constrictive pericarditis occurs when the pericardium becomes fibrosed and thickened and eventually restricts the filling of the heart during diastole. Causes are listed in Fig. 21.4.

Clinical features

The restricted filling of all four chambers of the heart results in low-output failure. Initially the right-sided component is more marked, resulting in a high venous pressure and hepatic congestion. Later left ventricular failure becomes apparent with dyspnea, orthopnea, and edema.

Examination

On examination the signs of right and left ventricular failure are evident, but these ventricles are not enlarged.

The single most important feature in the examination of such a patient is the jugular venous pressure (JVP), which is elevated as expected. Kussmaul's sign—an increase in the JVP during inspiration—may be evident. Since this sign is so strongly linked to constrictive pericarditis, patients who are hypovolemic need fluid administration before diagnosis can occur.

Another important feature of the JVP is a rapid x and y descent. This is an important differential diagnostic point when trying to exclude tamponade. There is no such feature in tamponade.

The heart sounds are often soft. Atrial fibrillation is common.

Investigation

Blood tests are carried out to exclude a possible underlying cause (e.g., leukocytosis in infection, viral titers).

On chest radiography the heart size is normal. There may be signs of a neoplasm or tuberculosis. Pleural effusions are not uncommon. Tuberculous pericarditis may be associated with radiographically visible calcification.

Echocardiography shows good left ventricular function.

Cardiac catheterization is diagnostic because it shows the classic pattern of raised left and right end-diastolic pressures with normal left ventricular function on the ventriculogram.

Management

The only definitive treatment is pericardectomy.

Antituberculous therapy may be required if the underlying cause is tuberculosis and should be continued for 1 year.

Pericardial effusion

A pericardial effusion is an accumulation of fluid in the pericardial space.

Cardiac tamponade describes the condition in which a pericardial effusion increases the intrapericardial pressure.

Causes

Causes of pericardial effusion (Fig. 21.5) include:

- Acute pericarditis (see Fig. 21.2).
- Myocardial infarction with ventricular wall rupture.
- Chest trauma.
- Cardiac surgery.
- Aortic dissection.
- Anticoagulation.

Causes of a pericardial effusion

Type of effusion	Examples
Transudate (<30g/L protein)	Congestive heart failure Hypoalbuminemia
Exudate (>30g/L protein)	Infection (viral, bacterial, or fungal) Post-myocardial infarction, malignancy (e.g., local invasion of lung tumor, systemic lupus erythematosus, Dressler's syndrome)
Hemorrhagic	Uremia, aortic dissection, trauma

Fig. 21.5 Causes of a pericardial effusion.

Clinical features

A pericardial effusion may remain asymptomatic, even if very large, if it accumulates gradually. As much as 2L of fluid can be accommodated without an increase in intrapericardial pressure if it accumulates slowly, but as little as 100mL can cause tamponade if it appears suddenly.

History

The only symptoms produced by a large chronic effusion may be a dull ache in the chest or dysphagia from compression of the esophagus.

If cardiac tamponade is present, however, the patient may complain of dyspnea, abdominal swelling (due to ascites), and peripheral edema.

Examination

The important examination findings in a patient who has tamponade are known as Beck's triad:

- Low blood pressure.
- Elevated JVP.
- In addition, the patient may have pulsus paradoxus—an exaggerated reduction of blood pressure (>10mmHg) during inspiration.
- Soft heart sounds (and rarely a pericardial rub).

Possible mechanisms for pulsus paradoxus

These are:

- Increased venous return during inspiration filling the right heart and restricting left ventricular filling because the pericardium forms a rigid sac with only limited space within it.
- Downward movement of the diaphragm causing traction on the pericardium and tightening it further (this theory is not widely supported).

Investigations

On the EKG a pericardial effusion results in the production of small voltage complexes with variable axis (electrical alternans is caused by the movement of the heart within the fluid). Low voltage in the presence of tachycardia or electrical alternans is highly specific for effusion or tamponade.

On chest radiography the heart may appear large and globular.

Echocardiography reveals the pericardial effusion. Right ventricular diastolic collapse is a classical echocardiographic sign of tamponade.

Management

The pericardial effusion should be drained.

If the patient is in cardiogenic shock due to tamponade, an emergency pericardial needle aspiration may be performed followed by formal drainage once the patient has been resuscitated.

Either technique involves insertion of the drain or needle just below the xiphisternum and advancing it at 45 degrees to the skin in the direction of the patient's left shoulder.

The fluid should be sent for cytology, microscopy, culture and biochemical analysis of protein content.

Long-term treatment depends upon the underlying cause.

22. Valvular Heart Disease

This topic has been touched upon in Chapters 6 and 10, but it is covered here in more detail. One way to learn valve disease in to learn it in parrot fashion. Once you know it, you will not forget it again, so it will be time well spent (Fig. 22.1).

Rheumatic fever

As mentioned in Chapter 23, rheumatic fever (RF) is much less common in the developed world than in developing countries due to better social conditions and antibiotic therapy and also because of a reduction in the virulence of beta-hemolytic streptococci. It is still a major problem in the developing world, where it is responsible for more heart disease than any other single entity.

Causes

RF is caused by a group A streptococcal pharyngeal infection. It occurs 2–3 weeks later in a small percentage of children aged 5–15 years. It is an antibody-mediated autoimmune response and occurs when antibodies directed against bacterial cell membrane antigens cross-react and cause multi-organ disease.

Clinical features

Diagnosis is entirely clinical. Diagnosis based on the Duckett–Jones criteria requires evidence of preceding beta-hemolytic streptococcal infection (e.g., increased anti-streptolysin O titers, positive throat cultures) plus two major criteria or the presence of one major criterion and two minor criteria. Major criteria are:

- Carditis—involves all layers (pancarditis) and is usually asymptomatic, although pleuritic chest pain and a friction rub can occur. In addition, the valves are often involved, and a new murmur may appear.
- Arthritis—a migrating polyarthritis affecting the larger joints, often the leg joints first. This is often the first manifestation of the disease.
- Sydenham's chorea—usually occurs months after the initial disease and is characterized by involuntary movements of the face and mouth (due to inflammation of the caudate nucleus), weakness, and emotional outbursts.
- Erythema marginatum—nonpruritic, seen mainly on the trunk; the rash has raised, sharp red edges and a clear center. The shape of the lesions changes with time.
- Nodules—hard, pea-sized subcutaneous nodules on the extensor surfaces that are painless. They are often seen over bony areas or tendons and rarely last for more than a month.

Minor criteria are:

- Fever.
- Previous rheumatic fever.
- Elevated erythrocyte sedimentation rate (ESR) or C-reactive protein (CRP).
- Long PR interval.
- Arthralgia.

Investigations

Blood tests reveal elevated inflammatory markers (ESR and CRP) and rising anti-streptolysin O (ASO) titers when taken 2 weeks apart. The throat swab may be positive.

Management

Treatment with high-dose benzylpenicillin is started immediately to eradicate the causative organism. Anti-inflammatory agents are given to suppress the autoimmune response. Aspirin is effective. Corticosteroids are used if carditis is present. Long-term follow-up is required, and any patients who have resulting valve damage need prophylactic antibiotics to prevent infective endocarditis. In addition, patients should be given antibiotic prophylaxis to prevent the recurrence of rheumatic fever, which can be common in the first 2 years following acute RF. The duration is unclear, but it is usually done until the patient is a young adult or for 10 years following the acute attack.

Acute rheumatic fever is extremely uncommon in the developed world, but it is a good idea to have a basic understanding of this disease because many elderly people still live with its after-effects. It is also important to recognize and treat acute rheumatic fever promptly.

Valve lesions and their abbreviations

Valve involved	Lesion
Mitral valve	Mitral stenosis (MS) Mitral regurgitation (MR) Mitral valve prolapse (MVP)
Aortic valve	Aortic stenosis (AS) Aortic regurgitation (AR)
Tricuspid valve	Tricuspid regurgitation (TR) Tricuspid stenosis (TS)
Pulmonary valve	Pulmonary stenosis (PS) Pulmonary regurgitation (PR)

Fig. 22.1 Valve lesions and their abbreviations.

Mitral stenosis

Causes

The most common cause of mitral stenosis (MS) is rheumatic fever (Fig. 22.2). Other causes are:

- Congenital (Lutembacher's syndrome—MS associated with an atrial septal defect).
- Malignant—carcinoid (rare).
- Annular calcification
- Systemic lupus erythematous and rheumatoid arthritis.
- Left atrial myxoma.

Rheumatic fever causes fusion of the cusps and commissures and thickening of the cusps, which then become immobile and stenosed in a fish-mouth configuration. An immobile valve often cannot close properly and is therefore often regurgitant as well. Rhuematic heart disease that leads to MS typically affects only women.

Clinical features

The main presenting features of MS are:

- Dyspnea—The stenotic mitral valve causes back pressure that results in pulmonary edema that can cause dyspnea. In addition, this chronic increase in

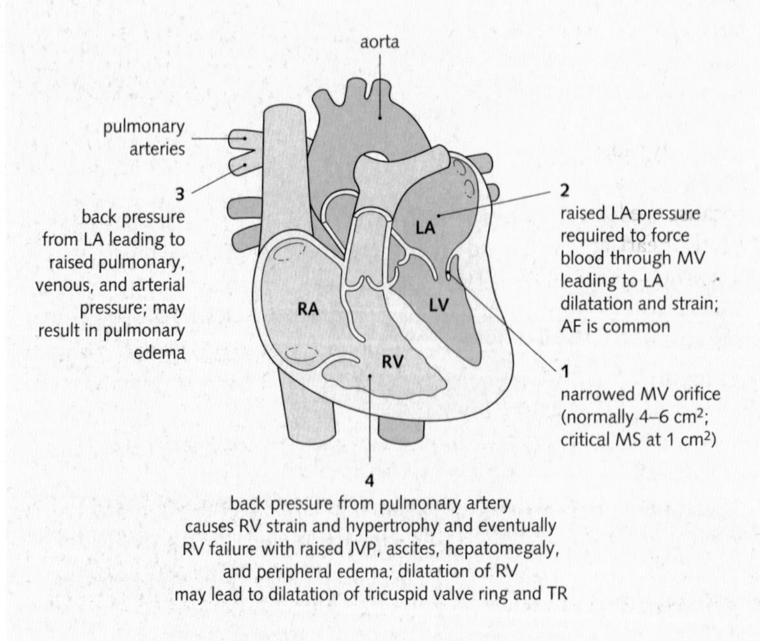
aorta
pulmonary arteries
3
back pressure from LA leading to raised pulmonary, venous, and arterial pressure; may result in pulmonary edema
LA
RA
LV
RV
2
raised LA pressure required to force blood through MV leading to LA dilatation and strain; AF is common
1
narrowed MV orifice (normally 4–6 cm^2; critical MS at 1 cm^2)
4
back pressure from pulmonary artery causes RV strain and hypertrophy and eventually RV failure with raised JVP, ascites, hepatomegaly, and peripheral edema; dilatation of RV may lead to dilatation of tricuspid valve ring and TR

Fig. 22.2 Pathophysiology of mitral stenosis. (LA, left atrium; LV, left ventricle; JVP, jugular venous pressure; MV, mitral valve; RA, right atrium; RV, right ventricle; TR, tricuspid regurgitation.)

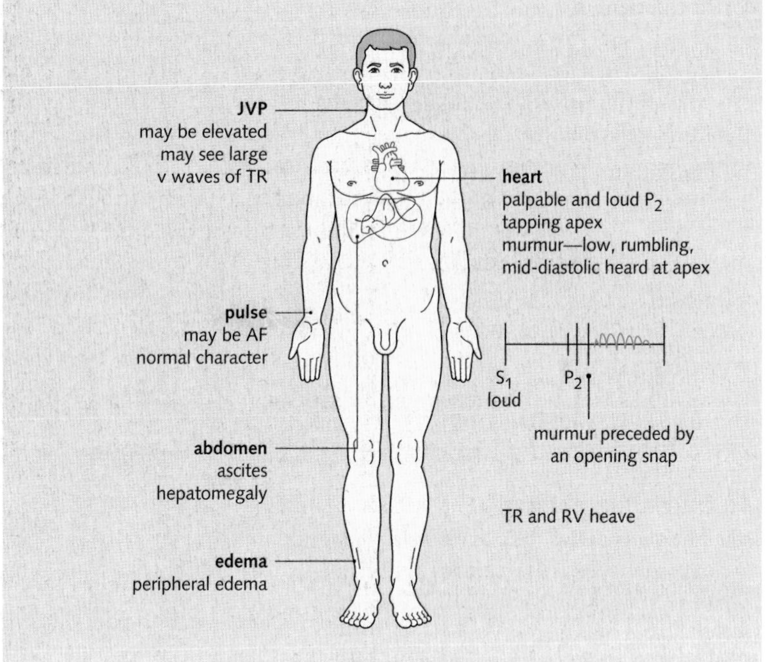

Fig. 22.3 Clinical findings in patients who have mitral stenosis. (AF, atrial fibrillation; S_1, first heart sound; P_2, pulmonary component of second heart sound.)

pulmonary venous pressure results in arterial changes that lead to pulmonary hypertension. Patients who have MS have an increased incidence of chest infections, which may cause dyspnea.

- Hemoptysis—there is an increased incidence of pulmonary vein and alveolar capillary rupture.
- Palpitations—atrial fibrillation is common in MS due to dilatation of the left atrium and may cause palpitations, which are often accompanied by a sudden worsening in the dyspnea because the loss of the atrial contraction (upon which the heart has become dependent) causes a considerable reduction in cardiac output.
- Systemic emboli—a recognized complication of atrial fibrillation.

Symptoms that are secondary to effects of left atrial enlargement include:

- Hoarseness due to stretching of the recurrent laryngeal nerve.
- Dysphagia due to esophageal compression.
- Left lung collapse due to compression of the left main bronchus.

> Mitral stenosis is a difficult murmur to hear. It is vital to listen for the murmur correctly (i.e., with the patient on his or her left side in full expiration). Unless you do this, you cannot say that you have excluded a diagnosis of mitral stenosis.

Examination

The principal clinical findings (Fig. 22.3) are:

- Loud first heart sound (S_1) due to the mitral valve slamming shut at the beginning of ventricular systole.
- A tapping apex beat that is not displaced.
- An opening snap after the second heart sound (S_2) followed by a low rumbling mid-diastolic murmur heard best at the apex with the patient on his or her left side and in expiration. If you have not listened in exactly this way, you cannot exclude MS.

- If the patient is in sinus rhythm, the mid-diastolic murmur has a presystolic accentuation; this is absent if the patient has atrial fibrillation. Severity is related to the duration, not the intensity of the mid-diastolic murmur.
- If pulmonary hypertension has developed, the pulmonary component of the second heart sound (P_2) is loud and palpable and there may be a right ventricular heave. Tricuspid regurgitation may be present.

Investigations

Investigations that may aid diagnosis include the following.

Electrocardiography

Atrial fibrillation may be seen. P mitrale is another feature and is seen only in sinus rhythm. The P wave in lead II is abnormally long (>0.12 sec) and may have an "M" shape.

Chest radiography

This shows the enlarged left atrium. The carina may be widely split. The mitral valve itself may be calcified and therefore visible. There may be prominent pulmonary vessels.

Doppler echocardiography

The mitral valve can be visualized and the cross-sectional area measured. The valve frequently has a "fish mouth" appearance on echocardiography. Pulmonary hypertension can also be measured. The degree of thickening, calcification, movement of valves, and regurgitation can also be measured. All of these factors influence the type and timing of a corrective procedure.

Cardiac catheterization

This is performed on most patients before valve replacement to exclude any coexistent coronary artery disease and evaluate any mitral regurgitation that may be present.

Management

Medical management

Medical treatment of MS may consist of:

- Digoxin or a small dose of a beta-blocker (beta-adrenoceptor antagonist)—may be used to treat atrial fibrillation. Direct current (DC) cardioversion may be successful in patients who have atrial fibrillation of recent onset, but only if they have been fully anticoagulated for at least 4 weeks. Digoxin is also appropriate if the patient is showing signs of heart failure. In addition, sotalol or amiodarone can be used to prevent the occurrence of atrial fibrillation, although this is often difficult given the frequent dilatation of the left atrium.
- Anticoagulation with warfarin is recommended in all patients who have MS and atrial fibrillation.
- Diuretics are used to treat the pulmonary and peripheral edema. Loop diuretics such as furosemide are especially important in the acute setting.

Surgical management

This is indicated in patients who have a mitral valve area of 1 cm^2 or less. Note that restenosis may occur after any valvuloplasty or valvotomy. In carefully selected patients this does not occur for many years; early restenosis within 5 years may occur in those who have thickened or rigid valves

Mitral valvuloplasty

Mitral valvuloplasty involves the passage of a balloon across the mitral valve and its inflation, thus stretching the stenosed valve. This procedure is carried out via a percutaneous route and requires only a local anesthetic and light sedation. The following features make a patient unsuitable for this procedure:

- Marked mitral regurgitation.
- A history of systemic emboli.
- Calcified or thickened rigid mitral valve leaflets.

Open mitral valvotomy

Open mitral valvotomy is performed under general anesthetic using a median sternotomy incision and requires cardiopulmonary bypass. It is used in patients who have already had a mitral valvuloplasty or who have mild mitral regurgitation.

Closed mitral valvotomy

This has now been superceded by mitral valvuloplasty. It does not require cardiopulmonary bypass. A curved incision is made under the left breast.

Mitral valve replacement

This is used for calcified or very rigid valves unsuitable for valvuloplasty or valvotomy.

Causes of mitral regurgitation (MR)	
Site of pathology	**Pathology**
Mitral annulus	Senile calcification Left ventricular dilatation and enlargement of the annulus Abscess formation during infective endocarditis
Mitral valve leaflets	Infective endocarditis Rheumatic fever Mitral valve prolapse Congenital malformation Connective tissue disorders—Marfan syndrome, Ehlers-Danlos syndrome, osteogenesis inperfecta, pseudoxanthoma elasticum
Chordae tendinae	Idiopathic rupture Myxomatous degeneration Infective endocarditis Connective tissue disorders
Papillary muscle	Myocardial infarction Infiltration—sarcoid, amyloid Myocarditis

Fig. 22.4 Causes of mitral regurgitation.

Mitral regurgitation

The mitral valve may become incompetent for four reasons (Fig. 22.4):

- Abnormal mitral valve leaflets or annulus.
- Abnormal myocardium surrounding the heart due to structural heart disease will also affect valve incompetence.
- Abnormal chordae tendinae.
- Abnormal papillary muscle function.

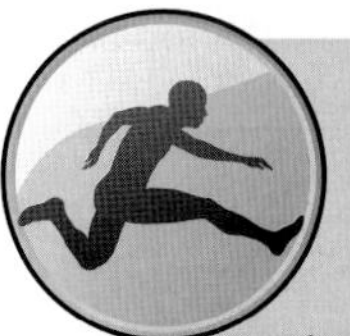

When considering the causes of regurgitation of any valve, it is useful to divide the causes into:

- Abnormalities of the valve ring.
- Abnormalities of the valve cusps and leaflets.
- Abnormalities of the supporting structures.

Pathophysiology

In mitral regurgitation (MR) the regurgitant jet of blood flows back into the left atrium, and with time the left atrium dilates and accommodates the increased volume and pressure. There is, however, also increased backpressure in the pulmonary veins, and as the MR worsens, pulmonary hypertension develops, which may eventually cause right ventricular hypertrophy and failure.

The left ventricle is dilated, because the blood entering from the left atrium with each beat is increased; this results in left ventricular hypertrophy and may, if severe, cause left ventricular dilatation and failure. Severe, chronic MR will, if not treated, results in biventricular failure. (Mitral stenosis differs because it does not cause left ventricular failure.)

Clinical features

These vary depending upon whether the MR is chronic or acute:

- Chronic MR develops slowly, allowing the heart to compensate, and usually presents with a history of fatigue, exercise intolerance, and dyspnea due to left ventricular dysfunction. Because of this compensation, symptoms usually do not present when with mild-to-moderate MR.
- Acute MR presents with severe dyspnea due to pulmonary edema. The left atrium has not had time to dilate to accommodate the increased volume due to regurgitation of blood back through the mitral valve. The pressure increase is therefore transmitted directly to the pulmonary veins, resulting in pulmonary edema.

Acute MR can be rapidly fatal and needs to be looked for in patients following myocardial infarction (papillary muscle rupture occurs at days 4–7 after myocardial infarction) and in patients who have infective endocarditis.

Examination

Features that may be seen are illustrated in Fig. 22.5 and include the following:

- Atrial fibrillation—an irregularly irregular pulse is common, especially in patients who have chronic MR and a dilated left atrium.
- Jugular venous pressure may be elevated—if the patient has developed pulmonary hypertension and right heart failure or fluid retention.

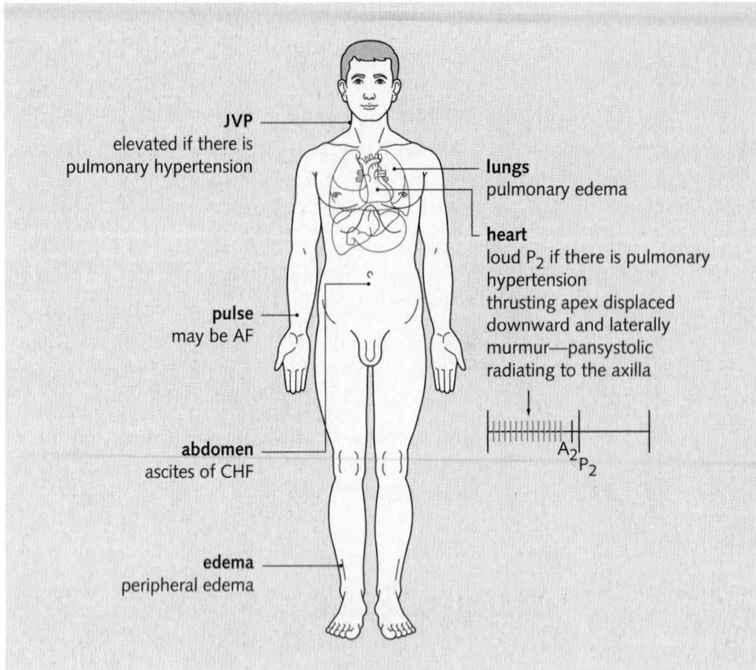

Fig. 22.5 Clinical findings in patients who have mitral regurgitation. (A_2, aortic component of second heart sound; AF, atrial fibrillation; CHF, congestive heart failure; P_2, pulmonary component of second heart sound.)

- The apex is displaced downward and laterally as the left ventricle dilates—eventually left ventricular failure may result. (Note that in MS the apex is not displaced because the left ventricle is protected by the stenosed mitral valve.)
- The murmur of MR is pansystolic and best heard at the apex. The murmur radiates to the axilla. Note that the loudness of the murmur is not an indicator of the severity of the MR. The murmur may increase with an increase in afterload, such as with squatting, and decrease with standing.
- Signs of congestive cardiac failure (i.e., third heart sound, bilateral basal inspiratory crepitations, ascites, peripheral edema).
- P_2 may be loud and there may be a right ventricular heave—if pulmonary hypertension has developed.

Investigations

The following investigations may aid diagnosis:

Electrocardiography

The EKG may show atrial fibrillation and left ventricular hypertrophy.

Chest radiography

An enlarged left ventricle may be seen as an increase in the cardiothoracic ratio. The mitral valve may be calcified and therefore visible.

Doppler echocardiography

The mitral valve can be clearly seen and the regurgitant jet visualized. The left atrium and ventricular sizes can be assessed.

Cardiac catheterization

Most patients have minimal MR on echocardiography and do not require catheterization. This is performed to assess the severity of the MR and to exclude other valve lesions and coronary artery disease.

Management

Patients who have a "compensated" form of MR, which is based on left ventricular dilatation, function, and clinical symptoms of heart failure, achieve the best results with surgical correction. Patients who have the "decompensated" form generally have poor alleviation of symptoms following intervention. It is important then to diagnose patients with MR early. In addition, if new-onset atrial fibrillation presents, it is generally better to perform surgery before this becomes chronic or resistant to electrical cardioversion.

Medical management

- Prophylaxis against infective endocarditis is indicated only in those patients who have MR.

- Most patients require no further treatment other than reassurance.

Medical management may consist of:
- Antiarrhythmics/anticoagulation to treat atrial fibrillation.
- Diuretics and angiotensin-converting enzyme (ACE) inhibitors to treat the congestive cardiac failure.

Surgical management
Patients are considered for surgery if the MR is severe at echocardiography and cardiac catheterization. Again, it is important to act before irreversible left ventricular damage has occurred.

Mitral valve repair
This may take the form of mitral annuloplasty, repair of a ruptured chordae, or repair of a mitral valve leaflet. These procedures are performed on patients who have mobile, noncalcified and nonthickened valves.

Mitral valve replacement
This is performed if mitral valve repair is not possible. Both repair and replacement of the mitral valve require a median sternotomy incision and cardiopulmonary bypass. The type of valve used depends on the age of the patient and risk of bleed on anticoagulation.

Mitral valve prolapse
Factors to consider are:
- This is a common disorder affecting approximately 4% of the population and more females than males.
- The mitral valve may merely prolapse minimally into the left atrium or cause varying degrees of MR.
- Most cases are idiopathic, but mitral valve prolapse is seen with greater frequency in certain conditions (e.g., Marfan syndrome and other connective tissue disorders). In addition, a familial form of MVP is also seen.
- Most patients are asymptomatic, the disorder being diagnosed at routine medical examination. Some patients present with fatigue, atypical chest pain, and palpitations.
- Examination reveals a mid-systolic click at the apex that moves closer to the first heart sound with standing or a reduction in afterload. This may or may not be followed by a systolic murmur of mitral regurgitation.

Causes of aortic stenosis (AS)

Type of AS	Cause
Valvular AS	Congenital; most common; males > females (deformed valve may be uni-, bi-, or tricuspid) Senile calcification Rheumatic fever Severe atherosclerosis
Subvalvular AS	Fibromuscular ring HOCM
Supravalvular AS	Associated with hypercalcemia in Williams's syndrome, a syndrome associated with elfin facies, mental retardation, strabismus, hypervitaminosis D, and hypercalcemia; the inheritance is autosomal dominant

Fig. 22.6 Causes of aortic stenosis. (HOCM, hypertrophic obstructive cardiomyopathy.)

Aortic stenosis

The most common form of aortic stenosis (AS) is valvular AS; however, aortic stenosis may also occur at the sub- or supravalvular level (Fig. 22.6).

Pathophysiology
The left ventricular outflow obstruction results in an increased left ventricular pressure. The left ventricle undergoes hypertrophy and more vigorous and prolonged contraction to overcome the obstruction and maintain an adequate cardiac output. Myocardial oxygen demand is increased, and because systole is prolonged, diastole is shortened. Therefore, myocardial blood supply from the coronary arteries is reduced (coronary artery flow occurs during diastole).

Clinical features
Patients are often asymptomatic for years before they present with symptoms. The most common valve abnormality associated with AS is a bicuspid aortic valve. In addition, certain risk factors accelerate the degree of stenosis, including: hypercalemia, hypercholesterolemia, exercise intolerance, renal

insufficiency, degree of calcification, and the velocity of the blood leaving the aortic root.

Patients are often asymptomatic; however, a number of symptoms are characteristic of AS, including:

- Dyspnea/congestive heart failure symptoms—may lead to orthopnea and paroxysmal nocturnal dyspnea as the left ventricle fails.
- Angina—due to the increased myocardial work and reduced blood supply (the coronary arteries may be normal).
- Dizziness and syncope—especially on exertion.
- Sudden death.
- Systemic emboli.

Patients who have aortic stenosis may present with angina, but an exercise test is absolutely contraindicated in patients with severe aortic stenosis because even the mildest exertion can cause syncope or sudden death. Therefore, it is crucial to examine every patient carefully before recommending an exercise EKG.

Examination

The following findings are common in valvular AS (Fig. 22.7):

- Pulsus tardus—A slow rising, small volume pulse, best felt at the carotid pulse.
- Low blood pressure.
- Heaving apex beat—rarely displaced.
- Harsh crescendo-decrescendo systolic "ejection" murmur at the aortic area, radiating to the carotids and accompanied by a palpable thrill.
- Signs of left ventricular or biventricular failure.

Investigations

Electrocardiography

This usually shows sinus rhythm and a picture of left ventricular hypertrophy with strain (tall R wave in lead V5 with deep S wave in lead V2 and T wave inversion in lateral leads).

Chest radiography

An enlarged cardiac shadow may occur due to left ventricular hypertrophy. The valve may be calcified and therefore visible. There may also be evidence of pulmonary edema.

Echocardiography

This will show the valve in great detail, including the number of cusps and their mobility and the presence

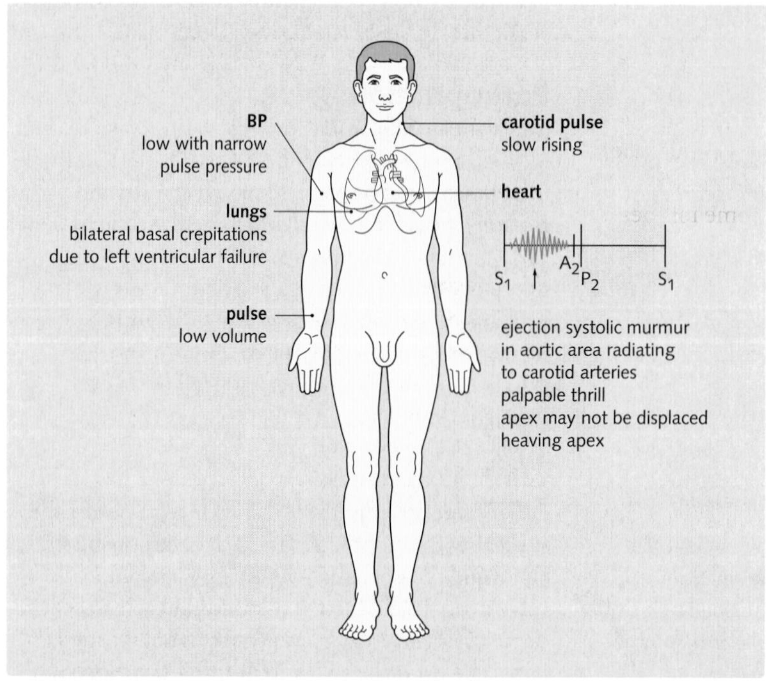

Fig. 22.7 Clinical findings in patients who have aortic stenosis.

of calcification. It will also show left ventricular hypertrophy or failure, and the aortic valve gradient can be measured using Doppler echocardiography.

Cardiac catheterization

This may provide information about the valve gradient and left ventricular failure, if not available from echocardiography. The coronary arteries are also assessed to rule out coronary artery disease that will require bypass grafting.

Management

Once the patient becomes symptomatic, survival is diminished. The median survival after angina presents is only 5 years. In addition, median survival after syncope occurs is three years, and after symptoms of heart failure occur, it is only two years. Surgical repair should be undertaken the minute any LV dysfunction occurs since this is often not reversible.

Medical management

Currently no medical therapy is available for AS. Apart from the use of diuretics to treat left ventricular failure, many antianginal drugs and ACE inhibitors are avoided in AS because:

- They may have a negative inotropic effect and result in acute pulmonary edema.
- They may vasodilate the patient, resulting in hypotension, because the left ventricle is unable to compensate by increasing cardiac output.

Surgical management

This is considered in all symptomatic patients who have marked stenosis (aortic valve gradient >50 mmHg). Without operation the outcome for these patients is very poor.

Aortic valve replacement is usually performed using a median sternotomy incision and requires cardiopulmonary bypass.

Aortic valvuloplasty is performed in children and rarely in the very elderly.

Aortic regurgitation

Aortic regurgitation (AR) may be due to an abnormality of the valve cusps themselves or dilatation of the aortic root and therefore the valve ring (Fig. 22.8).

Causes of AR

Type of disease	Cause
Valve disease	Congenital Rheumatic fever Infective endocarditis Rheumatoid arthritis SLE Connective tissue disease (e.g., Marfan syndrome, pseudoxanthoma elasticum)
Aortic root disease	Marfan syndrome Osteogenesis imperfecta Type A aortic dissection Ankylosing spondylitis Reiter's syndrome Psoriatic arthritis

Fig. 22.8 Causes of aortic regurgitation. (SLE, systemic lupus erythematosus.)

Pathophysiology

The regurgitation of blood back into the left ventricle after each systole results in an increased end-diastolic volume and an increased stroke volume. The left ventricle works harder and becomes hypertrophied. If the AR worsens, the left ventricle may no longer be able to compensate and left ventricular failure will result. If the situation deteriorates, further congestion results. The backpressure from the left ventricle may also cause pulmonary hypertension and right ventricular failure, but this is uncommon.

Clinical features

Moderate and mild cases of AR are often asymptomatic. Dyspnea is the main presenting feature (Fig. 22.9).

Symptoms

Patients often remain asymptomatic for years, despite moderate AR. Common symptoms when they do occur are:

- Palpitations.
- Atypical chest pain.
- A pounding heartbeat or awareness of heart beating.

Examination

Characteristic findings in aortic regurgitation are:

- A collapsing high-volume pulse (waterhammer pulse)—due to the increased stroke volume and

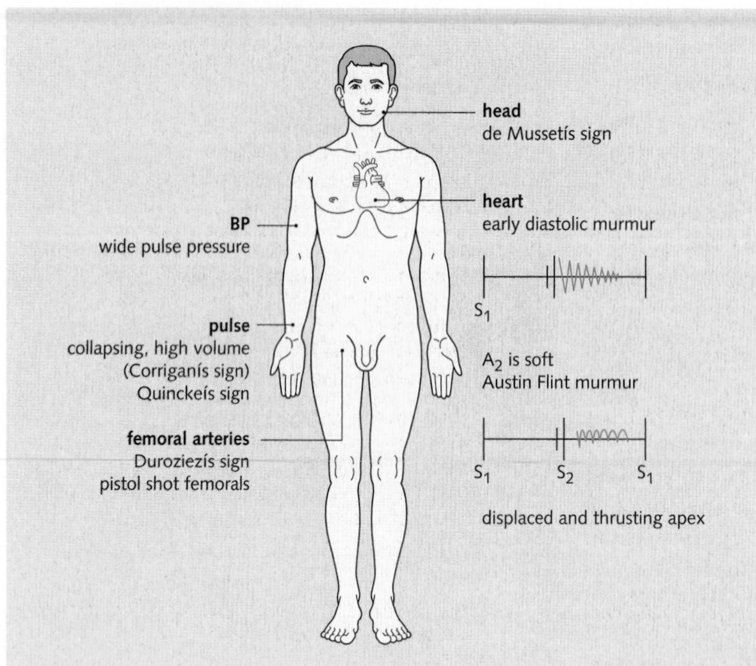

Fig. 22.9 Clinical findings in patients who have aortic regurgitation. (A_2, aortic component of second heart sound; S_1, first heart sound; S_2, second heart sound.)

the rapid run-off of blood back into the left ventricle after systole. This is better felt at the carotid pulse but can be felt at the radial pulse by lifting the arm and feeling the pulse with the fingers across it. The tapping quality is felt between the examiner's middle and distal interphalangeal joints.

- A wide pulse pressure on measuring blood pressure.
- Downward and laterally displaced apex, which has a thrusting nature.
- Murmur best heard at the left lower sternal edge with the patient sitting forward and in full expiration—it is a soft, high-pitched, early diastolic murmur, which is sometimes difficult to hear. Be sure to listen for it properly with a diaphragm.
- Increased flow across the aortic valve may produce an ejection systolic murmur.
- Signs of left ventricular or congestive failure may be present.
- Other signs include De Musset's sign (head bobbing with each beat), Quincke's sign (visible capillary pulsation in the nailbed), pistol shot femoral pulses (an audible femoral sound), and Duroziez's sign (another audible murmur over the femoral arteries—a to-and-fro sound).
- The Austin Flint murmur may be heard when the regurgitant jet causes vibration of the anterior mitral valve leaflet. The murmur is similar to that of MS but with no opening snap.

Investigations

Electrocardiography

The EKG shows left ventricular hypertrophy.

Chest radiography

The left ventricle may be enlarged, and pulmonary edema may be seen.

Echocardiography

The structure of the aortic valve and the size of the regurgitant jet may be seen. Left ventricular function can be assessed. Echocardiography usually results in the definitive diagnosis of AR.

Cardiac catheterization

This is the most accurate way to assess the severity of aortic regurgitation and also to assess the aortic root, although it is usually used only if less invasive testing is not conclusive. Left ventricular function can also be evaluated, as can the presence of coronary artery disease.

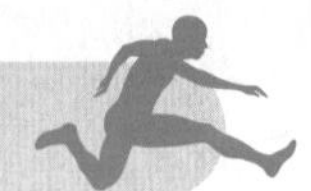

Management

Medical management

For acute management, the use of hydralazine, nitroprusside, or nifedipine will reduce the afterload or systolic resistance and allow more forward flow of blood. The use of diuretics and ACE inhibitors is valuable to treat cardiac failure in these patients. It is, however, important to make the diagnosis and surgically treat this condition before the left ventricle dilates and fails.

Surgical management

Aortic valve replacement is considered if the patient is symptomatic with severe AR, or if there are signs of progressive left ventricular dilatation. The aortic root may also need to be replaced if it is grossly dilated.

Assessing the severity of a valve lesion

Once a valve lesion has been diagnosed, it is useful to be able to comment on its severity. This is judged by clinical, echocardiographic, and angiographic means in most cases (Fig. 22.10).

Features indicating severity of valve disease

Valve	Features disease
MS	Proximity of opening snap to second heart sound and duration of murmur Valve area assessed on echocardiography Evidence of pulmonary hypertension on echocardiography and cardiac catheterization
MR	Symptoms and signs of pulmonary edema Size of regurgitant jet and poor left ventricular function on echocardiography Evidence of pulmonary hypertension on echocardiography and cardiac catheterization
AS	Presence of symptoms. Low volume pulse and BP Severity of aortic gradient and poor left ventricular function on echocardiography or cardiac catheterization
AR	Signs of LVF Left ventricular function and size of regurgitant jet at cardiac catheterization (echocardiography is useful but not as informative)

Fig. 22.10 Features indicating severity of valve disease. (AS, aortic stenosis; AR, aortic regurgitation; BP, blood pressure; LVF, left ventricular failure; MS, mitral stenosis; MR, mitral regurgitation.)

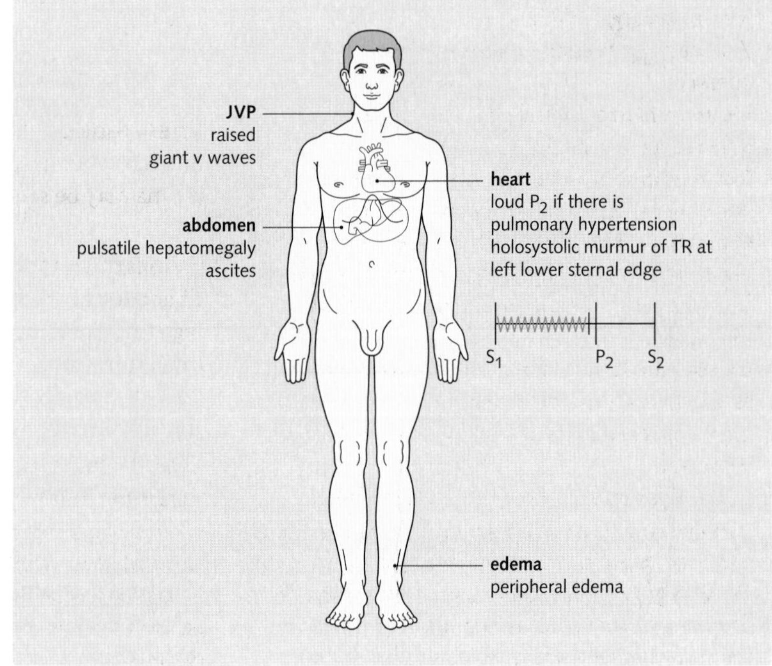

Fig. 22.11 Clinical findings in patients who have tricuspid regurgitation. Look out for signs of the underlying cause of right heart failure such as mitral valve disease or pulmonary disease. (JVP, jugular venous pressure; P_2, pulmonary component of second heart sound; S_1, first heart sound; S_2, second heart sound.)

Overview of other valve lesions			
Valve lesion	**Cause**	**Clinical features**	**Management**
Tricuspid stenosis	Rheumatic fever; rare	Venous congestion—JVP raised, large a waves, ascites, hepatomegaly, peripheral edema, soft diastolic murmur at left lower sternal edge	Treat pulmonary hypertension, valve replacement
Pulmonary stenosis	Congenital malformation—Noonan's syndrome, maternal rubella syndrome, carcinoid syndrome	If mild, asymptomatic; if severe—RVF and cyanosis, ejection systolic murmur in pulmonary area (2nd left ICS), wide splitting of second heart sound	Pulmonary valvuloplasty or pulmonary valve replacement
Pulmonary regurgitation (PR)	Dilatation of the valve ring secondary to pulmonary hypertension, infective endocarditis	RVF in severe cases, low-pitched diastolic murmur in pulmonary area, Graham Steell murmur—in severe PR the murmur is high-pitched due to the forceful jet and best heard at the left parasternal edge (i.e., similar to that in AR, but with signs of severe pulmonary hypertension and RVF)	Treat underlying disease

Fig. 22.12 Overview of other valve lesions. (ICS, intercostal space; JVP, jugular venous pressure; RVF, right ventricular failure.)

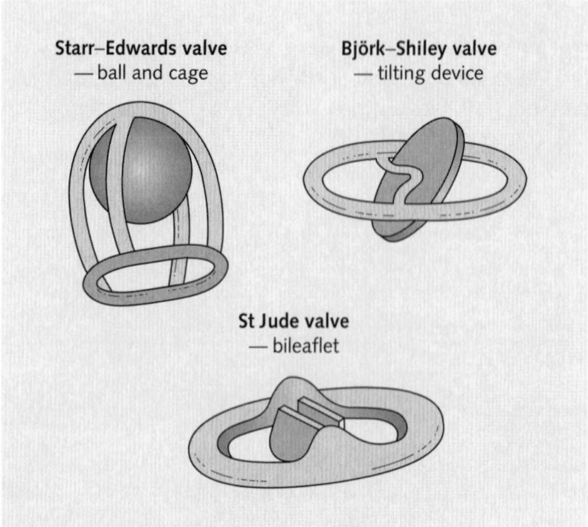

Fig. 22.13 Types of mechanical heart valve. Note that all patients must be anticoagulated for life, and the international normalized ratio (INR) must be kept at approximately 3–4. This lowers the risk of thromboembolism. Mechanical valves last for about 15 years. All patients who have prosthetic valves require antibiotic prophylaxis against infective endocarditis.

Types of biological heart valve	
Type of valve	**Features**
Xenograft	Manufactured from porcine valve or pericardium and mounted on a frame (on chest X-ray only the mounting ring can be seen) Lasts for about 10 years
Homograft	Cadaveric valve graft More durable than a xenograft

Fig. 22.14 Types of biological heart valve. Anticoagulation is necessary only if the patient has atrial fibrillation. All patients require antibiotic prophylaxis against infective endocarditis.

Tricuspid regurgitation

Causes

Most cases of tricuspid regurgitation (TR) result from dilatation of the tricuspid annulus due to dilatation of the right ventricle. This may be due to any cause of right ventricular failure or pulmonary hypertension.

Occasionally the tricuspid valve is affected by infective endocarditis (usually in intravenous drug abusers).

Rarer causes include congenital malformations and the carcinoid syndrome.

Ebstein's anomaly

This congenital malformation is caused by downward displacement of the tricuspid valve into the body of the right ventricle. The valve is regurgitant and malformed. The condition is associated with other structural cardiac abnormalities and a high incidence of both supraventricular and ventricular tachyarrhythmias.

Clinical features

The symptoms and signs are due to the backpressure effects of the regurgitant jet into the right atrium, which are transmitted to the venous system causing a prominent v wave in the jugular venous waveform (Fig. 22.11).

Fatigue and discomfort due to ascites or hepatic congestion are the most common feature. Patients usually present with symptoms of the disease causing the underlying right ventricular failure; the TR is often an incidental finding.

Management

The mainstay of management is medical with diuretics and ACE inhibitors to treat the right ventricular failure and fluid overload.

Tricuspid valve replacement is considered in very severe cases.

Other valve lesions

These are summarized in Fig. 22.12.

Prosthetic heart valves

Examples of mechanical and biological heart valves are shown in Figs 22.13 and 22.14.

23. Infective Endocarditis

Definition and diagnosis of infective endocarditis

Infective endocarditis refers to infection of the endothelial surface of the heart by a microorganism. Heart valves are most commonly affected, but any area causing a high-pressure jet through a narrow orifice may be involved (e.g., ventricular septal defect). Diagnostic criteria and causative organisms are listed in Fig. 23.1.

Epidemiology of infective endocarditis

Infective endocarditis is an evolving disease. Traditionally the main predisposing condition was rheumatic fever; however, in developed countries rheumatic fever is much less common due to better social conditions and antibiotic therapy. Now in developed countries different groups of patients are presenting with infective endocarditis for the following reasons:

- Increased number of prosthetic valve insertions.
- Increased number of patients who have congenital heart disease surviving to adulthood.
- Increasing elderly population.
- Increasing intravenous drug abuse.
- Antibiotic resistance.

With this change in the population affected by infective endocarditis, the organisms are also changing (Fig. 23.1). People who have certain conditions (Fig. 23.1) should be advised about the importance of antibiotic prophylaxis (often with 2g of amoxicillin prior to procedure) before certain procedures to prevent infective endocarditis. These procedures are as follows:

- Any dental work.
- Any operation.
- Any instrumentation of the urinary tract or gastrointestinal tract.
- Any transrectal procedure (e.g., prostatic biopsy, colonoscopy with biopsy).

The antibiotics used for prophylaxis vary. Advice should be sought from a microbiologist

Pathophysiology of infective endocarditis

The development of endocarditis depends upon a number of factors:

- Presence of anatomical abnormalities in the heart surface.
- Hemodynamic abnormalities within the heart.
- Host immune response.
- Virulence of the organism.
- Presence of bacteremia.

Transient bacteremia is a common occurrence, but infective endocarditis is rare; a healthy individual who has normal cardiac anatomy is well protected (Fig. 23.2).

Complications of infective endocarditis are potentially fatal and are as follows:

- Local destructive effects—valve incompetence, paravalvular abscesses, prosthetic valve dehiscence, and myocardial rupture. If they progress, the local effects lead to congestive heart failure and cardiogenic shock; sometimes this is very rapid.
- Embolization of infected or noninfected fragments—these can result in stroke or cerebral abscess, ischemic bowel, digital infarcts, renal and hepatic abscesses, renal infarcts (hepatic infarcts are rare because the liver is supplied by the hepatic artery and the hepatic portal system).
- Type III autoimmune reaction to the organism—resulting in the deposition of immune complexes (antibody plus antigen) and a subsequent inflammatory response. A diffuse or focal glomerulonephritis and arthritis may occur as a result.

Diagnostic criteria for infective endocarditis

Diagnosis of infective endocarditis requires 2 major criteria *or* 1 major plus 3 minor criteria *or* 5 minor criteria.

Major criteria:
- Persistently positive blood cultures
- Typical causative organisms: viridans streptococci, *Streptococcus bovis*, HACEK organisms (*Hemophilu paraninfluenzae*, *H. aphrophilus*, *Actinobacillus ectinomycetemcomitans*, *Cardiobacterium hominis*, *Eikinella corrodens*, *Kingellakingae*), community-acquired *Staphylococcus aureus*, or enterococci in the absence of primary focus
- Persistent bacteremia: ≥2 positive cultures separated by ≥12 hr or ≥3 positive cultures ≥1 hr apart or 70% blood culture samples positive if ≥4 are drawn
- Evidence of endocardial involvement
- Positive echocardiogram
- Oscillating vegetation
- Abscesses
- Valve perforation
- New partial dehiscence of prosthetic valve
- New valvular regurgitation

Minor criteria:
- Predisposing condition: mitral valve prolapse with mitral regurgitation (rare in isolated mitral valve prolapse), bicuspid aortic valve, rheumatic heart disease, complex congenital heart disease* (transposition of the great arteries, single ventricle states, tetralogy of Fallot), prosthetic valve (including bioprosthetic and homograft valves), intravenous drug abuse (most commonly affects tricuspid valve), recent myocardial infarction (mural thrombus may become infected), hypertrophic cardiomyopathy, surgically constructed systemic pulmonary shunts or conduits
- Fever
- Vascular condition: major arterial emboli, septic pulmonary emboli, mycotic aneurysm, intracranial hemorrhage, Janeway lesions
- Immunologic condition: glomerulonephritis, Osler's nodes, Roth spots, rheumatoid factor
- Positive blood cultures not meeting major criteria
- Positive echocardiogram not meeting major criteria

*Isolated secundum atrial defect and surgical repair of atrial septal defect, ventricular septal defect, or patent ductus arteriosus (without residua beyond 6 months) confer no additional risk.

Fig. 23.1 Diagnostic criteria for infective endocarditis.

Conditions predisposing to transient bacteremia

Dental work—the most common cause; note that any type of dental work may give rise to it (even cleaning)*
Intravenous drug abuse
Invasive procedures—intravenous cannulation, cystoscopy;* catheterization, surgery of any sort; any transrectal procedure*
Bowel sepsis

Fig. 23.2 Conditions predisposing to transient bacteremia. Note that upper gastrointestinal endoscopy and esophagogastroduodenoscopy are not thought to require antibiotic prophylaxis. *Procedures that are usually covered with prophylactic antibiotics.

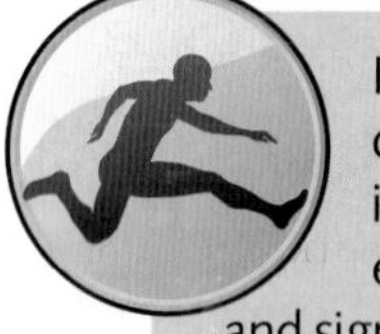

If you remember these three classes of complications of infective endocarditis, it is easy to fit actual symptoms and signs into each category. To classify signs according to the pathophysiology shows that you have a full understanding of the disease process.

Clinical features of infective endocarditis

History

The duration of the symptoms varies from a few days to several months. This tends to reflect the virulence of the organism—*Staphylococcus aureus* causes rapid

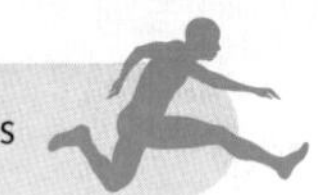

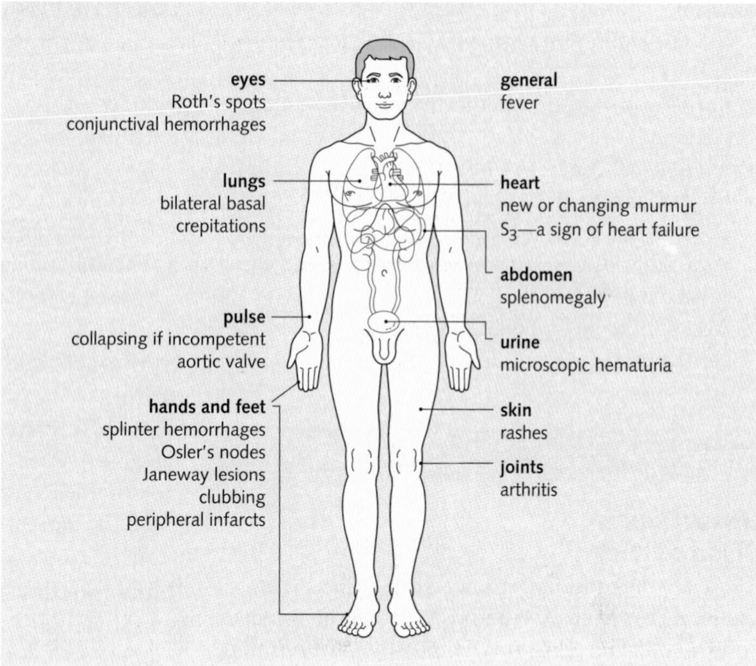

Fig. 23.3 Important clinical findings in patients who have infective endocarditis.

valvular destruction and presents early whereas a *Staphylococcus epidermidis* infection of a prosthetic valve may take a few months to present.

The following symptoms are common:

- Fever.
- Sweats.
- Anorexia and weight loss.
- General malaise.

Stroke is also seen as a presenting complaint, or myalgia and arthralgia. Important information to obtain from the patient for clues about the causative organism includes:

- A detailed history of any dental work, operations, or infections.
- Any history of rheumatic fever.
- Any history of intravenous drug abuse.

It is also important to find out about any drug allergies because long-term intravenous antibiotics may be needed.

Examination

A thorough examination is vital because it is sometimes possible to make the diagnosis on examination alone, which allows therapy to be started promptly. Failure to make the diagnosis early may have disastrous consequences because it is not uncommon to see this disease causing rapid valve destruction and cardiogenic shock. A full examination is required because the signs occur in all systems (Fig. 23.3).

The following signs are characteristic of infective endocarditis:

- A murmur—the heart murmur is usually that of an incompetent valve because the infection often prevents the valve from closing either due to perforation of the valve leaflets or vegetations and adhesions impeding valve movement. It is important to perform daily cardiac auscultation because the murmur may change due to progressive valve damage; this warns of imminent valve failure and an urgent echocardiogram is then necessary to evaluate the degree of valvular incompetence. The murmur of mitral regurgitation becomes louder as the regurgitation gets worse. The murmur of aortic regurgitation also gets louder and longer.
- Splenomegaly—a common finding, especially if the history is long.
- Clubbing—develops after a few weeks of infective endocarditis. Other causes of clubbing include cyanotic congenital heart disease, suppurative lung disease, squamous cell carcinoma of the lung, and inflammatory bowel disease.
- Splinter hemorrhages—more than four is pathological (remember that the most common cause of these is trauma).

- Osler's nodes (which are painful) and Janeway lesions—represent peripheral emboli (possibly septic).
- Roth's spots—retinal hemorrhages with a pale center.
- Evidence of congestive heart failure.
- Microscopic hematuria on urine dipstick—always ask to dipstick the urine if you suspect infective endocarditis. This is a very sensitive test and easily carried out.
- Also peripheral emboli, features of a cerebrovascular event, inflamed joints.

Investigations

Blood tests

Blood cultures

These are the most important investigations. Note the plural has been used because at least three sets of cultures must be performed. If possible, they should be taken at least 1 hour apart before commencing antibiotic therapy. (If the patient is very ill and there is a high index of suspicion of infective endocarditis, it is appropriate to start antibiotics after the first set has been obtained.)

Positive blood cultures are usually obtained in at least 95% cases of bacterial endocarditis if taken before antibiotic therapy. This allows therapy to be specifically directed according to the sensitivity of the organism. Remember that the HACEK organism (listed in Fig. 23.1) can also cause bacterial endocarditis. These are slow-growing and may delay the exact identification of the organisam via blood culture. In rare cases fungal organisms can cause endocarditis. In such cases surgery and antifungals are the appropriate therapy.

When taking blood cultures it is important to maintain a good aseptic technique to minimize the risk of contaminating the samples. Clean the skin with iodine-containing skin wash (or the equivalent if the patient has iodine allergy). Take the blood and then inject it into the culture bottles, using new needles.

Complete blood count

Anemia of chronic disease is common in patients who have less acute presentations. Other findings can include:

- Leukocytosis—may be seen as a sign of inflammation (usually a neutrophilia).
- Thrombocytopenia—may be an indication of disseminated intravascular coagulopathy.
- Thrombophilia—may be seen as part of the acute phase response.

Erythrocyte sedimentation rate and C-reactive protein

These are elevated as signs of inflammation. They are valuable markers of disease activity and repeated measurements every few days provide information about the patient's response to treatment.

Renal function tests

Renal function may be impaired due to infarction or immune complex-mediated glomerulonephritis. These tests also needsrepeating every few days during treatment as both aminoglycoside antibiotics and disease progression may cause renal impairment.

Liver function tests

These may be deranged due to septic microemboli.

Urinalysis

As well as the bedside urine dipstick, formal urine microscopy should be performed to look for casts as seen in glomerulonephritis.

Chest radiography

This may be clear or may show signs of pulmonary edema.

Echocardiography

Transthoracic echocardiography will reveal any valve incompetence and may also identify vegetations on the valve. This test is not very sensitive and cannot be used to exclude small vegetations.

Transesophageal echocardiography is over 90% sensitive in diagnosing vegetations.

Remember that echocardiography is not a diagnostic test in infective endocarditis. It may help confirm the diagnosis and give information about the severity of the valve damage, but blood cultures are the only specific diagnostic test of infective endocarditis.

Suggested antibiotic regimens

Staphylococcal endocarditis in the absence of prosthetic material
Methicillin-susceptible staphylococci
Nafcillin or oxacillin, 2 g IV every 4 hr for 4–6 wk, with optional addition of gentamicin, 1 mg/kg IM or IV every 8 hr for 3–5 days
For patients allergic to beta-lactam drugs: cefazolin, 2 g every 8 hr for 4–6 wk, with optional addition of gentamicin, 1 mg/kg IM or IV every 8 hr for 3–5 days
For patients allergic to penicillin: vancomycin, 30 mg/kg IV every 24 hr for 4–6 wk in two equally divided doses, not to exceed 2 g/day unless serum levels are monitored
Methicillin-resistant staphylococci
Vancomycin, 30 mg/kg IV every 24 hr for 4–6 wk in two equally divided doses, not to exceed 2 g/day unless serum levels are monitored

Native valve endocarditis due to viridans streptococci and *S. bovis(MIC≤0.1μg/mL)**
Four-week regimens
Aqueous crystalline penicillin G, 12–18 million U/24 hr IV continuously or in 6 equally divided doses (preferred in most patients over 65 and patients with impaired renal function) *or*
Ceftriaxone, 2 g once daily IV or IM
For patients allergic to beta-lactam drugs: vancomycin, 30 mg/kg IV every 24 hr in two equally divided doses, not to exceed 2 g/day unless serum levels are monitored
Two-week regimen
Aqueous crystalline penicillin G, dosed as above, with gentamicin, 1 mg/kg IM or IV every 8 hr

Endocarditis due to HACEK organisms
Ceftriaxone, 2 g once daily IV or IM for 4 wk
Ampicillin, 12 g/24 hr IV either continuously or in 6 equally divided doses with gentamicin, 1 mg/kg IM or IV every 8 hr for 4 wk

Fig. 23.4 Suggested antibiotic regimens. (Data from Wilson WR, Karchmer AW, Dajani AS, et al: JAMA 1995;274:1706.)

Management of infective endocarditis

There are two main aims in the management of infective endocarditis:

- To effectively treat the infection with appropriate antibiotics with the minimum of drug-related complications.
- To diagnose and treat complications of the endocarditis (e.g., congestive heart failure, severe valve incompetence, peripheral abscesses, renal failure).

Antibiotic therapy

If infective endocarditis is suspected, antibiotic therapy is started as soon as the blood cultures have been taken (Fig. 23.4). The choice of agent can then be modified once the organism is known.

Intravenous therapy is used initially in all cases. This may be via the central or peripheral route. It is vital that the intravenous access sites are changed regularly to prevent infection (peripheral lines every 3 days, non-tunneled central lines every 5–7 days). The sites should be inspected regularly and the line removed immediately if there is evidence of local infection.

Choice of antibiotic regimen

An infectious disease specialist is the best person to decide what the antibiotic regimen should be, and all cases of infective endocarditis should be reported to the infectious disease specialist as soon as possible, even if blood cultures are negative.

Duration of antibiotic therapy

This depends upon the organism and the clinical response to treatment. Most bacterial infections require at least 6 weeks of intravenous therapy, although in rare cases some centers change to oral therapy after 2 weeks if the response is good.

Another option is the placement of a PICC line for long-term IV antibiotics as an outpatient. Home nursing can usually be arranged to give the antibiotics through the PICC line at the patient's home. The most important thing to remember is that the patient must be closely monitored after changing to oral therapy and after stopping therapy. If there is any evidence of recurrent disease activity, intravenous therapy should be recommenced.

Monitoring antibiotic therapy

Blood should be taken for:

- Antibiotic levels (gentamicin, vancomycin).
- To calculate the minimum inhibitory concentration (MIC)—the MIC gives an indication of the sensitivity of the organism to the antibiotics used. If it is not satisfactory another antimicrobial may be added.

In addition to antibiotic therapy the source of infection should be sought—the patient needs a thorough dental examination and any infected teeth removed because this is a common cause of recurrent bacteraemia. Similarly recurrent urinary tract infections should be prevented with prophylactic antibiotics.

Complications of infective endocarditis

The following complications may occur:

- Congestive heart failure—the use of diuretics and angiotensin-converting enzyme inhibitors may be necessary. If heart failure remains severe due to profound valvular regurgitation, surgery to replace the valve is required.
- Thromboembolic complications—the use of anticoagulants is controversial; however, anticoagulation is used for patients who have thrombotic phenomena such as pulmonary embolus or deep venous thrombosis. Patients who have metal prosthetic valves should remain on their anticoagulation. Patients who have cerebral or peripheral arterial emboli are not anticoagulated because there is a risk of hemorrhage into the infarct.

Monitoring of patients with infective endocarditis

This should include:

- Daily examination—this is the most important aspect of monitoring. Look for worsening valvular incompetence, heart failure, new splinter hemorrhages, Roth's spots, Osler's nodes, etc., all suggestive of ongoing active disease.

Indications for valve replacement in infective endocarditis
Significant aortic or mitral regurgitation despite prolonged antibiotic therapy
Persistent infection despite prolonged antibiotic therapy
Large vegetations—these have a high incidence of embolization and can obstruct the valve orifice
Aortic root abscess
Unstable prosthetic valve (usually affects the sewing ring around prosthetic valves resulting in a perivalvular leak and occasionally dehiscence of the valve—this is an extremely dangerous condition and patients who have a significant perivalvular leak should be considered for valve replacement)

Fig. 23.5 Indications for valve replacement in infective endocarditis.

- Temperature chart—an increase in temperature after the patient has been afebrile for some time can represent reactivation of the infection and blood cultures should be sent immediately.
- Daily urine dipstick for microscopic hematuria—this is representative of disease activity.
- Daily blood tests for complete blood count, renal function, erythrocyte sedimentation rate, C-reactive protein, and liver function.
- Weekly EKG—look for lengthening of the PR interval. If an abscess develops around the aortic root or in the septum, this affects the atrioventricular node and may lead to complete heart block.
- Weekly echocardiography—to assess vegetation size if they are visible, but more importantly to assess left ventricular function and the severity of the valve incompetence.

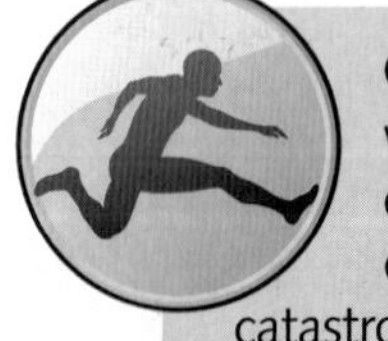

Close monitoring of patients with infective endocarditis is crucial because any deterioration can lead to catastrophic valve incompetence if missed.

Operative intervention in active infective endocarditis carries a high mortality rate and marked morbidity. Indications for replacement of the infected valve are listed in Fig. 23.5. The patient should receive a full course of intravenous antibiotic treatment (at least 6 weeks) postoperatively.

24. Hypertension

Hypertension is a major risk factor for cerebrovascular disease, myocardial infarction, heart failure, peripheral vascular disease, and renal failure. To reduce these risks, it is important to diagnose and adequately treat hypertensive patients.

Definition of hypertension

Normal blood pressure (BP) increases with age and varies throughout the day according to factors such as stress and exertion. There is also an underlying diurnal variation, with the lowest BP at around 4 AM. It is now thought that those who do not exhibit this diurnal variation are also hypertensive despite the fact that they may not fall into the categories listed below.

The definition of hypertension is that level of BP associated with an increased risk of complications. The new JNC 7 guidelines for hypertention define normal BP as less than 120/80mmHg, prehypertention as 120–139/80–89mmHg, stage I hypertension as 140–159/90–99mmHg, and stage II hypertension as >160/>100mmHg. In patients with DM or renal disease, the target BP is 130/80mmHg.

Causes of hypertension

Over 95% cases of hypertension are idiopathic and thus are termed essential hypertension.

Secondary causes of hypertension, although rare, are important to exclude because they may be curable (Fig. 24.1).

Whenever trying to learn a list of causes like the one in Fig. 24.1, most of your effort should be spent learning the main headings (i.e.. classification). This will trigger your memory, and you will be able to recall at least two conditions for each category.

Clinical features of hypertension

These are described in Chapter 7 and will not be repeated word for word here. The following is a summary of the clinical features of hypertension.

History

Most patients are entirely asymptomatic, but the presenting complaint may be headache, dizziness, or fainting.

There is no correlation between symptoms and severity of hypertension in the vast majority of patients.

When checking the past medical history, ask about other risk factors for ischemic heart disease such as:

- Smoking.
- Age/male sex.
- Diabetes mellitus.
- Hypercholesterolemia.
- Family history of heart disease.

Also be aware of the following:

- Evidence of cerebrovascular disease (cerebrovascular accident) or myocardial infarction in the past.
- If the patient is young, think about possible secondary causes (e.g., recurrent urinary tract infections).

When checking the drug history, ask about all current medications including over-the-counter analgesics and the oral contraceptive pill.

With regard to the family history:

- Ask about family history of hypertension.
- If the patient is young think about possible secondary causes (e.g., family history of renal problems or cerebrovascular disease in polycystic kidney disease).

Causes of secondary hypertension	
Classification	**Examples of cause**
Renal	Renovascular disease, renal parenchymal diseases (e.g., polycystic kidney disease, glomerulonephritis, diabetic nephropathy—basically any significant renal disease), renin-producing tumors
Endocrine	Adrenal—Cushing's syndrome, congenital adrenal hyperplasia, Conn's syndrome, pheochromocytoma Acromegaly Carcinoid Hyper- or hypothyroidism Hypercalcemia Oral contraceptive pill
Vascular	Coarctation of the aorta
Drugs	Oral contraceptive pill, corticosteroids, monoamine oxidase inhibitors
Pregnancy	Pregnancy-induced hypertension
Neurological	Increased intracranial pressure, sleep apnea, acute porphyria, Guillain–Barré syndrome (may be associated with very large swings in blood pressure and heart rate)
Alcohol	Common cause (alcohol intake is an important part of the history)

Fig. 24.1 Causes of secondary hypertension.

An assessment of social history should take into account:

- Smoking.
- Alcohol intake.
- Level of stress at work.
- Likelihood of non-compliance with medication.

Examination

Hypertension is diagnosed after three readings over 140/90mmHg have been taken on separate occasions over a period of at least 3 months. Severe hypertension (e.g., >200/100mmHg) does not require three such readings for diagnosis).

Fig. 24.2 shows the important features to note on examination of a patient who has hypertension. Remember to look for signs of end-organ damage and signs of possible underlying causes of secondary hypertension.

The following are examples of end-organ damage secondary to hypertension:

- Ischemic heart disease.
- Heart failure.
- Left ventricular hypertrophy.
- Cerebrovascular disease.
- Peripheral vascular disease.

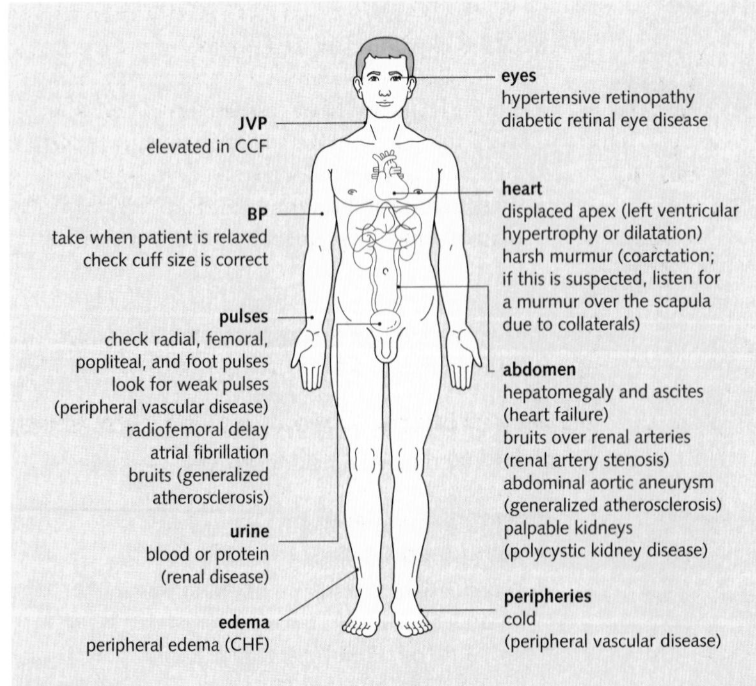

Fig. 24.2 Important clinical findings in hypertensive patients. Look for signs of end-organ damage and signs of the underlying cause of hypertension. It is essential to keep an open mind. This illustration is only a guide; there are many other possible findings (e.g., signs of thyroid disease or Cushing's syndrome). (CHF, congestive cardiac failure; JVP, jugular venous pressure.)

- Renal impairment (judged by a patient's creatinine leel and urine dipstick looking for protein (such as albumin).
- Hypertensive retinopathy.

Investigation of patients with hypertension

Investigations, as listed in Fig. 24.3, should be performed at presentation and repeated on a yearly basis as a measure of how well the hypertension is responding to treatment. For example, left ventricular hypertrophy should gradually regress once hypertension has been successfully controlled.

These investigations are also directed towards looking for evidence of end-organ damage and possible causes of secondary hypertension.

If the patient is at high risk of having secondary hypertension, further investigations are indicated. The criteria for excluding secondary hypertension are as follows:

- Under 35 years of age.
- Symptoms and signs of malignant hypertension (i.e., blood pressure >180/100mmHg, grade 3 or 4 hypertensive retinopathy, heart failure at a young age).
- Symptoms of an underlying cause (e.g., pheochromocytoma—sweating, dizzy spells, tachycardia).
- Signs of an underlying cause (e.g., differential blood pressure in both arms, hyperkalemia in the absence of diuretics, Cushingoid appearance).

Investigations for hypertension

Blood tests—renal function and electrolytes, blood lipid profile, blood glucose

EKG—may provide evidence of LVH (i.e., R wave in V5 > 25mm, deep S wave in V2 or R wave in V5 added to S wave in V2 greater than 50mm, R wave in AVL > 11mm, lateral T-wave inversion)

Echocardiogram—LVH, usually concentric in nature (i.e., left ventricular wall thickness >1.1cm); performed routinely at some centers because LVH is thought to be a valuable indicator of prognosis

Fig. 24.3 Investigations for hypertension. (LVH, left ventricular hypertrophy.)

Investigation of secondary hypertension

All patients should have the investigations listed in Fig. 24.3. For patients at high risk of secondary hypertension, the following screening tests should exclude most causative conditions:

- 24-hour urine protein and creatinine clearance to exclude marked renal pathology.
- 24-hour urine catecholamines or vanillylmandelic acid (VMA) and 5-hydroxy indole acetic acid (5HIAA) to exclude pheochromocytoma and carcinoid syndrome, respectively. (Three sets of urinary catecholamines should be tested.)
- 24-hour urine cortisol excretion and dexamethasone suppression test to exclude Cushing's syndrome.
- Renal ultrasound—to reveal any overt structural abnormality (e.g., pheochromocytoma, small kidney, or polycystic kidneys). Doppler images added to this study can also show obstruction of arterial and venous vessels.
- Magnetic resonance angiogram (MRA) is now becoming the major investigation (vs. renal perfusion scans) to determine renal blood flow and to diagnose renal artery stenosis.
- Renal perfusion scan (diethylenetriamine pentaacetic acid, DTPA) with and without angiotensin-converting enzyme (ACE) inhibition to exclude renal artery stenosis. The kidney in renal artery stenosis depends heavily upon increased levels of angiotensin II to provide adequate blood pressure for renal perfusion. This is abruptly stopped by the administration of an ACE inhibitor and the reduction in renal blood flow that results can be detected by the scan. If this test is positive, renal angiography is the gold standard investigation to confirm the diagnosis.

Management of hypertension

Importance of treating hypertension

Hypertension is a common disorder that, if left untreated, damages a number of systems. Complications of hypertension include:

- Heart failure.
- Renal failure.
- Stroke.
- Ischemic heart disease.
- Peripheral vascular disease.

This end-organ damage can largely be prevented by adequate blood pressure control.

Hypertension is, however, difficult to diagnose because patients are often asymptomatic; treatment is therefore difficult because patients are less likely to comply with drug regimens or follow-up visits to their doctor.

Nonpharmacological management

This is important because in patients who have mild hypertension it may result in a moderate decrease in blood pressure of 11/8mmHg, and this may be sufficient to avoid the need for drug therapy. The following nonpharmacological treatments are recognized:

- Weight loss.
- Reduction in alcohol consumption.
- Reduction in salt intake.
- Regular exercise.

All other risk factors for ischemic heart disease should be sought and treated in these patients as a matter of routine.

Pharmacological management

There are many effective agents (Fig. 24.4). The main categories are as follows:

- Diuretics.
- Antiadrenergic agents—beta-blockers, alpha blockers (alpha-adrenoceptor antagonists), and centrally acting agents.
- Calcium channel blockers.
- Angiotensin-converting enzyme (ACE) inhibitors and angiotensin II receptor blockers.
- Vasodilators.

These agents may be used alone or in combination to achieve good blood pressure control. Remember that patient compliance is likely to be better if:

- The disease and its complications have been fully explained.
- The treatment options have been discussed with the patient.
- The drugs used have been explained and common side effects discussed.
- Once-daily preparations are used.
- Polypharmacy is avoided (i.e., the drug regimen is kept as simple as possible by using a higher dose of a single agent before adding another drug).

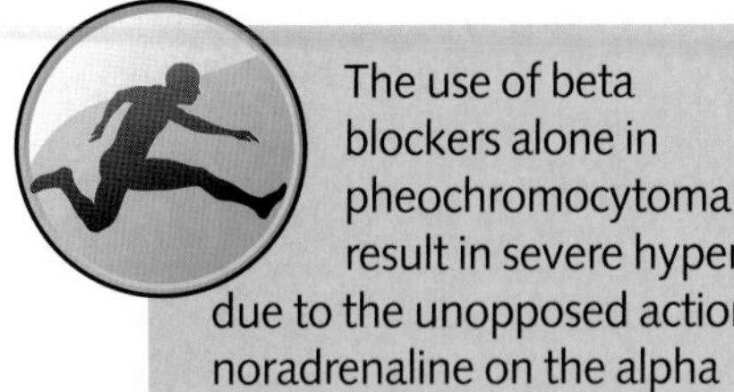

The use of beta blockers alone in pheochromocytoma may result in severe hypertension due to the unopposed action of noradrenaline on the alpha receptors.

Most patients with hypertension need multiple medications to reach the goal blood pressure.

Recommended treatment of hypertension

The following recommendations are taken from the Seventh Report of the Joint National Committee on Prevention, Detection, Evaluation, and Treatment of High Blood Pressure and the National Heart, Lung, and Blood Institute (NHLBI):

- In persons older than 50 years, systolic blood pressure greater than 140mmHg is a much more important risk factor for cardiovascular disease (CVD) than diastolic blood pressure.
- The risk of CVD beginning at 115/75mmHg doubles with each increment of 20/10mmHg; individuals who are normotensive at age 55 have a 90% lifetime risk for developing hypertension.
- Individuals with a systolic blood pressure of 120–139mmHg or a diastolic blood pressure of 80–89mmHg should be considered as prehypertensive and require health-promoting lifestyle modifications to prevent CVD.
- Thiazide-type diuretics should be used in drug treatment for most patients with uncomplicated hypertension, either alone or combined with drugs from other classes. Certain high-risk conditions are compelling indications for the initial use of other antihypertensive drug classes (ACE inhibitors, angiotensin receptor blockers, beta-blockers, calcium channel blockers).
- Most patients with hypertension require two or more antihypertensive medications to achieve goal blood pressure (<140/90mmHg, or <130/80mm Hg for patients with diabetes or chronic kidney disease).

Overview of drugs used to treat hypertension				
Class of drug	**Examples**	**Indications**	**Contraindications**	**Adverse effects**
Diuretics	Thiazides (e.g., hydrochlorothiazide), loop diuretics (e.g., furosemide)	Mild hypertension or in conjunction with other agents for more severe hypertension	Thiazides exacerbate diabetes mellitus; all diuretics should be avoided in patients who have gout if possible	Hypokalemia, dehydration, exacerbation of renal impairment, gout
Antiadrenergic agents	Beta-blockers (e.g., atenolol, propanolol, metoprolol)	Moderate-to-severe hypertension (note that they are antianginal)	Asthma, heart failure, severe peripheral vascular disease	Postural hypotension, bronchospasm, fatigue, impotence, cold extremities
	Alpha-blockers (e.g., prazosin, doxazosin)	Moderate-to-severe hypertension	Postural hypotension	
	Centrally acting agents (e.g., methyldopa)	Moderate hypertension (safe during pregnancy)	Postural hypotension, galactorrhoea, gynecomastia, hemolytic anemia	
Calcium channel blockers	Nifedipine, amlodipine, verapamil, diltiazem	Moderate hypertension*	Cardiac failure, heart block (2nd or 3rd degree)—these are contraindications mainly for verapamil and diltiazem	Postural hypotension, headache, flushing, ankle edema
ACE inhibitors	Captopril, enalapril, lisinopril	Moderate-to-severe hypertension, especially with cardiac failure	Renal artery stenosis, pregnancy	Postural hypotension, dry cough, loss of taste, renal failure, hyperkalemia
Angiotensin-II receptor blockers	Losartan, valsartan	Moderate-to-severe hypertension, especially with cardiac failure	Renal artery stenosis, pregnancy	Postural hypotension, renal failure, hyperkalemia
Vasodilators	Hydralazine	Moderate-to-severe hypertension	SLE	Postural hypotension, headache, lupus-like syndrome
	Sodium nitroprusside (as an IV infusion)	Malignant hypertension	Weakness, cyanide toxicity if drug not protected from light	

Fig. 24.4 Overview of drugs used to treat hypertension. (ACE, angiotensin-converting enzyme; SLE, systemic lupus erythematosus; *diltiazem and verapamil are less commonly used for hypertension because they have a more pronounced action on heart muscle and conductive tissue, respectively; diltiazem is used predominantly for angina and verapamil for its antiarrhythmic affects.)

- If blood pressure is >20/10 mmHg above goal blood pressure, consideration should be given to initiating therapy with two agents, one of which usually should be a thiazide-type diuretic.
- The most effective therapy prescribed by the most careful clinician will control hypertension only if patients are motivated. Motivation improves when patients have positive experiences with, and trust in, the clinician. Empathy builds trust and is a potent motivator.

In presenting these guidelines, the committee recognizes that the responsible physician's judgment remains paramount. Fig. 24.5 summarizes the above recommendations; Fig. 24.6 summarizes the recommendations for treatment of hypertension in patients with compelling indications.

Follow-up of patients who have hypertension

Follow-up is every bit as important as the initial treatment. Remember: if the patient is to measure

JNC 7 outline for treatment of hypertension
1. Begin with lifestyle modifications. 2. If the patients does not reach the goal blood pressure (<140/90mmHg; <130/80mmHg for patients with diabetes or chronic kidney disease), initiate drug therapy. 3. For most patients with stage 1 hypertension (systolic BP of 140–59mmHg or diastolic BP of 90–99mmHg) and no compelling indications, begin with a thiazide diuretic. You may also consider an ACE inhibitor, angiotensin II receptor blocker, beta-blocker, calcium channel blocker, or combination therapy. 4. For most patients with stage 2 hypertension (systolic BP ≥ 160mmHg or diastolic BP ≥ 100mmHg), two-drug therapy is recommended; begin with a thiazide diuretic plus an ACE inhibitor or an angiotensin II receptor blocker or a beta blocker or a calcium channel blocker. 5. For patients with compelling indications, use combination therapy as summarized in Fig. 24.6. 6. If patients with stage 1 hypertension, stage 2 hypertension, or compelling indications still do not reach the goal blood pressure, optimize dosages or add additional drugs until BP goal is achieved. Consider consultation with a hypertension specialist.

Fig. 24.5 JNC 7 outline for treatment of hypertension.

JNC 7 recommendations for treatment of hypertensive patients with compelling indications	
Indication	**Recommended drugs**
Heart failure	Diuretic, beta blocker, angiotensin II receptor blocker, aldosterone antagonist
Post-myocardial infarction	Beta-blocker, ACE inhibitor, aldosterone antagonist
High coronary artery disease risk	Diuretic, beta-blocker, Ace inhibitor, calcium channel blocker
Diabetes	Diuretic, beta-blocker, ACE inhibitor, antiotensin II receptor blocker, calcium channel blocker
Chronic kidney disease	ACE inhibitor, angiotensin II receptor blocker
Recurrent stroke prevention	Diuretic, ACE inhibitor

Fig. 24.6 JNC 7 recommendations for treatment of hypertensive patients with compelling indications.

blood pressure at home, have the BP cuff calibrated in an office setting to verify the patient's ability to take accurate home measurements. Patients should be seen on a 1- or 2-monthly basis until the blood pressure is less than 140/90mmHg and then on a yearly basis. The yearly follow-up should involve:

- Examination to look for evidence of end-organ damage—especially cardiovascular system and retinas.
- EKG.
- Blood tests for urea, creatinine, and electrolytes—these may be deranged due to renal damage secondary to hypertension or to the drug therapy or both.
- Echocardiography if the patient had left ventricular hypertrophy at diagnosis—it is appropriate to repeat the echocardiography until the hypertrophy has resolved.
- A screen of risk factors for ischemic heart disease (i.e., blood lipid profile and blood glucose) and lifestyle advice if necessary.

Pheochromocytoma

Pheochromocytoma is a tumor of the chromaffin cells—90% occur within the adrenal medulla and 10% are extramedullary; 10% are malignant.

Clinical features

Paroxysmal catecholamine secretion results in a variety of signs and symptoms, including:

- Hypertension.
- Headaches.
- Sweating attacks.
- Postural hypotension.
- Acute pulmonary edema.

These symptoms are characteristically paroxysmal, but patients may have persistent hypertension.

Investigations

Investigations include:

- EKG—ST elevation or T-wave inversion may be seen transiently.

- Echocardiography—shows left ventricular hypertrophy or dilated cardiomyopathy.
- 24-hour urinary catecholamines or VMA—these are elevated. (At least three measurements should be taken due to the intermittent nature of the catecholamine excretion.)
- Computed tomography scan of the adrenals or meta-iodobenzylguanidine (MIBG) scan if the tumor is extra-adrenal.
- Selective venous sampling.

Management

Careful blood pressure control is vital before any invasive procedure, as follows:

- Initially an alpha blocker is used (phenoxybenzamine, an irreversible alpha blocker, is commonly used).
- Beta blockade may then be added if required. The use of beta blockers alone may result in severe hypertension due to the unopposed action of norepinephrine on the alpha receptors.

The tumor is then removed surgically.

25. Congenital Heart Disease

Definition of congential heart disease

Congenital heart disease refers to cardiac lesions present from birth.

Causes of congenital heart disease

Many factors both genetic and environmental affect cardiac development in the uterus; therefore, not surprisingly, no one cause can explain all cases (Fig. 25.1). These factors include:

- Maternal rubella—in addition to cataracts, deafness, and microcephaly, this can cause patent ductus arteriosus (PDA) and pulmonary stenosis.
- Fetal alcohol syndrome—associated with cardiac defects (as well as microcephaly, micrognathia, microphthalmia, and growth retardation).
- Maternal systemic lupus erythematosus—associated with fetal complete heart block (due to transplacental passage of anti-Ro antibodies).

There are many genetic associations with congenital heart disease, including:

- Trisomy 21—endocardial cushion defects, atrial septal defect (ASD), ventricular septal defect (VSD), tetralogy of Fallot.
- Turner's syndrome (XO)—coarctation of the aorta.
- Marfan syndrome—aortic dilatation and aortic and mitral regurgitation.
- Kartagener's syndrome—dextrocardia.

Complications of congenital heart disease

Before discussing individual lesions, it is important to have a grasp of the significance of congenital heart disease. Lesions have effects depending upon their size and location. These effects include:

- Cyanosis—defined as the presence of more than 5g/dL of reduced hemoglobin in arterial blood. Central cyanosis can be caused by congenital heart disease due to shunting of venous blood straight into the arterial circulation bypassing the lungs. This type of cyanosis does not therefore respond to increasing the concentration of inspired oxygen.
- Congestive heart failure—this occurs due to the inability of the heart to maintain sufficient tissue perfusion as a result of the cardiac lesion. This may occur in infancy (e.g., due to a large VSD or transposition of the great arteries) or in adulthood in less severe conditions.
- Pulmonary hypertension—this occurs as a result of an abnormal increase in pulmonary blood flow due to a left-to-right shunt (e.g., ASD, VSD, PDA). This increased flow results in changes to the pulmonary vessels with smooth muscle hypertrophy and obliterative changes. The pulmonary vascular resistance increases causing pulmonary hypertension. Eventually pulmonary pressure exceeds systemic pressure causing reversal of the shunt and this results in a syndrome of cyanotic heart disease called Eisenmenger's syndrome.
- Infective endocarditis—congenital heart disease may result in lesions prone to bacterial colonization. Appropriate antibiotic prophylaxis should be taken to prevent this.
- Sudden death—this may be due to arrhythmias (more common in these disorders) or outflow tract obstruction as seen in aortic stenosis.

Notes on cyanosis:

- Central cyanosis is cyanosis of the tongue.
- Peripheral cyanosis is cyanosis of the peripheries (e.g., lips, feet, hands).
- Cyanosis caused by pulmonary disease or heart failure improves on increasing inspired oxygen.
- Cyanosis caused by a right to left shunt bypassing the lungs does not improve on increasing inspired oxygen.

Cardiac malformations
Ventricular septal defect (VSD)
Atrial septal defect (ASD)
Patent ductus arteriosus (PDA)
Pulmonary stenosis—causes cyanosis if severe
Coarctation of the aorta
Aortic stenosis
Tetrology of Fallot—causes cyanosis
Transposition of the great arteries—causes cyanosis
Other causes of cyanotic congenital heart disease—pulmonary atresia, hypoplastic left heart, severe Ebstein's anomaly with ASD

Fig. 25.1 Cardiac malformations (in descending order of incidence).

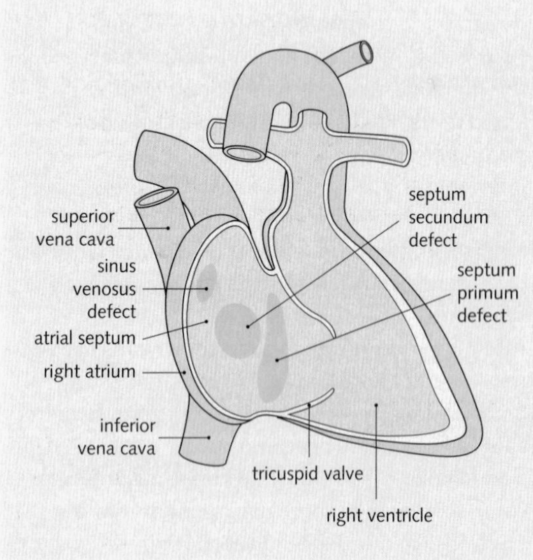

Fig. 25.2 Location of the three main types of atrial septal defect. Here the heart is viewed from the right side. The right atrial and ventricular walls have been omitted to reveal the septum.

Atrial septal defect

There are three main types of ASD based on the location of the defect in the atrial septum (Fig. 25.2):

- Septum primum (also called ostium primum ASD)—this defect lies adjacent to the atrioventricular valves, which are often also abnormal and incompetent.
- Septum secundum (also called ostium secundum ASD)—the most common form of ASD, it is midseptal in location.
- Sinus venosus ASD—this lies high in the septum and may be associated with anomalous pulmonary venous drainage (in which one of the pulmonary veins drains into the right atrium instead of the left).

Clinical features

The magnitude of the left-to-right shunt depends upon the size of the defect and also the relative pressures on the left and right sides of the heart.

History

In early life patients are usually asymptomatic. In adult life, however, symptoms of dyspnea, fatigue, and recurrent chest infections occur.

As time goes by, the increased pulmonary blood flow results in pulmonary hypertension and eventually reversal of the shunt and Eisenmenger's syndrome.

Examination

The findings on examination of a patient who has an ASD (Fig. 25.3) depend upon the following factors:

- Size of the ASD.
- Presence or absence of pulmonary hypertension.
- Presence of shunt reversal.

The second heart sound is widely split because closure of the pulmonary valve is delayed due to increased pulmonary blood flow. The splitting is fixed in relation to respiration because the communication between the atria prevents the normal pressure differential between right and left sides that occurs during respiration. This is referred to as fixed splitting of the second heart sound.

The increased pulmonary blood flow causes a mid-systolic pulmonary flow murmur.

If pulmonary hypertension has developed, there is reduction of the left-to-right shunt and the pulmonary flow murmur disappears; instead there is a loud pulmonary component to the second heart sound because the increased pressure causes the pulmonary valve to slam shut.

If Eisenmenger's syndrome occurs, the patient becomes centrally cyanosed and develops finger clubbing.

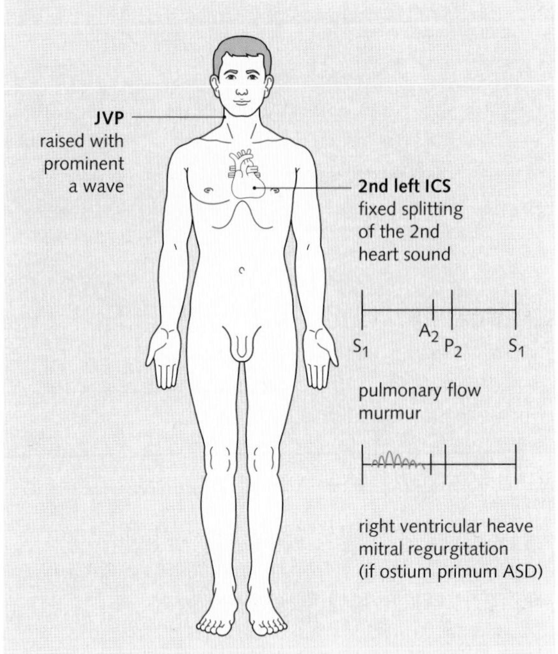

Fig. 25.3 Physical findings in all patients who have an atrial septal defect (ASD). If the ASD is large and pulmonary hypertension is present, check for loud P_2 at the second left intercostal space (ICS) and a prominent right ventricular heave. If there is shunt reversal, you will find clubbing, central cyanosis, and signs of congestive heart failure (i.e., peripheral edema, ascites, and bilateral basal crackles). (A_2, aortic component of second heart sound; JVP, jugular venous pressure; S_1, first heart sound.)

Investigations

Electrocardiography

Patients who have ostium secundum ASD usually have right axis deviation. Those who have an ostium primum defect have left axis deviation.

Chest radiography

The pulmonary artery appears dilated, and its branches are prominent. The enlarged right atrium can be seen at the right heart border and the enlarged right ventricle causes rounding of the left heart border.

Echocardiography

The right side of the heart is dilated, and the pulmonary artery is dilated. The ASD may be directly visualized and a jet of blood may be seen passing through it. Associated mitral or tricuspid valve incompetence may be seen.

Cardiac catheterization

This again reveals the ASD because the catheter can be passed across it. Serial oxygen saturation measurements are made at different levels from the superior vena cava through the atrium and the right ventricle into the pulmonary artery. At the level of the left-to-right shunt there will be a step up increase of the oxygen saturation as blood from the left side enters the right. This measurement can be used to calculate the size of the shunt, which helps decide on whether operative correction of the ASD is required.

Eisenmenger's syndrome can occur in any condition involving a left-to-right shunt. With worsening pulmonary hypertension the shunt eventually reverses (changes to right to left), causing blood to bypass the lungs and resulting in profound cyanosis that is not responsive to oxygen therapy. There is no treatment at this late stage.

Management

If there are signs of congestive heart failure, diuretics and angiotensin-converting enzyme (ACE) inhibitors may be of benefit.

Because an ASD carries a risk of infective endocarditis, the appropriate prophylactic measures should be taken.

The primary aim in these patients is to diagnose the ASD early and evaluate its severity to be able to repair the defect before pulmonary hypertension occurs. Once the patient has developed pulmonary hypertension, repair does not stop its deterioration.

All ASDs with pulmonary to systemic flow ratios exceeding 1.5:1 should be repaired.

Operative closure requires cardiopulmonary bypass and involves a median sternotomy scar.

A new technique has been developed where the ASD is closed using a clam shell-shaped device that can be introduced via a cardiac catheter and involves only an arterial and a venous puncture.

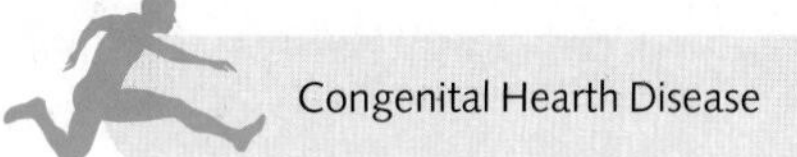

When asked about the management of any valve disease or congenital defect, many students forget that antibiotic prophylaxis is probably one of the most important aspects of management. Don't forget to put it high on your list of priorities.

Ventricular septal defect

This is the most common congenital cardiac abnormality.

The ventricular septum is made up of two main components:

- The membranous septum—situated high in the septum and relatively small. This is the most common site for a VSD.
- The muscular septum—this is lower and defects here may be multiple.

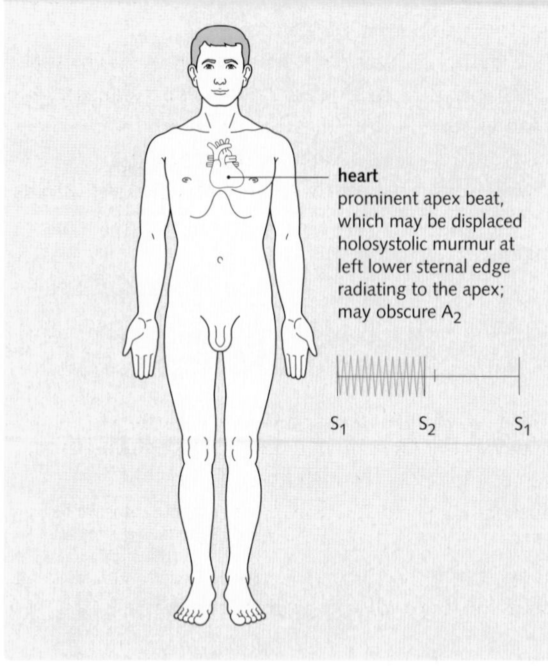
heart
prominent apex beat, which may be displaced
holosystolic murmur at left lower sternal edge radiating to the apex; may obscure A2
S1
S2
S1

Fig. 25.4 Physical findings in all patients who have a ventricular septal defect (VSD). If the VSD is large, the apex is displaced and pulmonary hypertension may develop, resulting in a loud P_2 and right ventricular heave. Eisenmenger's syndrome may also develop with clubbing and cyanosis and disappearance of the holosystolic murmur. (A_2, aortic component of second heart sound.)

Clinical features

History

In the neonate a small VSD isasymptomatic, but a large VSD results in the development of left ventricular failure (LVF). This occurs because in the neonate pulmonary pressures are very high (because they are in utero), and a right-to-left shunt occurs via the VSD. If this is very large, the left ventricle cannot cope and fails. The signs of LVF in a neonate are as follows:

- Failure to thrive, feeding difficulties, and sweating on feeding.
- Tachypnea and intercostal recession.
- Hepatomegaly.

The adult who has a VSD may be asymptomatic or may present with dyspnea due to pulmonary hypertension (which develops as a consequence of the left-to-right shunt) or Eisenmenger's syndrome.

Examination

The findings on examination of a patient who has a VSD (Fig. 25.4) vary according to the following criteria:

- Size of the VSD—a small VSD causes a loud holosystolic murmur that radiates to the apex and axilla. A very large VSD causes a less loud holosystolic murmur but may be associated with signs of left ventricular and right ventricular hypertrophy.
- Presence or absence of pulmonary hypertension.
- Presence of shunt reversal.

Investigations

Chest radiography

This may show an enlarged left ventricle with prominent pulmonary vascular markings. Pulmonary edema may be seen in infants.

Echocardiography

This shows the VSD and its size and location.

Management

Approximately 30% of cases close spontaneously, most of these by the time the child is 3 years of age. Some do not close until the child is 10 years old.

Defects near the valve ring or near the outlet of the ventricle do not usually close.

Operative closure is the treatment of choice and is recommended for all lesions that have not undergone spontaneous closure. Some small lesions are left; such patients have a loud holosystolic murmur.

A VSD is a risk factor for infective endocarditis so the appropriate prophylactic measures should be taken.

Patent ductus arteriosus

In the fetus most of the output of the right ventricle bypasses the lungs via the ductus arteriosus. This vessel joins the pulmonary trunk (artery) to the descending aorta distal to the left subclavian artery (Fig. 25.5). The ductus arteriosus normally closes about 1 month after birth in full-term infants and takes longer to close in premature infants.

Clinical features

The factors that determine the nature of the clinical features are the same as in VSD and ASD (i.e., the size of the defect, the presence of pulmonary hypertension, and the development of Eisenmenger's syndrome).

A patent PDA is more likely in babies born at high altitude, probably due to the low atmospheric oxygen concentration. This lesion is also common in babies who have fetal rubella syndrome.

History

A small PDA is asymptomatic, but a large defect causes a large left-to-right shunt and may lead to left ventricular failure with pulmonary edema causing failure to thrive and tachypnea.

Adults who have undiagnosed PDA may develop pulmonary hypertension and present with dyspnea.

Differential cyanosis occurs in adults with reversal of the shunt as the venous blood enters the systemic circulation below the subclavian arteries, causing cyanosis of the lower extremities. The arms remain pink.

Examination

The classic findings in a patient who has PDA (Fig. 25.6) are:

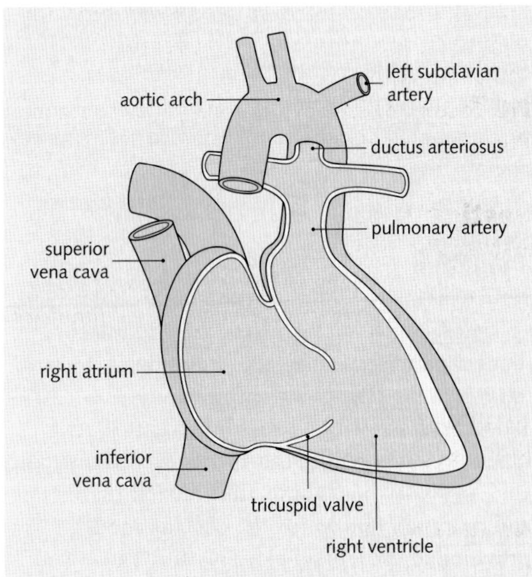

Fig. 25.5 Position of the ductus arteriosus.

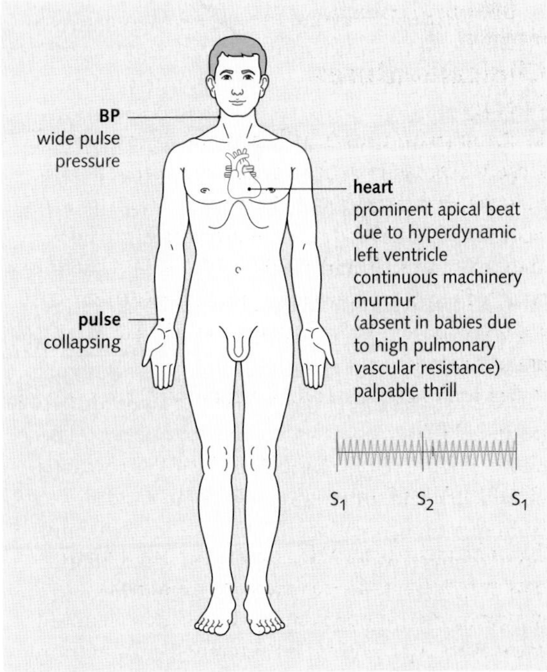

Fig. 25.6 Physical findings in all patients who have patent ductus arteriosus (PDA). In patients who have a large PDA there is a loud pulmonary component of the second heart sound (P_2) due to pulmonary hypertension and the murmur is soft or absent. In those who have Eisenmenger's syndrome there is differential cyanosis and the toes are clubbed.

- Collapsing high-volume pulses—this is due to the effect of the run-off of blood back down the ductus.
- A loud continuous machinery murmur.

Management

The management of PDA involves two stages:

- Pharmacological closure in neonates—indomethacin may induce closure if given early.
- Operative closure of the PDA—this can be performed as an open procedure in which the PDA is ligated or divided. Alternatively, a percutaneous approach can be performed with introduction of an occluding device via a cardiac catheter. Antibiotic prophylaxis is required for all patients before operative correction because PDA is a risk factor for infective endocarditis.

Coarctation of the aorta

In this condition there is a congenital narrowing of the aorta, usually beyond the left subclavian artery.

There are two main types:

- Infantile type—this presents soon after birth with heart failure.
- Adult type—the obstruction develops more gradually and presents in early adulthood. This type is associated with a high incidence of bicuspid aortic valve.

An adaptive response to the coarctation develops in patients who do not present in infancy. This involves the development of collateral blood vessels, which divert blood from the proximal aorta to other peripheral arteries bypassing the obstruction. These collaterals are seen around the scapula as tortuous vessels that can sometimes be palpated and as prominent posterior intercostal arteries that cause rib notching that is visible on a chest radiograph. These collaterals take some years to develop and are rarely seen before 6 years of age.

Clinical features

History

Infants may present with failure to thrive and tachypnea secondary to left ventricular failure. Alternatively, coarctation may present as rapid severe cardiac failure with the infant in extremis.

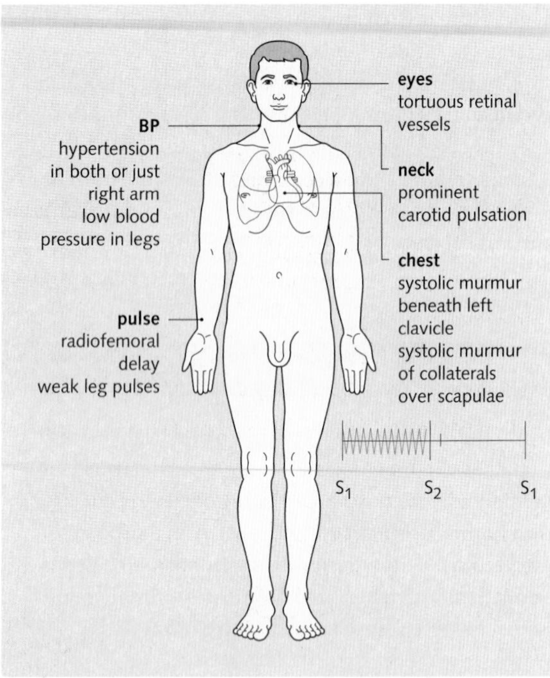

Fig. 25.7 Physical findings in patients who have coarctation of the aorta. If the coarctation is severe, there is a continuous murmur beneath the left clavicle and there are signs of left ventricular failure (bilateral basal crackles and audible third heart sound.)

Adults whose condition is not diagnosed in childhood may present with:

- Hypertension diagnosed at routine medical testing.
- Symptoms of leg claudication.
- Left ventricular failure.
- Subarachnoid hemorrhage from associated berry aneurysm.
- Angina pectoris due to premature heart disease.

Examination

Careful examination of these patients is vital because the diagnosis must not be missed. The physical findings in patients who have coarctation of the aorta are shown in Fig. 25.7. Check for:

- Blood pressure—it is always important to take blood pressure in both arms whenever performing the cardiovascular examination. Aortic dissection and coarctation in which the obstruction is proximal to the left subclavian artery cause a pressure differential between the arms. The blood pressure in the legs is also lower than in the arms.

Uncommon causes of congenital cardiac abnormalities			
Congenital cardiac defect	**Anatomic abnormality**	**Clinical features**	**Treatment**
Congenital aortic stenosis (acyanotic)	Stenosis may be valvular (most common), subvalvular, or supravalvular; note Williams syndrome—autosomal dominant condition with hypercalcemia and supravalvular aortic stenosis	More common in males; child may be hypotensive, dyspneic, and sweaty; increased incidence of angina and sudden death, especially on exertion; ejection systolic murmur heard in the 2nd right ICS; may be signs of left ventricular strain (heaving apex) and failure (S_2, tachycardia, and bilateral basal crackles)	Operative correction of the stenosis is the treatment of choice; in very small infants valvuloplasty is preferred in the first instance
Hypoplastic left heart (cyanotic)	Underdevelopment of all or part of the left side of the heart	Heart failure occurs in the 1st week of life; echocardiography is diagnostic	Surgical treatment is the only option and the mortality rate is extremely high
Pulmonary artery stenosis (cyanotic only if severe)	Stenosis at one or many points along the pulmonary arteries; associated with tetralogy of Fallot in some cases; complication of maternal rubella infection	If mild, the patient may be asymptomatic with signs of RVH (i.e., left parasternal heave) and a pulmonary ejection systolic murmur. If severe, blood flows from the right side to the left through the foramen ovale, and the child is cyanosed and dyspneic	Diagnosis is confirmed by echocardiography; pulmonary angioplasty may provide a definitive cure; if there is a recurrence or the lesion is not suitable for pulmonary angioplasty, the obstruction may be removed surgically
Tetralogy of Fallot (cyanotic)	Four components: VSD, pulmonary stenosis, overriding aorta, and RVH. Therefore, blood flow passes from the right ventricle through the VSD and through the aorta, resulting in a right-to-left shunt	Most children present with cyanosis within the first year of life; patients may have "spells" of intense cyanosis from time to time due to a sudden increase in the right-to-left shunt. These attacks may be terminated by squatting, which increases systemic resistance and therefore reduces the right-to-left shunt	Total surgical correction is the treatment of first choice; in very young infants with severe pulmonary atresia, a palliative operation to reduce the pulmonary obstruction usually provides relief, and a definitive procedure can be done later when the risk is lower
Complete transposition of the great arteries (cyanotic)	The aorta arises from the right ventricle and the pulmonary artery arises from the left ventricle. The two circulations are thus parallel; death is rapid if there is no communication between them. Therefore, it is common to see an ASD, VSD, or PDA in these infants	Early cardiac failure and cyanosis are the most common presenting features; symptoms are less severe in infants with a large communication between the two sides; diagnosis is made by echocardiography and cardiac catheterization	Medical treatment of cardiac failure and the use of prostaglandin E_1 to prevent postnatal closure of the ductus may help; operative procedures to create a large ASD may also help in the short term; surgical correction of the transposition is the definitive treatment

Fig. 25.8 Uncommon causes of congenital cardiac abnormalities. (ASD, atrial septal defect; ICS, intercostal space; PDA, patent ductus arteriosus; RVH, right ventricular hypertrophy; S_3, third heart sound; VSD, ventricular septal defect.)

- Radiofemoral delay and weak leg pulses—it is always important to look for radiofemoral delay because it is diagnostic of this condition.
- Murmurs—the coarctation may cause a systolic murmur (or a continuous murmur if the narrowing is very tight). This is located below the left clavicle. The collaterals around the scapulas cause an ejection systolic murmur that can be heard over the scapulas. There may be a murmur associated with a bicuspid aortic valve, which is ejection systolic in nature and is located over the aortic area.

Investigation

Electrocardiography

EKG reveals left ventricular hypertrophy and often right bundle-branch block.

Chest radiography

Rib notching may be seen in children over 6 years of age. (Because the first and second intercostal arteries arise from the vertebral arteries, there is no rib notching on these ribs.) The aortic knuckle is absent, and a double knuckle is seen (made up of the dilated subclavian artery above and the poststenotic dilatation of the aorta below).

Echocardiography

The coarctation can be visualized as can any associated lesion. Coarctation is associated with a number of other congenital abnormalities (e.g., transposition of the great arteries, septum primum ASD, mitral valve disease, bicuspid aortic valve).

Cardiac catheterization

This localizes the coarctation accurately and also provides more information about associated lesions.

Management

The most popular first-line treatment is an operation to relieve the obstruction. Without correction the prognosis is extremely poor and most patients die by 40 years of age.

Balloon angioplasty is another option, but this is usually reserved for the treatment of postsurgical restenosis.

Coarctation may be complicated by infective endocarditis; antibiotic prophylaxis should be used.

Other causes of congenital heart disease

A number of less common congenital cardiac abnormalities are discussed in Fig. 25.8.

Notes on pulmonary hypertension and Eisenmenger's syndrome

Pulmonary hypertension

This causes mild dyspnea when the shunt is from left to right and severe dyspnea on shunt reversal.

Signs on examination include:

- Dominant a wave in the jugular venous pulse.
- Palpable and loud pulmonary component of second heart sound.
- Ejection systolic murmur in pulmonary area due to increased flow.
- Right ventricular heave.
- Tricuspid regurgitation if the right ventricle dilates.

The investigation of choice is echocardiography, which allows assessment of the pulmonary pressures. This is vital because an operation should be performed before significant pulmonary hypertension develops.

Eisenmenger's syndrome

This refers to the situation in which a congenital cardiac abnormality initially causes acyanotic heart disease, but cyanotic heart disease develops as a consequence of raised pulmonary pressure and shunt reversal.

These clinical features are also seen in patients who have cyanotic congenital heart disease (i.e., when the lesion results in a right-to-left shunt from the outset). Cyanosis develops when the level of reduced hemoglobin is over 5g/dL.

Dyspnea is usually relatively mild considering the profound hypoxia (oxygen saturations of 50% are not uncommon).

Complications include:

- Clubbing—develops in the fingers and toes.
- Polycythemia and hyperviscosity—with resulting complications of stroke and venous thrombosis. Regular phlebotomy is the treatment of choice.
- Cerebral abscesses—especially in children.
- Paradoxical emboli—emboli from venous thrombosis may pass across the shunt and give rise to systemic infarcts.

Index

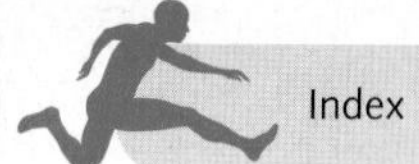

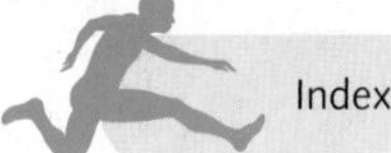

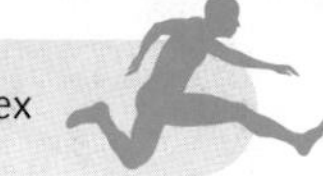

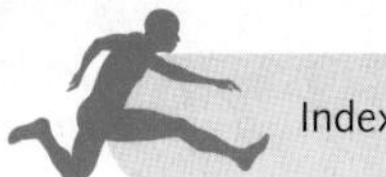

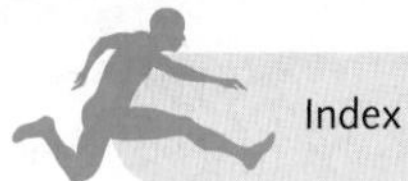

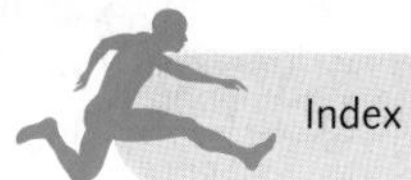